New Drugs for Malignancy

Guest Editor

FRANCO MUGGIA, MD

HEMATOLOGY/ONCOLOGY CLINICS OF NORTH AMERICA

www.hemonc.theclinics.com

Consulting Editors
GEORGE P. CANELLOS, MD
NANCY BERLINER, MD

June 2012 • Volume 26 • Number 3

SAUNDERS an imprint of ELSEVIER, Inc.

W.B. SAUNDERS COMPANY
A Division of Elsevier Inc.

1600 John F. Kennedy Blvd. ● Suite 1800 ● Philadelphia, PA 19103-2899

http://www.theclinics.com

HEMATOLOGY/ONCOLOGY CLINICS OF NORTH AMERICA Volume 26, Number 3
June 2012 ISSN 0889-8588, ISBN 13: 978-1-4557-3876-2

Editor: Patrick Manley
Developmental Editor: Donald Mumford

Hematology/Oncology Clinics (ISSN 0889-8588) is published bimonthly by Elsevier Inc., 360 Park Avenue South, New York, NY 10010-1710. Months of issue are February, April, June, August, October, and December. Business and Editorial Offices: 1600 John F. Kennedy Blvd., Ste. 1800, Philadelphia, PA 19103–2899. Customer Service Office: 3251 Riverport Lane, Maryland Heights, MO 63043. Periodicals postage paid at New York, NY and at additional mailing offices. Subscription prices are $353.00 per year (domestic individuals), $576.00 per year (domestic institutions), $173.00 per year (domestic students/residents), $401.00 per year (Canadian individuals), $705.00 per year (Canadian institutions) $477.00 per year (international individuals), $705.00 per year (international institutions), and $233.00 per year (international and Canadian students/residents). International air speed delivery is included in all *Clinics* subscription prices. All prices are subject to change without notice. **POSTMASTER:** Send address changes to *Hematology/Oncology Clinics of North America*, Elsevier Health Sciences Division, Subscription Customer Service, 3251 Riverport Lane, Maryland Heights, MO 63043. Customer Service (orders, claims, online, change of address): Elsevier Health Sciences Division, Subscription Customer Service, 3251 Riverport Lane, Maryland Heights, MO 63043. Tel: 1-800-654-2452 (U.S. and Canada); 314-447-8871 (outside U.S. and Canada). Fax: 314-447-8029. E-mail: journalscustomerservice-usa@elsevier.com (for print support); journalsonlinesupport-usa@elsevier.com (for online support).

Reprints. For copies of 100 or more, of articles in this publication, please contact the Commercial Reprints Department, Elsevier Inc., 360 Park Avenue South, New York, New York 10010-1710; Tel.: 212-633-3813, Fax: 212-462-1935, E-mail: reprints@elsevier.com.

Hematology/Oncology Clinics of North America is covered in *MEDLINE/PubMed (Index Medicus), EMBASE/ Excerpta Medica, and BIOSIS.*

Printed and bound by CPI Group (UK) Ltd, Croydon, CR0 4YY
Transferred to Digital Print 2012

Contributors

CONSULTING EDITORS

GEORGE P. CANELLOS, MD
William Rosenberg Professor of Medicine, Department of Medical Oncology, Dana-Farber Cancer Institute, Boston, Massachusetts

NANCY BERLINER, MD
Chief, Division of Hematology, Brigham and Women's Hospital; Professor of Medicine, Harvard Medical School, Boston, Massachusetts

GUEST EDITOR

FRANCO MUGGIA, MD
Professor of Medicine, New York University School of Medicine, New York, New York

AUTHORS

MARK J. ADLER, MD
Director, UC San Diego Cancer Center, Department of Medicine, University of California Health Systems; San Diego Cancer Research Institute, Encinitas, California

FERNANDA I. ARNALDEZ, MD
Pediatric Oncology Branch, Center for Cancer Research, National Cancer Institute, National Institutes of Health, Bethesda, Maryland

SUSANA M. CAMPOS, MD, MPH
Assistant Professor, Harvard Medical School, Program in Gynecologic Oncology, Department of Medical Oncology, Dana-Farber Cancer Institute, Boston, Massachusetts

ALICE CHEN, MD
Medical Officer, Investigational Drug Branch, Cancer Therapy Evaluation Program, Division of Cancer Treatment and Diagnosis, National Cancer Institute, Rockville, Maryland

DEIRDRE J. COHEN, MD
Assistant Professor of Medicine, Division of GI Oncology, New York University Cancer Institute, New York, New York

ROBERT L. COLEMAN, MD
Department of Gynecologic Oncology and Reproductive Medicine; Center for RNA Interference and Non-Coding RNAs, The University of Texas MD Anderson Cancer Center, Houston, Texas

DIMITER S. DIMITROV, PhD, ScD
Frederick National Laboratories for Cancer Research, National Institutes of Health, Frederick, Maryland

DON S. DIZON, MD, FACP
Associate Professor, Warren Alpert Medical School of Brown University, Medical Oncology, Program in Women's Oncology, Women and Infants' Hospital, Providence, Rhode Island

ANNA C. FERRARI, MD
Professor of Medicine, Director, Genitourinary Oncology Program, Department of Medicine, New York University Cancer Institute, New York University School of Medicine, New York, New York

GIUSEPPE GIACCONE, MD, PhD
Chief, Medical Oncology Branch and Thoracic Oncology Section, National Cancer Institute, Bethesda, Maryland

I. DAVID GOLDMAN, MD
Professor, Departments of Medicine and Molecular Pharmacology; Director, Albert Einstein Cancer Center, The Albert Einstein College of Medicine, Bronx, New York

ALEJANDRO GOMEZ-PINILLOS, MD
Postdoctoral Research Fellow, Department of Medicine, New York University Cancer Institute, New York University School of Medicine, New York, New York

LEE J. HELMAN, MD
Pediatric Oncology Branch, Center for Cancer Research, National Cancer Institute, National Institutes of Health, Bethesda, Maryland

JULIA MOUKHARSKAYA, MD
Fellow, Department of Medicine, Vermont Cancer Center, Burlington, Vermont

SOOK RYUN PARK, MD, PhD
Visiting Fellow, Division of Cancer Treatment and Diagnosis, National Cancer Institute, Bethesda, Maryland

ARUN RAJAN, MD
Staff Clinician, Medical Oncology Branch, National Cancer Institute, Bethesda, Maryland

ANIL K. SOOD, MD
Department of Gynecologic Oncology and Reproductive Medicine; Center for RNA Interference and Non-Coding RNAs; Department of Cancer Biology, The University of Texas MD Anderson Cancer Center, Houston, Texas

ANISH THOMAS, MD
Clinical Fellow, Medical Oncology, National Cancer Institute, Bethesda, Maryland

CLAIRE VERSCHRAEGEN, MD
Professor of Medicine, Department of Medicine, Vermont Cancer Center, Burlington, Vermont

MICHELE VISENTIN, PhD
Postdoctoral Fellow in Molecular Pharmacology, Departments of Medicine and Molecular Pharmacology and the Albert Einstein Cancer Center, The Albert Einstein College of Medicine, Bronx, New York

JASMINE ZAIN, MD
Director, Bone Marrow Transplant Program; Assistant Professor, Division of Hematologic Malignancies and Medical Oncology, New York University Langone Medical Center, New York, New York

BEHROUZ ZAND, MD
Department of Gynecologic Oncology and Reproductive Medicine, The University of Texas MD Anderson Cancer Center, Houston, Texas

RONGBAO ZHAO, PhD
Assistant Professor of Medicine, Departments of Medicine and Molecular Pharmacology and the Albert Einstein Cancer Center, The Albert Einstein College of Medicine, Bronx, New York

Contents

Antibody-based therapeutics against cancer are highly successful and currently enjoy unprecedented recognition of their potential; 13 monoclonal antibodies (mAbs) have been approved for clinical use in the European Union and in the United States. Bevacizumab, rituximab, and trastuzumab had sales in 2010 of more than $5 billion each. Hundreds of mAbs, including bispecific mAbs and multispecific fusion proteins, mAbs conjugated with small-molecule drugs, and mAbs with optimized pharmacokinetics, are in clinical trials. However, deeper understanding of mechanisms is needed to overcome major problems including resistance to therapy, access to targets, complexity of biological systems, and individual variations.

Mammalian target of rapamycin (mTOR) is a serine/threonine protein kinase. It is ubiquitously expressed in cells and is a therapeutic target for the cancer treatment arsenal. Despite the great responses obtained in tumors addicted to specific mutations or overactivation of key members of the mTOR pathway (HiF1α in RCC, cyclin D1 in MCL, or TSC in SEGA), mTOR inhibitors as single agents have modest activity. Dual PI3K/mTOR kinase inhibitors have been developed with the idea of overcoming resistance to the mTOR inhibition through preventing the activation of PI3/Akt as a result of release negative feedback loops.

Topoisomerase 1 inhibitors cure human cancer xenografts in animal models, more so than most other chemotherapy agents. However, their activity in patients with cancer is modest. Ongoing research is studying the optimal analogues that could reproduce animal data in the cancer population. This article analyzes the clinical research with topoisomerase 1 inhibitors in ovarian cancer.

The IGF axis is a tightly controlled endocrine system that regulates cell growth and development, known to have an important function in cancer biology. IGF1 and IGF2 can promote cancer growth in a GH-independent manner both through paracrine and autocrine secretion and can also confer resistance to chemotherapy and radiation. Many alterations of this system have been found in neoplasias, including increased expression of ligands and receptors, loss of heterozygosity of the IGF2 locus and increased IGF1R gene copy number. The IGF1 network is an attractive candidate for targeted therapy, including receptor blockade with monoclonal antibodies and small molecule inhibitors of receptor downstream signaling. This article reviews the role of the IGF axis in the initiation and progression of cancer, and describes the recent advances in IGF inhibition as a therapeutic tool.

Gynecologic malignancies carry an estimated incidence of 83,750 cases per year and estimated mortality rate of more than 27,000 women per year. New therapies and therapeutic approaches are needed to improve the outlook for women with gynecologic cancers. Recent insights at the molecular and cellular levels are paving the way for a more directed approach to target mechanisms driving tumorigenesis. This article reviews the roles of new and emerging antiangiogenesis drugs, summarizes the data obtained from clinical trials of antiangiogenic agents, and discusses trials under way to address the role of such strategies in gynecologic cancers.

The Hedgehog (Hh) pathway is a signaling cascade that is evolutionally highly conserved and plays an important role in embryonic pattern formation and stem cell response to tissue damage. Given the pivotal role the Hh pathway plays in embryonic development in terms of proliferation and differentiation, it is not surprising that it has also been implicated in tumorigenesis and tumor growth acceleration in a vast variety of malignancies. This article summarizes the mechanism of Hh pathway signal transduction, discusses the models of pathway activation, reviews the clinical data using Hh inhibitors, and discusses challenges to the development of pathway inhibitors.

Identification of driver mutations in growth related protein kinases, especially tyrosine kinases, has led to clinical development of an array of tyrosine kinase inhibitors in various malignancies, including lung cancer. Improved understanding of tyrosine kinase biology has led to faster drug development, identification of resistance mechanisms, and ways to overcome resistance. This review discusses the clinical data supporting the use and practical aspects of management of patients on epidermal growth factor receptor and anaplastic lymphoma kinase tyrosine kinase inhibitors.

Of the agents available in the treatment of both solid and hematologic cancers, microtubule-targeted agents are among the most widely used and exploiting other mechanisms involving the microtubule and its role in mitosis is an area of continued interest. This review will focus on novel microtubule-targeted agents, both recently approved (eg, ixabepilone and eribulin) and in later-stage clinical trials, and kinase inhibitors that aim to directly inhibit the mitotic spindle, such as the aurora kinase, pololike kinase, and kinsein-spindle protein inhibitors.

New Drugs for Malignancy

HEMATOLOGY/ONCOLOGY CLINICS OF NORTH AMERICA

Preface

Clinical Drug Development in 2012

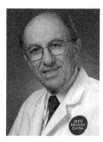

Franco Muggia, MD
Guest Editor

Hosting as editor this 2012 issue of *Hematology Oncology Clinics of North America* is an opportunity to reflect on trends in clinical drug development. In particular, awareness of the incredible possibilities that our "new biology" conveys should not preclude continuing exploitation of "conventional" chemotherapy.

Advances are noted in the management of patients with highly responsive lymphomas to refractory solid tumors such as pancreatic cancer. Three articles illustrate how developments may take place even more than five decades from initial observations[1]: *mitotic inhibitors*—long since Greenspan's interest in podophyllotoxins and witnessing tumor lysis from leurocristine (later renamed vincristine) in two patients with hematologic malignancies; *the antifolates* aminopterin and later amethopterin (methotrexate) effect against acute lymphoblastic leukemia shortly after identification on folate pathways[2]; and *topoisomerase-interacting drugs*, joining 5-fluorouracil in showing benefit against gastrointestinal cancers—a decade before topoisomerases were identified. In fact, these old chemotherapies have proven to be quite "targeted." A fourth article deals with PARP inhibitors with their effects on specific DNA repair pathways. Their role, alone or in combination, relies on selective enhancement of the consequence of DNA damage—often produced by a number of established anticancer drugs.

Kohler and Milstein were awarded the Nobel Prize in 1984 for hybridomas enabling production of monoclonal antibodies[3] that gave rise to hopes for "magic bullets" against cancer. These molecules have moved slowly from diagnostics to a platform for therapeutic developments including diverse actions such as pathway inhibition, immune activation, and immunotoxins. Pioneering efforts of Judah Folkman[4] on tumor angiogenesis resulted in the development of bevacizumab and has impacted on the treatment of several malignancies, but particularly on ovarian cancer. The role of anti-angiogenic including angiopoietin-targeted peptibodies is further covered in this issue. Monoclonal antibodies (such as cetuximab and panitumumab) and small molecules targeting the epidermal growth factor receptor as well as newly identified signal

Hematol Oncol Clin N Am 26 (2012) xi–xii
doi:10.1016/j.hoc.2012.03.003
0889-8588/12/$ – see front matter

transduction pathways in lung cancer have changed systemic approaches to this most common of malignancies. The mTOR/PI3 kinase pathways activated via cell membrane receptor or by hypoxia, cellular metabolism, and proliferation provide new targets for treating Ewing's sarcoma and renal cancer, among others. Inhibitors or the hedgehog pathway—responsible for key steps in stem cell biology and cellular remodeling—have already yielded remarkable clinical results in basal cell cancers and medulloblastoma. Finally, reprogramming of the genome by DNA methylation (by drugs such as azacytidine,[5] initially developed as "cytotoxic" chemotherapy) is part of exciting new strategies against hematologic malignancies. As this issue attests, Louis Pasteur's dictum "serendipity favors the prepared mind" certainly applies to clinical drug development 2012.

Franco Muggia, MD
NYU School of Medicine
550 First Avenue
New York, NY 10016, USA

E-mail address:
Franco.Muggia@nyumc.org

REFERENCES

1. Muggia FM. Platinum compounds: the culmination of the era of cancer chemotherapy. In: Bonetti A, Leone R, Muggia FM, et al, editors. Platinum and other heavy metal compounds in cancer chemotherapy. Humana Press, Springer Science; 2009. p. 1–7.
2. Goldin A, Mantel N, Greenhouse SW, et al. Estimation of the antileukemic potency of the antimetabolite aminopterin, administered alone and in combination with citrovorum factor or folic acid. Cancer Res 1953;13(12):843–50.
3. Köhler G, Milstein C. Continuous cultures of fused cells secreting antibody of predefined specificity. Nature 1975;256:495–7.
4. Folkman J. Angiogenesis: an organizing principle for drug discovery. Nat Rev Drug Discov 2007;6:273–86.
5. Von Hoff DD, Slavik M, Muggia FM. 5-Azacytidine. A new anticancer drug with effectiveness in acute myelogenous leukemia. Ann Intern Med 1976;85:237–45.

Therapeutic Antibodies Against Cancer

Mark J. Adler, MD[a,b,]*, Dimiter S. Dimitrov, PhD, ScD[c]

KEYWORDS

- Therapeutics • Antibodies • Cancer • Immunogenicity • Safety • Efficacy

KEY POINTS

- Antibody-based therapeutics against cancer are highly successful in the clinic and currently enjoy unprecedented recognition of their potential.
- Hundreds of mAbs, including bispecific mAbs and multispecific fusion proteins, mAbs conjugated with small-molecule drugs, and mAbs with optimized pharmacokinetics, are in clinical trials.
- Challenges remain, and deeper understanding of mechanisms is needed to overcome major problems including resistance to therapy, access to targets, complexity of biological systems, and individual variations.

Antibody therapy has its roots thousands of years ago; early forms of vaccination against infectious diseases were developed in China as early as 200 BC. However, the history of true antibody therapy began much more recently with the discovery that serum from animals immunized with toxins, for example, diphtheria toxin or viruses, is an effective therapeutic against the disease caused by the same agent in humans. This discovery resulted in the development of the serum therapy, which saved thousands of lives; von Behring, who in the 1880s developed an antitoxin that did not kill the bacteria but neutralized the toxin released into the body by the bacteria, was awarded the first Nobel Prize in Medicine in 1901 for his role in the discovery and development of a serum therapy for diphtheria. Although historically success with antibody (serum) therapy was initially mostly in the treatment of patients with infectious diseases, currently there is only one monoclonal antibody (mAb) approved for treatment of any infectious disease (palivizumab [Synagis]), which is for prevention of the infection and not for treatment of the already established

This study was supported by the NIH NCI CCR intramural program.

[a] UC San Diego Cancer Center, Department of Medicine, University of California Health Systems, 1200 Garden View, Encinitas, CA 92024, USA

[b] San Diego Cancer Research Institute, Encinitas, CA 92024, USA

[c] Frederick National Laboratories for Cancer Research, National Institutes of Health, Building 469, Room 150B, Frederick, MD 21702, USA

* Corresponding author. UC San Diego Cancer Center, Department of Medicine, University of California Health Systems, 1200 Garden View, Encinitas, CA 92024.

E-mail address: oncologic@gmail.com

infection. Initial attempts with serum therapy to treat patients with cancer were not successful. It was not until several decades ago that several revolutionary scientific discoveries were made, which allowed the development of recombinant therapeutic antibodies leading to the approval of the first anticancer therapeutic antibody, the mAb rituximab, in 1997 (**Table 1**). Since then 13 mAbs have been approved for clinical use against cancer in the European Union and the United States, and 12 are on the market in August 2011; one of these, gemtuzumab ozogamicin (Mylotarg), has been withdrawn (see **Table 1**); by contrast, the first approved mAb-based therapeutic against an infectious disease (Synagis is for prevention) is still awaited. In 2010 sales of the top 4 recombinant therapeutic antibodies (bevacizumab, rituximab, trastuzumab, cetuximab) exceeded US$20 billion (**Table 2**).

Dating back to mummies and up to the recent successes with ipilimumab, it has become axiomatic that the human immune system has an inherent capacity for anti-tumor activity. This notion was bolstered in the 1900s by the finding of spontaneous remissions recorded, often in sparse anecdotal findings, in nearly every stage and form of cancer, by the more common observation of spontaneous regressions of melanoma and renal carcinoma, the success of nonspecific immune-stimulants such as bacillus Calmette-Guérin or Coley toxin, and the increasingly targeted use of antibodies against antigens more specific to certain cell types.[1] Indeed, the antibody specificity was perhaps the first and still the most powerful story supporting the ubiquitous catch-call of personalized medicine.

With all of the elegance of the specificity story and more than 35 years since the recipe for generating monoclonal antibodies by Kohler and Milstein,[2] the clinical promise has been largely disappointing. With rare exceptions, these molecular missiles have not annihilated their target tumors and have fallen far short of the marvel of the antibiotic revolution. The rarity of cures should not dampen the substantial, if incremental, progress that has been made. Even in the age of single-nucleotide etiologies there is a strong case that cancer, by the time of its clinical visibility, consists of many broken parts; hence the growing argument that targeted therapies may parallel the breakthrough to cure with chemotherapy in the 1970s with the move toward not one, but a cocktail of simultaneous, combined agents. As in the case of combination chemotherapy, antibody therapy may come to use different effector pathways in this assault.

Therapeutic mAbs and other therapeutic proteins have been reviewed previously (see recent reviews[1,3–15] and articles cited therein). Therefore, here the authors review the monoclonal antibodies used directly in treatment, shed some light on presumed primary mechanism of action, and survey use, from initial indication to the wider adoption based principally on clinical trials and trends. This line-up, with its wide spectrum of targets and mechanisms, may give some hope that the long trek may yet reach the originally envisioned summit. If not, these agents are undoubtedly part of the solution. This article focuses mainly on those native, unconjugated antibodies that directly affect solid tumors. Bevacizumab, though its antivascular action is indirect, has gained such wide application for solid tumors (and has been the subject of much controversy) that its inclusion seemed important. Although immune-conjugates have been well reviewed elsewhere[16–18] and are not the present focus, brentuximab vedontin, as the first new indication for Hodgkin lymphoma in 30 years, warranted special inclusion. Its success represents a partial rescue of a paradigm after the first approved antibody-drug conjugate, gemtuzumab, was withdrawn in 2010 because of lack of efficacy and increased mortality.[19] In the context of the present review it may also point to some limiting aspects of unconjugated tumor-directed antibodies which, as has been stated, have not delivered their quarter-century promise.

Table 1
Therapeutic monoclonal antibodies against cancer approved or in review in the European Union (EU) or United States (US) (information current as of August 2011)

Name	Trade Name	Type	Indication First Approved	First EU (US) Approval Year
Rituximab	MabThera, Rituxan	Anti-CD20; chimeric IgG1	Non-Hodgkin lymphoma	1998 (1997)
Trastuzumab	Herceptin	Anti-HER2; humanized IgG1	Breast cancer	2000 (1998)
Gemtuzumab ozogamicin	Mylotarg	Anti-CD33; humanized IgG4	Acute myeloid leukemia	NA (2000[a])
Alemtuzumab	MabCampath, Campath-1H	Anti-CD52; humanized IgG1	Chronic myeloid leukemia	2001 (2001)
Tositumomab + ^{131}I-tositumomab	Bexxar	Anti-CD20; murine IgG2a	Non-Hodgkin lymphoma	NA (2003)
Cetuximab	Erbitux	Anti-EGFR; chimeric IgG1	Colorectal cancer	2004 (2004)
Ibritumomab tiuxetan	Zevalin	Anti-CD20; murine IgG1	Non-Hodgkin lymphoma	2004 (2002)
Bevacizumab	Avastin	Anti-VEGF; humanized IgG1	Colorectal cancer	2005 (2004)
Panitumumab	Vectibix	Anti-EGFR; human IgG2	Colorectal cancer	2007 (2006)
Catumaxomab	Removab	Anti-EpCAM/CD3; rat/mouse bispecific mAb	Malignant ascites	2009 (NA)
Ofatumumab	Arzerra	Anti-CD20; human IgG1	Chronic lymphocytic leukemia	2010 (2009)
Ipilimumab	Yervoy	Anti-CTLA-4; human IgG1	Metastatic melanoma	2011 (2011)
Brentuximab vedotin	Adcetris	Anti-CD30; chimeric IgG1; immunoconjugate	Hodgkin lymphoma, systemic ALCL	NA (2011)

Abbreviations: ALCL, anaplastic large-cell lymphoma; CD, cluster of differentiation; CTLA-4, cytotoxic T-lymphocyte antigen 4; EGFR, epidermal growth factor receptor; EpCAM, epithelial cell adhesion molecule; NA, not approved; VEGF, vascular endothelial growth factor.
 [a] Voluntarily withdrawn from market in 2010.
Data from Dimitrov DS, Marks JD. Therapeutic antibodies: current state and future trends—is a paradigm change coming soon? Methods Mol Biol 2009;525:1–27.

Table 2
The 4 top-selling therapeutic antibodies in 2010 (in billion US$)

Rank (2009)	Name	Target	Type	Company	Sales
2 (3)	Bevacizumab	VEGF	Humanized IgG	Genentech Roche Chugai	6.973
3 (4)	Rituximab	CD20	Chimeric IgG	Genentech Biogen-IDEC Roche	6.859
6 (7)	Trastuzumab	HER2	Humanized IgG	Genentech Chugai Roche	5.859
18 (19)	Cetuximab	EGFR	Chimeric IgG	Eli Lilly BMS Merck Serono	1.791

The numbers denote ranking out of all therapeutic proteins in 2010; numbers in parentheses are for 2009. Currencies as of March 2012: 1 € = 1.33 US$; 1 CHF = 1.11 US$; 1 Yen = 0.01 US$; 1 DKK = 0.18 US$; 1 SEK = 0.15 US$.
Data from LaMerie Business Intelligence, Barcelona.

mAbs APPROVED FOR CLINICAL USE

At present 13 mAbs are approved for clinical use in the European Union or the United States (see **Table 1**). One of the approved mAbs, gemtuzumab ozogamicin (Mylotarg), was withdrawn from the market because of lack of clinical benefit and safety reasons after a clinical trial in which a greater number of deaths occurred in the group of patients with acute myeloid leukemia (AML) who received Mylotarg compared with those receiving chemotherapy alone. Mylotarg, catumaxumab (Removab) (not yet approved in the United States), and the two radiotherapeutic mAbs, tositumomab (Bexxar) and ibritumomab tiuxetan (Zevalin), are not reviewed here.

Rituximab

The first candidate remains in many ways the poster child for both specificity and efficacy. Rituximab (MabThera, Rituxan), initially developed in San Diego in the late 1980s, and father to that region's biotech explosion, was based on the finding of CD20 antigen on normal and malignant lymphocytes; it is not appreciably expressed at either pole of lymphocyte ontogeny—stem cells and plasma cells—or on other nonlymphoid cellular compartments. In contrast to many emerging cancer targets clearly connected with signal transduction circuitry, there is no clear consensus on the function of CD20. Nonetheless, the chosen antigen-antibody duo in CD20/rituximab rendered a striking clinical success and ushered in a continuing wave of similarly conceived agents, albeit with variant tactical goals and mechanisms of effect. It is interesting that only after many years afterward were clinical agents developed to target perhaps the ultimate tissue-specific bull's eye: the individual epitope of each B-lymphocyte population, separating the malignant fiend from more than a million brethren lymphocytes by one signature antigen expressed on one malignant subspecies.

In 1997 rituximab was approved by the US Food and Drug Administration (FDA) for the treatment of relapsed indolent B-cell non-Hodgkin lymphoma (NHL). The antibody is a mouse-human chimera using murine variable regions to effect anti-CD20 specificity and human immunoglobulin (Ig) G1k constant region to facilitate effector function, including complement-mediated lysis and antibody-directed cellular cytotoxicity.[20,21] Additional mechanisms include caspase activation,[22] a "vaccinal effect" based on increased idiotype-specific T-cell response to follicular lymphoma,[23] and upregulation of proapoptotic proteins such as Bax.[24,25]

Rituximab's well-known, early recognized, and sometimes fatal chief toxicity has been acute infusion reactions. Rare fatalities, occurring mainly during first infusion, have been considered secondary to a cytokine reaction; generally associated with flu-like symptoms, they may progress to life-threatening hypotension, bronchospasm, and hypoxia, but can usually be controlled by stopping or adjusting of rates of infusion and proper premedication.[26] Black-box events include tumor lysis syndrome, severe mucocutaneous reactions, and progressive multifocal leukoencephalopathy (PML) resulting in death.[27,28]

Rituximab has demonstrated clinical activity across the spectrum of lymphoprolifer-ative disorders, but the greatest impact has been in NHL, for which combinations and optimizations have sought to raise RRs and, ultimately, cure. Since its 1997 start with relapsed indolent NHL, rituximab has obtained the following additional indications for lymphoma per package insert: relapsed and refractory, follicular or low-grade, CD20-positive, B-cell NHL as single agent; previously untreated CD20-positive, follicular, B-cell NHL in combination with first-line chemotherapy; as single-agent maintenance therapy for patients achieving a partial or complete response to rituximab in combina-tion with chemotherapy; for nonprogressing (including stable), CD20-positive, low-grade, B-cell NHL, as a single agent after first-line combination of cyclophosphamide, vincristine, and prednisone (CVP) chemotherapy; previously untreated CD20-positive, diffuse large B-cell NHL in combination with anthracycline-based chemotherapy, for example, in the workhorse, R-CHOP.[29] It also has an oft-used indication for treatment of previously treated or untreated patients with CD20 chronic lymphocytic leukemia (CLL) in combination with fludarabine and cyclophosphamide (FC).[30]

Rituximab has found off-label use in the clinic in all or nearly all malignant (and many nonmalignant) settings where B cells are presumed to participate in pathogenesis, and has been the subject of many scholarly reviews. Common use spans from aggressive to low-grade lymphoproliferative disorders including: combination with chemotherapy for induction in second-line therapy for relapsed lymphoma anticipating autologous transplant[31]; combination with chlorambucil for indolent and with bendamustine in treat-ment of relapsed or refractory CLL[32]; induction for Burkitt lymphoma; use for gastric and nongastric mucosa-associated lymphoid tissue (MALT tumors),[33,34] mantle cell tumor,[35] primary cutaneous B cell,[36] splenic marginal zone NHL,[37] Waldenström's macroglobuli-nemia/lymphoplasmacytic lymphoma.[38] Its uses have been tailored to mutational status of del(17p) and del(11q) with refractory CLL (National Comprehensive Cancer Network [NCCN] guidelines: http://www.nccn.org/index.asp) and combined in cocktail fashion with other antibodies such as alemtuzumab for refractory lymphoid malignancies.

The evolution of treatment for CLL mirrors, in many ways, that of NHL as it leads from purines to chemoimmunotherapy, and most recently to novel anti-CD20 anti-bodies. Conventional treatment of CLL evolved from alkylators to purine analogues when it was demonstrated that fludarabine (F) yielded greater efficacy with better complete response (CR), progression-free survival (PFS), and overall survival (OS) rates than with chlorambucil as primary therapy.[39] Subsequently, the combination of fludarabine with cyclophosphamide (FC) showed better CR and PFS than F.[40] Based on the activity of rituximab (R) alone as a front-line agent, it was added to FC (ie, FCR) and compared with FC alone; in a phase III randomized trial the combination FCR demonstrated better OR, CR, and PFS, establishing both the regimen and the concept of chemoimmunotherapy in this setting as the upfront standard of care.[41]

Ofatumumab

Unfortunately, the activity of rituximab as a single agent is only modest,[42] and duration of response in relapsed disease is generally measured in months.[43] This shortcoming was part of the impetus to develop newer anti-CD20 targeted antibodies with a goal of improving such characteristics as binding affinity, specificity and effector function, and efficacy.[44] Ofatumumab (ofa), a fully human monoclonal IgG1 antibody, binds to a unique epitope,[45] induces considerably higher complement-dependent cytotoxicity (CDC) than rituximab,[46] and shows activity in rituxan-refractory B-cell lymphoma.[47]

Based on these potential biological advantages and modest early-phase clinical activity,[48] ofa was tested against CLL, which was either refractory to fludarabine and alemtuzumab or refractory to fludarabine with disease considered too bulky for efficacy with alemtuzumab.[49] The drug was well tolerated, though complicated by infections in 25% of the patients, but the impressive clinical results including median OS of 13.7 or 15.4 months, within 2 high-risk groups, respectively, contributed to the approval of ofa for disease refractory to fludarabine and for those who have failed alemtuzumab.[50,51]

Given the potential advantages of ofa versus rituximab and with FCR established as standard of care in the front line, substituting ofa for rituxan in the so-called O-FC regimen was tested in a multinational, randomized phase II trial in treatment-naïve patients.[52] Of the 2 tested doses, the higher dose arm yielded a CR rate of 50%. It remains unclear as to how this should be positioned with respect to such other findings as the initial randomized phase III trial that established FCR as standard of care. The precedent of combining permutations of purine analogues, alkylators, and antibodies including newer regimens such as ofa/bendamustine continues to inform ongoing studies.[53]

Ipilimumab

The novel treatment agents for melanoma, vemurafenib (a B-raf inhibitor) and ipilimumab (an antibody against cytotoxic T-lymphocyte antigen 4 [CTLA-4]), represent perhaps the most significant advance in oncology in several years. How they will fit into tactical treatment strategies and with respect to conventional dacarbazine, interleukin (IL)-2, and a new gp100-based vaccine is a welcome and exciting challenge after decades without appreciable progress.[54] Blockade of the CTLA-4 has been the subject of long and intensive investigation.[55,56]

Among the most active immune inhibitory pathways is the CD28/CTLA-4:B7-1/B7-2 receptor/ligand grouping, which modulates peripheral tolerance to tumors and outgrowth of immune-evasive clones. Inhibition is both toward the overexpressed self targets and via upregulation of inhibitory ligands on lymphocytes. Thus, blockade of CTLA-4 has potential for both monotherapy and in synergy with other therapies that enhance presentation of tumor epitopes to the immune system.[56] Genetic ablation of CTLA-4 leads to a massive and lethal lymphoproliferative disorder.[57] Antibody blockade of CTLA-4 induces potent antitumor activity through enhancing effector cells and concomitantly inhibiting T-cell regulatory activity.[58]

Given that this inhibition is not tumor specific, it is not surprising that other tumors including ovarian cancer, prostate cancer, and renal cell cancer have demonstrated durable remissions.[59]

In a recent phase III trial, patients with melanoma refractory to chemotherapy or IL-2 who received ipilimumab had improved OS compared with those receiving the gp100 peptide vaccine, and on this basis received FDA approval in 2011.[60]

Ipilimumab holds an FDA indication for the treatment of unresectable or metastatic melanoma, with NCCN guidelines that largely elucidate specific contexts consistent with this approval, including use as single agent for unresectable stage III in-transit metastases, local/satellite and/or in-transit unresectable recurrence, incompletely resected nodal recurrence, limited recurrence or metastatic disease, and disseminated recurrence of metastatic disease in patients with good performance status.

Based on its mechanism of unleashing the immune recognition and effector system, there was rationale to test the interactive effects with tumor-specific antigen. Specifically, the melanoma antigen, gp100, overexpressed on this tumor and among the antigens presented in the appropriate genetic major histocompatibility complex (MHC) context (HLA*A201), represented a prime vaccine candidate. In a phase III randomized trial, increased RRs were seen when vaccine was added to IL-2 compared with IL-2 alone (16% vs 6%, P = .03); PFS was also significantly improved with a trend toward improved OS.[61] Questions arose, nonetheless, as to whether gp100 vaccine was an appropriate control in the aforementioned phase III trial for ipilimumab. Another phase III randomized clinical trial treating previously untreated patients with metastatic melanoma compared ipilimumab (every 3 weeks for 4 doses followed by maintenance every 3 months) with and without dacarbazine as the standard control; improved OS was seen, including a difference at 3 years of nearly 21% versus 12%.[62]

The cluster of well-identified side effects induced by CTLA-4 inhibition has been referred to as immune-related adverse events (IRAEs). These unique adverse effects are likely a direct effect of impairing immune tolerance, and include colitis/diarrhea, dermatitis, hepatitis, uveitis, nephritis, inflammatory myopathy, and endocrinopathies. Although these reactions have gained a black-box designation for occasional severe and even fatal instances, they are generally manageable and reversible with treatment guidelines that include systemic corticosteroids.[63] These toxicities may be prolonged, suggestive of sustained release from immune tolerance, and perhaps a different response profile including long periods of stable disease, and correlation of toxicity with efficacy. In one report with high-risk melanoma, ipilimumab-treated patients who experienced high-grade IRAEs had a significantly higher rate of tumor regression than those without IRAEs (36% vs 5% of patients).[64]

Based on a mechanism of action clearly different from IL-2, which increases responsiveness to immune targets and is nonoverlapping with chemotherapy, earlier phase trials and future efforts will focus on combinations of vaccines, chemotherapy, and other immune modulators.[59] Furthermore, given the prolonged time course of side effects and the resulting requirement for prolonged steroids, timing of its use with respect to IL-2 and vaccines will be the subject of much attention.[65]

Trastuzumab

The human epidermal growth factor receptor 2 (HER2) is overexpressed in 20% to 30% of invasive breast cancers and is associated with a worse prognosis.[66] Trastuzumab is a humanized mAb targeting HER2, which was approved by the FDA in 1998 as the first monoclonal for a solid tumor indicated for patients with invasive breast cancer that overexpresses HER2. It is now a standard part of the treatment of HER2-positive tumors in both metastatic and adjuvant settings. Because tumors that overexpress HER2 receptor respond better across the range of studies, considerable effort has been expended to accurately assess receptor status.[67–69]

HER2 is part of a family of transmembrane tyrosine kinase receptors that normally regulate cell growth and survival, differentiation, and migration.[70] It consists of an extracellular binding domain, a transmembrane segment, and an intracellular tyrosine kinase domain. The receptor is activated generally by homodimerization or heterodimerization, but not always activated through ligand binding; it can dimerize and thus activate, independent of ligand[71] through either overexpression or mutation.[72] Thus activated by overexpression, signal-transduction cascades act to promote a host of progrowth activities including proliferation, survival, and invasion. Such signal transduction is mediated through the RAS-MAKP pathway, inhibiting cell death through the m-TOR pathway.[73] In addition, it inhibits the PI3K pathway, reducing PTEN phosphorylation and AKT dephosphorylation and thus increasing cell death.[74,75]

The human IgG1 is capable of inducing antibody-dependent cell-mediated cytotoxicity (ADCC) in vitro[76] and of recruitment of effector cells in animal studies.[77] An immune mechanism is suggested by the increased lymphoid infiltration into tumor after preoperative administration of trastuzumab.[78] There is also evidence that it causes regression of vasculature by modulating angiogenic factors.[79]

As a single agent in metastatic breast cancer, and receptor status using earlier immunohistochemistry (IHC) expression criteria, trastuzumab produced RRs of 11% to 26%.[80] From the earliest studies, though time has sharpened the assessment, it has been clear that the best results occur in tumors that overexpress HER2. The breakthrough trial for trastuzumab in metastatic disease came in a randomized phase III trial when it was used in combination with chemotherapy for HER2-positive patients.[81] As first-line therapy for metastatic disease, patients were given either chemotherapy alone or in combination. Patients were given an anthracycline and cyclophosphamide or, paclitaxel (if they had previous anthracycline in an adjuvant setting). Results showed not only improvement in response rate (RR) and progression-free interval but also in OS. Trastuzumab was subsequently showed to have efficacy and safety with a variety of other chemotherapeutics including docetaxel,[82] vinorelbine,[83] and doxil[84] in nonrandomized trials.

As for the adjuvant setting, large randomized trials established significant benefits from the addition of trastuzumab to both anthracycline and nonanthracycline regimens for early breast cancer.[85] Four major adjuvant trials including more than 13,000 women with HER2-positive early breast cancer used different adjuvant regimens with trastuzumab; in these studies overall, trastuzumab reduced the 3-year risk of recurrence by about half in this population.[86] On this basis, trastuzumab has become part of standard adjuvant therapy. Both the international Consensus Group and NCCN recommend its use for women with HER2-positive, node-positive tumors as well as for node-negative disease when the primary tumor is larger than 1 cm.

Trastuzumab combined with chemotherapy has also shown improvement in pathologic responses and event-free survival when used in the neoadjuvant setting before surgery.[87] In a randomized phase III trial, patients with advanced gastroesophageal and gastric adenocarcinoma tumors that overexpressed HER2 showed a significant increase in OS when trastuzumab was added to their chemotherapy.[88] Trastuzumab now has an FDA indication for use in combination with cisplatin and fluorouracil (5FU) or capecitabine for first-line treatment of gastric and gastroesophageal tumors that overexpress HER 2.

The most significant toxicity associated with trastuzumab is cardiomyopathy, ranging from subclinical decreases in left ventricular ejection fraction to cardiac failure manifesting as congestive heart failure. The risk is greatest when administered concurrently with anthracyclines.[81] Use following anthracyclines was associated commonly with asymptomatic cardiac dysfunction, but most severe decreases recovered with time.[89] Close monitoring of clinical status and cardiac function, sequential rather than concomitant use, and development of nonanthracycline regimens[90,91] have all been objectives.

Bevacizumab

The discussion of bevacizumab here is asymmetric in bulk and breadth compared with the other antibodies, owing to its conceptual and actual application in many tumor types, its unique mechanism, and toxicity profile. Bevacizumab is a humanized IgG1 mAb that binds to and neutralizes the ligand vascular endothelial growth factor (VEGF) rather than binding the cell-surface receptor. In fact many tissues and most malignancies produce VEGF whose native function, whether acting from a distance or in an autocrine loop, operates through binding and activation of the VEGF receptor.[91] The latter includes an extracellular binding domain and a cytoplasmic kinase domain. Following VEGF binding, the otherwise inactive monomer receptor undergoes dimerization, autophosphorylation of the tyrosine kinase domain, and downstream activation of many of the usual signal transduction suspects including MAPK and protein kinase C pathways, which mediate proliferative events—in this setting, endothelial proliferation and angiogenesis[92]; such neoangiogenesis is required by tumors once they grow to greater than 2 mm.[93]

Many of this antibody's common toxicities are related to its impact on microvasculature, including hypertension, proteinuria, rare bowel perforation, impaired wound healing, and bleeding.[94] Other than the rare bowel perforation, these can generally be managed without necessitating cessation of therapy. Although there will naturally be some specificity of side effects and adverse reactions dependent on the drugs with which bevacizumab is paired, with some notable exceptions toxicities are generally neither drug-combination specific nor tumor specific.

More severe and fatal consequences of bevacizumab have been the subject of several meta-analyses and reports of large-institution experience. In perhaps the largest of these, fatal adverse events (FAEs) were considered in a meta-analysis of more than 10,000 patients with various solid tumor types, comparing regimens with and without the addition of bevacizumab. The overall incidences of FAEs were 2.5%, and among these nearly a quarter were attributable to hemorrhage, about half related to neutropenia, and a smaller amount to perforation. There was increased RR attributable to combining bevacizumab with taxanes or platinum but not with other agents, nor were there significant tumor-specific increases. In another large meta-analysis bevacizumab was associated with high-grade congestive heart failure in breast cancer, with an overall incidence of 1.6%.[95] Yet a third large meta-analysis identified a 12% risk of thromboembolic events.[96] Of note, a pooled analysis of phase II and phase III trials did not show an increase in venous thromboembolic events (VTEs), which is important to recognize given a baseline of tumor-associated VTEs of around 10% with or without this agent.[97] Massive hemoptysis, which has been linked to large central lesions at risk for cavitation,[98] was avoided in these circumstances, and more generally in squamous cancer where this risk is increased. Bowel perforation occurred with an incidence of less than 2% in a large institution with a treated population of more than 1400 patients; it was generally managed without the need for surgical intervention.[99]

Bevacizumab demonstrated no[100] to small[101] RRs as monotherapy and, with such exceptions as maintenance regimens and single-agent use with recurrent glioblastoma, its predominant clinical role lies in combination with chemotherapy. In 2004, based on improvement of RRs, PFS, and OS, bevacizumab, when combined with chemotherapy in metastatic colorectal cancer,[102] became the first antiangiogenic agent approved for clinical use. Since then it has gained indications for metastatic breast cancer, metastatic renal cancer, metastatic (as well as advanced or recurrent) non–small cell lung cancer (NSCLC), and glioblastoma. Increasing use of bevacizumab is also being seen with hepatocellular and ovarian cancer.

Colorectal cancer
At this time bevacizumab has an indication in metastatic colorectal cancer in both first-line and second-line settings. The initial approval followed its use with bolus irinotecan, 5FU, and leucovorin (IFL) whereby addition of bevacizumab significantly improved RR and median survival (20 vs 16 months) compared with chemotherapy only.[102] While

bolus IFL has fallen out of general use because of its toxicity profile, studies have supported the value of bevacizumab in combination with more widely used treatments including FOLFIRI (FOL, leucovorin plus F, 5FU and IRI, irinotecan [Camptosar]),[103,104] and 3 oxaliplatin-containing regimens.[105] In addition, when bevacizumab was added to 5FU/leucovorin in the absence of irinotecan or oxaliplatin, RRs were approximately doubled and median survival improved in comparison with chemotherapy alone.[106,107]

Efforts to apply bevacizumab in the adjuvant setting for colorectal cancer moved from initial enthusiasm to disappointment. As already noted, bevacizumab had shown favorable impact in metastatic disease in several settings including in combination with IFL (irinotecan, 5FU, and leucovorin) for metastatic colorectal cancer. Borrowing the prevailing paradigm for chemotherapy, which attempts to apply results in metastatic disease to adjuvant use on the presumption of potential elimination of micrometastases, bevacizumab was studied in the adjuvant setting for colorectal cancer. Two recently published phase III trials, unfortunately, did not show the sought-for benefit. When bevacizumab was added (for 12 months) to FOLFOX (folinic acid [FOL], fluorouracil [F], and oxaliplatin [OX]) (for 6 months), it failed to meet its primary end point of improving 3-year disease-free survival.[108] In a second phase III trial the combination of bevacizumab with FOLFOX actually led to a slight but significant decrease in OS.[109]

Non–small cell lung cancer

The role of bevacizumab in NSCLC was initially established in a phase III trial as first-line therapy for advanced, nonsquamous NSCLC including those with malignant effusions and metastatic disease.[110] Patients received paclitaxel and carboplatin with or without bevacizumab; those patients receiving bevacizumab then continued it as monotherapy for an additional 6 cycles unless disease progressed. The objective RR more than doubled, and there was an increase in PFS and OS. At 2 years, the survival rate was 23% in the group treated with bevacizumab versus 15% without. In another phase III trial with a similarly defined patient population, on the addition of bevacizumab to gemcitabine and cisplatin (also with maintenance bevacizumab in the concurrent bevacizumab group) an increase in PFS did not translate into improved OS[111]; the investigators suggested this may have been due to the wide availability of secondary therapies. Testing with a current standard, pemetrexate, is under way but has not yet ripened to a point to give clinical guidance.[112,113]

The story for use of bevacizumab in advanced metastatic breast cancer (MBC) has been tumultuous, tracking a course from early excitement and widespread use to an FDA withdrawal; understandably this raised public furor from a highly engaged population. In the first phase III trial to assess impact in newly diagnosed patients with MBC, bevacizumab was either added to chemotherapy (weekly paclitaxel) or not; the bevacizumab arm doubled the PFS and significantly improved RR.[114] These striking results led to accelerated FDA approval and its wide adoption. Unfortunately, neither of 2 phase III postapproval studies, one trial with docetaxel and the other with capecitabine, a taxane, or an anthracycline, confirmed this magnitude of benefit, and no trial has shown an improvement in OS.[115,116]

Renal cancer

For metastatic renal cancer, 2 phase III trials demonstrated improved OS when bevacizumab was added to interferon-α in first-line treatment.[117,118] In one of these trials the initially reported PFS with bevacizumab of 10.2 months was nearly doubled,[117] but only a nonsignificant and clinically small difference of OS was reported in the final analysis.[119] In the second phase III trial, with a similar dose schedule as the first, bevacizumab plus interferon-α improved RR and PFS compared with monotherapy with interferon, but did not reach significance for OS.[118,120]

Glioblastoma

For recurrent glioblastoma, adding bevacizumab to irinotecan increased RR.[121,122] Nevertheless, in the notoriously difficult setting of recurrent glioblastoma both alone and in combination with irinotecan, bevacizumab showed respectable RRs of 28% and 38%, respectively[123]; it holds an indication for use as monotherapy in this setting despite the absence of a demonstrated improvement in OS.

Ovarian cancer

The benefit of bevacizumab in ovarian cancer was assessed in the setting of first-line use with paclitaxel and carboplatin in a large trial for stage III or IV epithelial ovarian, primary peritoneal, or fallopian tube cancer following maximal cytoreduction.[124] Of the 3 arms in this phase III trial, representing chemotherapy only, concurrent bevacizumab and chemotherapy, and concurrent bevacizumab and chemotherapy followed by maintenance bevacizumab, the latter improved PFS but not OS. First-line use for advanced and high-risk early-stage disease treated with paclitaxel and carboplatin, with and without bevacizumab, showed significant improvement in median survival without improving OS; a subset analysis suggested that adding bevacizumab may be more beneficial among women with a poorer prognosis.[125]

Small studies in hepatocellular with bevacizumab alone[126] or with gemcitabine and oxaliplatin[127] showed RRs sufficient to generate further interest and more definitive study.

Bevacizumab has a unique profile of toxicities and adverse reactions. Some preclinical studies had suggested that VEGF-targeted therapies could unfavorably alter the biology of the neoplasms, for example, by upregulating proinflammatory pathways and factors that are associated with metastasis,[128] but a pooled meta-analysis of 5 randomized phase III trials did not show altered disease progression following bevacizumab.[129] Although the clinical data are too scant to explain the unpredicted disappointments such as failure in the adjuvant setting for colorectal cancer, numerous hypotheses such as the foregoing, some readily testable, have been suggested.[130] As in most contexts in oncology, risk/benefit analysis is important to decision making, and the risk in some clinical settings where bevacizumab is considered often pits treatment against the prospect and probability of imminent death. It is notable, therefore, that while a recent meta-analysis of 16 randomized trials in advanced cancer showed nearly a 1.5-fold increase in fatal adverse events, the absolute values were 2.5% versus 1.7% in the respective presence or absence of bevacizumab.[131] Nevertheless, these same numbers gather increased clinical sway in adjuvant settings where the risks and benefits are markedly different.

Cetuximab

Cetuximab is a recombinant chimeric antibody that derives specificity from its murine Fv portion and effector functions from human IgG1 constant regions. The primary mechanism of impact is through disruption of the signal transduction pathway of the endothelial growth factor receptor (EGFR).[132] Nevertheless, selection based on IHC expression of EGFR expression or somatic mutations[133,134] of the EGFR tyrosine kinase domain,[135] as in the response of NSCLC to small-molecule tyrosine kinase inhibitors, do not predict response of colorectal cancer to EGFR antibodies. Wild-type K-ras, on the other hand, is necessary for effect.[136]

Cetuximab has been studied alone and in combination, predominantly with colorectal cancer and head and neck cancer. In colorectal cancer, cetuximab as monotherapy showed improvement in OS compared with best supportive care (BSC) in patients previously treated with a fluoropyrimidine, irinotecan, and oxaliplatin.[137] This study also demonstrated improved quality of life and the association of rash with a favorable outcome. Cetuximab as monotherapy or combined with irinotecan both showed clinically significant activity in patients with metastatic disease who were refractory to irinotecan, but the combination showed superior RR, time to progression, and median survival.[138] In another study, the combination of cetuximab and irinotecan also showed improvement in RR and PFS in patients previously treated with oxaliplatin and fluoropyrimidines for metastatic disease.[139] In combination with FOLFIRI as first-line therapy for metastatic disease it showed increased OS in patients with wild-type K-ras.[140] The data showing advantage in the first line when combined with oxaliplatin are not as clear. In one study the addition of cetuximab to FOLFOX showed significant improvement of RR only in the wild type K-ras subpopulation[141] but in another, more recent trial, no advantages were shown when added to oxaliplatin, even in the wild-type K-ras group.[142]

In squamous cell head and neck cancer, cetuximab showed improvement in OS when added to radiation compared with radiation alone for locally and regionally advanced disease.[143,144] The advantage did not extend to those with marked functional compromise or who were older than 65 years. Here, too, response was improved in those with acneiform rash.

As first-line treatment in patients with recurrent or metastatic squamous cell carcinoma of the head and neck, cetuximab plus platinum-5FU chemotherapy improved OS compared with platinum-based chemotherapy plus fluorouracil alone.[145]

Despite 2 recent phase III trials in NSCLC, the role of cetuximab in lung cancer remains unclear. These randomized trials compared doublets of standard chemotherapy with and without cetuximab in the first-line setting for metastatic disease, and may suggest different clinical guidance. In the FLEX trial, a randomized phase III multinational study, patients with IIIB (malignant pleural effusion) and IV, who expressed EGFR, received cisplatin and vinorelbine with or without cetuximab. Patients who received cetuximab had significant but clinically modest increased OS at 11.3 months versus 10.3 months with chemotherapy alone.[146] First-cycle rash in this study was substantially associated with OS, with the median with rash at 15 months compared with 8.8 months without the rash.[147] In another phase III randomized trial studying same-stage patients in first-line treatment, without restrictions on EGFR expression, cetuximab combined with taxol/carboplatin did not improve PFS compared with chemotherapy alone; a small increase in OS for cetuximab of less than 2 months did not reach statistical significance.[148]

Panitumumab

Panitumumab, an IgG2 class antibody to the EGFR receptor, was the first fully human antibody to be approved by the FDA in 2006 for the treatment of patients with EGFR-expressing, metastatic colorectal carcinoma with disease progression on or following fluoropyrimidine-, oxaliplatin-, and irinotecan-containing chemotherapy regimens. It received regulatory approval for use as monotherapy in refractory disease based on prolonging disease-free survival.[149] Given the similarities to cetuximab, efforts have focused on where to place each and in which clinical contexts and sequences, although they have notably not been compared in a face-to-face randomized phase III trial. The close relation to cetuximab, both biological and clinical, provides a helpful context for review. Like cetuximab, panitumumab binds to the receptor, the dyad is internalized, and the downstream signal transduction is blunted. Its activity cannot be reliably shown to depend on the overexpression of EGFR.[150–152] However, downstream signal transduction by constitutively activated K-ras abrogates its effect, and its use according to American Society of Clinical Oncology guidelines, consistent with clinical trials,[141,153] is limited to tumors with wild-type K-ras. There is more recent evidence that mutations in B-raf may also predict no response to either cetuximab or panitumumab.[154] Biologically, its difference from cetuximab in being fully human may underlie its significant reduction in infusion reactions. Despite its design to be more activating of cell-mediated cytotoxicity and ADCC, neither of these activities nor its efficacy compared with cetuximab has been demonstrated.[1] Its toxicities, which include a predictable rash in almost all cases, as well as frequent diarrhea and malaise, parallel those of cetuximab, as does the positive association of rash with clinical impact.[153]

Panitumumab has shown activity when used both in monotherapy and in combination. A large phase III trial showed improved RR and decreased tumor progression when used as monotherapy compared with BSC in patients refractory to oxaliplatin and irinotecan-based therapies.[155] In combination chemotherapy with FOLFOX, panitumumab in the first line improved both RR and PFS[156] in contrast to cetuximab, which had mixed results as previously noted. When combined with FOLFIRI versus FOLFIRI alone after failure with 5FU-based chemotherapy (the majority with oxaliplatin), addition of panitumumab significantly improved PFS.[157]

Brentuximab Vedotin

The first-in-class antibody drug conjugate (ADC), brentuximab vedontin, received accelerated FDA approval in August 2011 for treatment of relapsed or refractory Hodgkin lymphoma and systemic anaplastic large-cell lymphoma (ALCL). Approval was based on impressive RR rather than demonstrable survival improvement in rather dire clinical circumstances: in Hodgkin lymphoma after failure of at least 2 prior systemic regimens in autologous stem cell candidates, and for ALCL after failure of at least 1 multiagent regimen.

The antibody is a chimerized IgG, which targets CD30 and thus delivers its antimitotic payload, monomethyl auristatin (vedontin). CD30 is only minimally expressed in normal tissue but densely expressed in both Hodgkin lymphoma and ALCL.[158]

As optimistically as progress with treatment of Hodgkin disease (HD) is viewed, approximately 15% to 30% of patients do not achieve long-term remissions on conventional therapy, and despite autologous stem cell transplantation (ASCT) many of these subsequently perish while still in young adulthood.[159]

In the pivotal phase I[160] and subsequent phase II trials[161] RR data were rightly greeted with excitement. In the phase II trial, for patients with HD, all with prior transplants, 75% achieved an objective response including 32% complete responders who have not yet reached median duration of response. For 58 patients with relapsed or refractory systemic ALCL, a CR was reached in 56% of patients the median duration of which, likewise, has not yet been reached. Moreover, retreatment has been successfully used to maintain complete remissions[162] and, though the number of patients was small, a retrospective look across 3 studies demonstrated provocatively high responses with retreatment.[163]

It has been suggested that these impressive results may include several mechanisms, from apoptosis by ligating CD30, to cytotoxic, to the bystander effect on surrounding tissue.[160,164] The remarkable results with HD were particularly impressive considering the minimal responses achieved using the unconjugated anti-CD30 antibody. Beyond the direct impact on the malignant cell, it has been suggested that the local effect on the tumor-supporting cellular milieu was also a factor. By bulk, malignant Reed-Sternberg cells represent a minority of the masses in HD, which otherwise consist largely of inflammatory cells recruited by chemokines that in turn support the tumor cells that recruited them.[165] The shrinkage of these masses might thus be understood, in part, to be due to the bystander effect caused by local diffusion of the cytotoxic agent into this local environment. Although other differences no doubt exist, this may be one factor to explain greater responses than achieved for similar antibody-toxin conjugates, for example, with trastuzumab in HER2-positive cancer[166] where tumor masses are predominantly composed of malignant cells.

Alemtuzumab

Alemtuzumab is a humanized anti-CD52 IgG1 monoclonal antibody. Early studies demonstrated its efficacy in refractory disease, leading initially to approval by the FDA in 2001 for treatment of fludaribine-refractory CLL; subsequent trials demonstrated its use as front-line monotherapy for B-cell CLL.[167] Antibodies to CD52 induce complement-mediated lysis and antibody-directed cellular toxicity through this target that is not only expressed on CLL and lymphomas but also on both normal B cells and normal T cells, neutrophils, and monocytes.[168] This large spectrum of targets accounts not only for positive aspects such as off-label uses with T-cell lymphoproliferative disorders such as peripheral T-cell lymphoma, T-cell prolymphocytic leukemia, cutaneous T-cell lymphoma,[169–171] mycosis fungoides, and Sezary syndrome,[172] but also for negative consequences such as heightened infusion reactions and significant vulnerability to opportunistic infections.

Based on increased acute toxicity and prolonged myelosuppression, alemtuzumab has not supplanted the more B-cell–specific rituximab either as monotherapy or in combination with cytotoxic chemotherapy. First-line treatment for CLL generally uses fludaribine as the cornerstone, often in combination with cyclophosphamide and rituximab.[173] Second-line therapy with alemtuzumab added to fludarabine and cyclophosphamide demonstrated substantial efficacy in a recently reported phase II trial.[174] Response rates have ranged in the area of 30% to 50% in the relapsed setting and 80% to 90% in previously untreated patients with CLL.[1] In a large multicenter study, patients with refractory or relapsed CLL, previously exposed to alkylating agents and having failed fludarabine, had an overall RR of about one third, nearly all partial responses; median survival for responders was 32 months.[49] Alemtuzumab has received particular attention in high-risk settings, including 17p deletions and p53 defects[175,176] known to be resistant to standard agents including chlorambucil, purine analogues and rituximab. One study demonstrated nearly 50% overall RRs and favorable OS[177] in the 17p-deletion cytogenetic group. Alemtuzumab has been shown to achieve CR in the setting of p53 mutation and resistance to chemotherapy,[178] and in one study of fludarabine-refractory disease, even within a small subset with the presence of p53 mutations or deletions (predictors of poor response to conventional therapy), responses occurred in 40% with a median response duration of 8 months.[179] In a phase II trial with subcutaneous alemtuzumab, efficacy with fludarabine-refractory CLL did not vary with 17p deletion, mutated p53, 11q deletion, or mutated p53.[180]

Combination of alemtuzumab with rituximab has not gained traction, based on results of FCR that are hard to compete with and significant infectious complications. In a study of 32 patients with relapsed or refractory disease, for example, while slightly more than 50% showed response a similar percentage also developed infections, including 27% cytomegalovirus antigenemia.[181] In a recent phase II trial, alemtuzumab was added to conventional FCR yielding 70% CR and 18% partial response in high-risk patients, results considered comparable with historic FCR-treated high-risk patients. Based on nearly 60% CRs in the subset with 17p deletion it was suggested, however, that this may nonetheless have a useful front-line role before allogeneic stem cell transplantation.[182]

The general use of alemtuzumab for consolidation in the community setting cannot yet be recommended, although the question remains to be settled and is the subject of significant investigation.[183] A phase III trial in which alemtuzumab was used as consolidation to fludarabine $\pm$ cyclophosphamide was stopped prematurely because of severe infections; nevertheless, minimal residual disease was durably reduced by consolidation and PFS was significantly improved after median follow-up of 48 months.[184] Although there was a trend toward shorter response duration in comparison with historic groups receiving intravenous alemtuzumab, patients receiving subcutaneous treatment showed reliable decreases in graded measures of residual disease.[185] Although alemtuzumab consolidation improved both CR and minimal residual disease (MRD)-negative rates, in a study of 102 patients initially treated with induction fludarabine and rituxan there were 5 deaths from infection, and 2-year PFS and OS were not improved.[186] Efforts have been under way over the past decade to unravel genomic complexity in CLL.[187,188] Such understanding will inform trial design and, undoubtedly, the value of consolidation will depend on identification of molecular diagnostic settings where improvements of MRD-negative status translate into improved OS.

mAbs IN CLINICAL AND PRECLINICAL DEVELOPMENT

Hundreds of mAbs are in thousands of clinical trials[14]; 2239 entries for planned, ongoing, or completed clinical trials were retrieved from http://www.clinicaltrials.gov by searching with cancer AND therapy AND monoclonal antibodies as of August 2011, of which 270 are in phase III. A significant number of all new medicines are mAbs against cancer (see also http://www.phrma.org/research/new-medicines). At least 1 to 3 different antibodies are being developed at different companies for each relevant therapeutic target. However, some molecules are targeted by many more mAbs; for example, the insulin-like growth factor receptor type I (IGF-IR) is targeted by more than 10 different mAbs.[189] During the last decade and especially in the last several years, the number of clinical trials with therapeutic antibodies has increased dramatically. However, this increase has been largely due to an increase in the number of indications for the same antibodies, especially in combination with other therapeutics. The number of targets and corresponding antibodies in preclinical development and in the discovery phase has also increased significantly during the past decade.

Second- and third-generation mAbs are being developed against already validated targets. The improvement of already existing antibodies also includes an increase (to a certain extent) of their binding to Fc receptors for enhancement of ADCC and half-life, selection of appropriate frameworks to increase stability and yield, decrease of immunogenicity by using in silico and in vitro methods, and conjugation to small molecules and various fusion proteins to enhance cytotoxicity. A major lesson from the current state of antibody-based therapeutics is that gradual improvement in the properties of existing antibodies and identification of novel antibodies and novel targets is likely to continue in the foreseeable future.

One area where one could expect conceptually novel antibody-based candidate therapeutics, even though within the current paradigm, is going beyond traditional antibody structures. At present, all FDA-approved anticancer therapeutic antibodies (see **Table 1**) and the vast majority of those in clinical trials are full-size antibodies, mostly in IgG1 format of about 150 kDa. A fundamental problem for such large molecules is their poor penetration into tissues (eg, solid tumors) and poor or absent binding to regions on the surface of some molecules (eg, on the human immunodeficiency virus envelope glycoprotein) that are accessible by molecules of smaller size. Therefore much work, especially during the last decade, has been aimed at developing novel scaffolds of much smaller size and higher stability (see, eg, recent reviews in Refs.[11,190,191]). Such scaffolds are based on various human and nonhuman molecules of high stability and could be divided into 2 major groups for the purposes of this review: antibody-derived and others. Here the advantages of antibody-derived scaffolds, specifically those derived from antibody domains, and binders selected from libraries based on engineered antibody domains (eAds) are briefly discussed; an excellent recent review describes the second group.[190]

First, their size (12–15 kDa) is about an order of magnitude smaller than the size of an IgG1 (about 150 kDa). The small size leads to relatively good penetration into tissues and the ability to bind into cavities or active sites of protein targets that may not be accessible to full-size antibodies. Second, eAds may be more stable than full-size antibodies in the circulation and can be relatively easily engineered to further increase their stability. For example, some eAds with increased stability could be taken orally or delivered via the pulmonary route, or may even penetrate the blood-brain barrier, and retain activity even after being subjected to harsh conditions such as freeze-drying or heat denaturation. In addition, eAds are typically monomeric, of high solubility, and do not significantly aggregate or can be engineered to reduce aggregation. Their half-life in the circulation can be relatively easily adjusted from minutes or hours to weeks by making fusion proteins of varying size and changing binding to the neonatal Fc receptor (FcRn). In contrast to conventional antibodies, eAds are well expressed in bacterial, yeast, and mammalian cell systems. Finally, the small size of eAds allows for higher molar quantities per gram of product, which should provide a significant increase in potency per dose and reduction in overall manufacturing cost. However, despite all these advantages there is still no candidate therapeutic based on such scaffolds in phase III clinical trial as of August 2011.

Research on novel antibody-derived scaffolds continues. The authors identified a scaffold based on the variable region of heavy chain that is stable and highly soluble.[192] It was used for construction of a large-size (20 billion clones) eAd phage library by grafting complementarity-determining regions (CDR3s and CDR2s) from 5 of the authors' other Fab libraries and randomly mutagenizing CDR1. It was also proposed to use engineered antibody constant domains (C_H2 of IgG, IgA and IgD, and C_H3 of IgE and IgM) as scaffolds for construction of libraries.[193] Because of their small size and the domain's role in antibody effector functions, these have been termed nanoantibodies, the smallest fragments that could be engineered to exhibit simultaneous antigen binding and effector functions. Several large libraries (up to 50 billion clones) were constructed and antigen-specific binders successfully identified.[194] The authors have recently engineered C_H2-based scaffolds with high stability by introducing an additional disulfide bond[195] and by shortening C_H2.[196] It is possible that these and other novel scaffolds under development could provide new opportunities for identification of potentially useful therapeutics.

SAFETY, EFFICACY, AND QUALITY OF CANDIDATE THERAPEUTIC mAbs

The success of antibody-based therapeutics is mostly attributable to the use of concepts and methodologies developed during a paradigm change decades ago that resulted in dramatic improvement of 3 key features in candidate therapeutics required for FDA approval: safety, efficacy, and quality. These factors are critical for the success of any drug, and are discussed in more detail as regards antibody-based therapeutics.

Safety

Side effects caused by therapeutic antibodies may be divided into 2 large groups: (1) interactions with intended targets and (2) interactions with unintended targets. Binding to an intended target can lead to undesirable side effects, for example, by immuno-modulatory antibodies that could be suppressory or stimulatory. Administration of suppressory therapeutic antibodies could lead to a wide range of side effects related to decreased function of the immune system. An important example is the use of the best-selling antibody-based therapeutics targeting tumor necrosis factor α (TNFα) (infliximab, certolizumab pegol, and adalimumab), which can lead to infectious compli-cations.[197] The overstimulation of the immune system can also produce life-threatening illness. In one case, which gained wide publicity, administration of a single dose of the stimulatory anti-CD28 mAb TGN1412 resulted in induction of a systemic inflammatory response characterized by a rapid induction of proinflammatory cyto-kines in all 6 volunteers, leading to critical illness within 12 to 16 hours.[198] One impor-tant difference between antibody-based therapeutics containing Fc and other therapeutic proteins (not conjugated with toxic molecules) is that the antibody effector functions including ADCC and CDC could lead to toxicities after binding to intended target molecules, but on tissues other than those intended. An example of this is the trastuzumab-associated cardiotoxicity that is potentiated when the antibody is used concurrently or sequentially with an anthracycline.[199]

Interactions with unintended targets can lead to a wide range of side effects, in many cases with poorly understood mechanisms. An important example is the adverse acute infusion reactions after administration of antibodies whereby cytokine release plays a pivotal role but whereby other not fully explained mechanisms could also be involved; such reactions were reported for many antibodies including inflixi-mab, rituximab, cetuximab, alemtuzumab, trastuzumab, and panitumumab.[200] Infu-sion side effects for rituximab can result from release of cellular contents from lysed malignant B cells.[201] Administration of antibodies can also lead to hypersensitivity reactions, including anaphylactic shock and serum sickness.[197] Preexisting IgEs that cross-react with therapeutic antibodies can increase the number and severity of such reactions, which can occur even with the first protein infusion. A notable example of this occurred with administration of cetuximab.[200] Hypersensitivity is frequently associated with immunogenicity.

Immunogenicity

Immunogenicity of antibodies can be a significant issue in safety and effi-cacy.[197,202–207] For example, the success of the mAb-based therapeutics was criti-cally related to the development of less immunogenic proteins. Murine mAbs were used initially as candidate therapeutics in the 1980s, but their high immunogenicity resulted in high titers of human antimouse antibodies (HAMAs), and related toxicities and low potency. Development of the less immunogenic chimeric mAbs, which contain human Fc fragments, and humanized mAbs, which contain mouse CDRs grafted into a human antibody framework, was critical for the clinical success of the products. Human antibodies exhibit low immunogenicity on average, and are currently the favored type of antibody in development, although most of the therapeutic anti-bodies approved for clinical use are still chimeric and humanized mAbs.

Immunogenicity can be influenced by factors related to protein structure, composition, posttranslational modifications, impurities, heterogeneity, aggregate formation, degradation, formulation, storage conditions, as well as properties of its interacting partner, the patient's immune system and disease status, concomitant medications, dose, route, and time and frequency of administration, especially when administered as multiple doses over prolonged periods.[203] Even human proteins can elicit human antihuman antibodies. In one of the most studied cases of anti-TNFα mAbs, treatment with the human mAb adalimumab resulted in antibodies against the therapeutic that varied from less than 1% to up to 87% for different cohorts of patients, protocols, diseases, and methods of measurement.[208]

A likely mechanism for the immunogenicity of human mAbs involves the unique antibody sequences that confer antigen binding and specificity, but may appear foreign. Human therapeutic proteins can also break immune tolerance, and aggregation can be a major determinant of antibody elicitation.[203] Aggregation can result in repetitive structures that may not require T-cell help.[209] Antibody immunogenicity may also affect efficacy through either the pharmacokinetic or neutralizing effects of the antibody responses that are dependent on several factors, including the affinity, specificity, and concentration of the induced antibodies.[202] Because immunogenicity is an important factor in both safety and efficacy, significant efforts to predict and reduce immunogenicity of therapeutic antibodies are ongoing.[204–207]

Individual immune responses to therapeutic antibodies vary widely. A key, and largely unanswered, question is what determines these variations. Despite extensive laboratory and clinical studies that were instrumental in delineating general concepts about critical factors involved in immunogenicity, it is impossible to predict the extent to which a novel therapeutic protein will be immunogenic in human patients. Little is known about the individual antibodies that compose the polyclonal response to therapeutic proteins. The germline antibody repertoire at any given time could be a major determinant of individual differences, so knowledge of large portions of antibodies generated by the human immune system, preferably the complete set, that is, the antibodyome,[8] could ultimately help to predict individual immune responses to therapeutic antibodies.

Despite the possibility for immunogenicity and other side effects, antibody therapeutics are relatively safe, primarily because of their high specificity. This advantage is fundamental in comparison with small-molecule drugs, which on average are less specific and can bind nonspecifically to a large number of molecules. However, in some cases there are significant side effects, and safety concerns can lead to the withdrawal of therapeutic antibodies from the market (eg, Mylotarg). Thus, choosing the most appropriate animal model for toxicity testing is very important and species cross-reactivity should be included when identifying new candidate mAb therapeutics. If such a model does not exist, transgenic animals expressing the human target and surrogate protein that is cross-reactive with the human homologous target in relevant animals can be used.[210]

Efficacy

After safety, efficacy is the most important parameter considered by the FDA for approval. Many therapeutic antibodies are highly effective in vivo and have revolutionized the treatment of cancer (eg, rituximab for NHL).[201] Alemtuzumab plays an important role in therapy for hematological malignancies.[211] Another example is trastuzumab as adjuvant systemic therapy for HER2-positive breast cancer.[212] Results from 6 trials randomizing more than 14,000 women with HER2-positive early breast cancer to trastuzumab versus nontrastuzumab-based adjuvant chemotherapy demonstrate that the addition of trastuzumab reduces recurrence by approximately 50% and improves OS by 30%.[213]

On average, the efficacy of therapeutic mAbs is not high, and there is substantial individual variability. One prominent example is trastuzumab (Herceptin), which has clearly revolutionized the treatment of HER2-positive patients; however, half of the patients still have nonresponding tumors, and disease progression occurs within a year in most cases.[214] For patients with disease progression, combination with small molecules could be useful; for example, the addition of a the dual tyrosine kinase inhibitor of EGFR and HER2 lapatinib to capecitabine was shown to provide superior efficacy for women with HER2-positive, advanced breast cancer progressing after treatment with anthracycline-, taxane-, and trastuzumab-based therapy.[215] Current data do not support the use of trastuzumab for more than 1 year; the appropriate length of treatment, optimum timing, and administration schedule are not known.[212] Like other therapeutic proteins, trastuzumab does not appear to efficiently cross the blood-brain barrier, and it is unclear whether the current practice of local therapy for the central nervous system and continued trastuzumab is optimal.[214]

Antiangiogenic therapies that target the VEGF, for example, bevacizumab, and the VEGF receptor (VEGFR), are effective adjuncts for the treatment of solid tumors, and are commonly administered in combination with cytotoxic chemotherapy. However, at least half of patients fail to respond to antiangiogenic treatment of gliomas, and the response duration is modest and variable.[216] The use of bevacizumab plus paclitaxel as a first-line treatment for patients with MBC doubled median PFS (11.8 months vs 5.9 months; hazard ratio = 0.60; $P<.001$) compared with paclitaxel alone; however, a statistically significant improvement in OS was not provided by the addition of bevacizumab, although a post hoc analysis demonstrated a significant increase in 1-year survival for the combination arm.[217]

The anti-EGFR mAbs cetuximab and panitumumab, either as single agents or in combination with chemotherapy, have demonstrated clinical activity against metastatic colorectal cancer, but seem to benefit only select patients with predictive markers of efficacy, including EGFR overexpression, development of rash, and the absence of a K-ras mutation.[218] In general, as single agents or in combination, therapeutic mAbs and other proteins have produced only modest clinical responses in solid tumors.[219] There are no mAbs approved for the treatment of several tumors (eg, prostate cancer). However, for prostate cancer there are 30 candidates in the pipeline (16 vaccines and 14 antibodies), and one FDA-approved prostate cancer vaccine (Provenge); of these candidates, 19 are in phases II and III (9 vaccines and 10 antibodies) and 8 are in phase I clinical trials.

The mechanisms underlying the relatively low efficacy of some therapeutic antibodies and the high variability of responses to treatment are not well known, but are likely to involve multiple factors. Preexisting resistance or development of resistance is a fundamental problem for any therapeutic. Various mechanisms, including mutations, activation of multidrug transporters, and overexpression or activation of signaling proteins, are exemplified as EGFR-targeted therapies.[220] Another major problem is poor penetration into tissues (eg, solid tumors).

New approaches are being developed to increase efficacy of mAbs, including enhanced effector functions, improved half-life, increased tumor and tissue accessibility, and greater stability; the methods used involve both protein engineering and glycoengineering, and results to date are encouraging.[221,222] mAbs that do not engage the innate immune system's effector functions are being developed when binding is sufficient.[223] Multitargeted antibodies are being developed and tested in clinical trials, for example, an antibody targeting HER2/neu and CD3 with preferential binding to activating Fcγ type I/III receptors, resulting in the formation of tri-cell complexes between tumor cells, T cells, and accessory cells.[224] A similar bispecific (targeting CD3 and EpCAM) trifunctional mAb, catumaxomab, was approved in the European Union for the treatment of malignant ascites in 2009 (see **Table 1**), and is the first bispecific mAb approved for clinical use. This antibody binds to cancer cells expressing epithelial cell adhesion molecule (EpCAM) on their surface via one arm, to a T-lymphocyte–expressing CD3 via the other arm and to an antigen-presenting cell like a macrophage, a natural killer cell, or a dendritic cell via the Fc. This process initiates an immunologic reaction leading to the removal of cancer cells from the abdominal cavity, thus reducing the tumor burden that is considered the cause of ascites in cancer patients. Bispecific and multispecific mAbs and other therapeutic proteins are currently being developed to be aimed at several targets.

A promising line of enquiry is the modulation of immune responses by mAbs targeting regulators of T-cell immune responses. The cytotoxic T-lymphocyte antigen 4 (CTLA-4), present on activated T cells, is an inhibitory regulator of such responses. Human antibodies and Fc fusion proteins that abrogate the function of CTLA-4 have been tested in the clinic and have been found to have clinical activity against melanoma.[225,226] It appears that CTLA-4 blockade also enhanced the cancer-testis antigen NY-ESO-1–specific B-cell and T-cell immune responses in patients with durable objective clinical responses and stable disease, suggesting immunotherapeutic designs that combine NY-ESO-1 vaccination with CTLA-4 blockade.[226] Ipilimumab, which targets CTLA-4, was approved by the FDA in 2011 for the treatment of metastatic melanoma (see **Table 2**). Therapeutic mAbs that mimic the natural ligand, for example, the TNF-related apoptosis inducing ligand (TRAIL), have also been developed.[227,228]

Second- and third-generation mAbs against already validated targets, for example, HER2, CD20, and TNFα, are currently under clinical study or already approved. Various approaches have been used to discover novel, relevant targets, but progress has been slow. Modifications of the standard panning procedures have been reported, including enhanced selection of cross-reactive antibodies by sequential antigen planning[229] and competitive antigen panning for focused selection of antibodies targeting a specific protein domain or subunit.[230,231] To ensure better tissue penetration and hidden epitope access, a variety of small engineered antibody domains (about 10-fold smaller than IgG) are being developed.[191,192] Knowledge of antibodyomes could be used for generation of semisynthetic libraries for selection of high-affinity binders of small size and minimal immunogenicity.[8]

A major lesson from the current state of antibody-based therapeutics is that gradual improvement in the properties of existing therapeutic proteins and identification of novel proteins and targets is likely to continue in the foreseeable future. A fundamental challenge has been to increase dramatically the efficacy of therapeutic antibodies and to apply them to many more diseases. Other major challenges are the development of effective personalized antibody-based therapeutics, and prediction of toxicity or potentially low efficacy in vivo.

Quality

Quality is a very important parameter for approval of any drug by the FDA. A specific fundamental feature that distinguishes mAbs and other biologics from small-molecule drugs is their heterogeneity. Heterogeneity of mAbs is due to modifications such as incomplete disulfide bond formation, glycosylation, N-terminal pyroglutamine cyclization, C-terminal lysine processing, deamidation, isomerization, oxidation, amidation of the C-terminal amino acid, and modification of the N-terminal amino acids by maleuric acid, as well as noncovalent associations with other molecules, conformational diversity, and aggregation.[232] Tens of thousands of variants with the same sequence may coexist.

Development of high-quality protein therapeutics with minimal heterogeneity and contamination is essential for their safety and approval by the FDA. Process development for production of a therapeutic protein is a complex operation involving recombinant DNA technologies, verification of a strong expression system, gene amplification, characterization of a stable host-cell expression system, optimization and design of the mammalian cell-culture fermentation system, and development of an efficient recovery process resulting in high yields and product quality.[233] Titers in the range of 5 to 10 g/L or even higher, cell densities of more than 20 million cells/mL, and specific productivity of more than 20 pg/cell/d (even up to 100 pg/cell/d) have been achieved.[234]

Genetic delivery of therapeutic antibodies by in vivo production offers a new way of increasing quality and reducing cost. Three approaches can be used for the stable long-term expression and secretion of therapeutic proteins in vivo: (1) direct in vivo administration of integrating vectors carrying the gene, (2) grafting of ex vivo genetically modified autologous cells, and (3) implantation of an encapsulated antibody producing heterologous or autologous cells. Another promising direction is the prospect of using molecular farming methods to create relatively low-cost therapeutic proteins in plants, for example, in genetically engineered tobacco leaves.

BIOSIMILAR AND BIOBETTER THERAPEUTIC ANTIBODIES

A major goal of current activity is to develop therapeutic antibodies that are similar but cheaper than the currently existing ones, or are better in terms of efficacy and safety. By 2015 biologics worth $60 billion in annual sales will lose patent protection, bolstering hopes for the rapid growth of the biosimilars as generics companies elbow their way into a large new market. Rituxan/MabThera and Remicade are on the top of the list for biosimilars. Sandoz, for example, which is leading the pack of generic companies angling to get into the market, expects to see biosimilar revenue jump from $250 million in 2011 to $20 billion by 2020. Over the next 5 years, the market for biosimilars will increase to $10 billion, but only a handful of big pharmaceutical companies and world-class R&D facilities will be able to take part, meaning that most small and medium-sized drug developers will never have a chance of getting into the new market for follow-on biologics.

The niche for most small biotech companies is taking a preclinical or very early-stage candidate to proof of concept, at which point they can make the sale to bigger companies. With biosimilars, the developer will start with proof-of-concept data and then ramp up the most expensive stage of clinical development, with the added charge of running a likely comparison study with the marketed therapeutic; such a process will not be cheap. It could take 8 years to run a biosimilar program, with development costs sliding from $100 million to $150 million. With that much time and money at stake, most biotech companies may never be competitive.

SUMMARY

The rapid progress made in the last few decades toward the development of potent therapeutic antibodies raises several questions for the future directions of this field. A key question is whether there are any indications of a paradigm change that could lead to radically different therapeutics, as occurred 2 to 3 decades ago, and which resulted in an explosion of antibody therapeutics approved for clinical use during the last decades. If history provides an answer and such a paradigm shift occurs, it will probably take decades before the fruition of such a shift in terms of new licensed protein therapeutics is witnessed. Meanwhile, gradual improvements in the characteristics of existing antibody therapeutics, discovery of novel antibody-based drugs and novel targets, combining therapeutics and conjugating them with drugs, nanoparticles, and other reagents, using integrative approaches based on cell biology, bioengineering and genetic profiling as well as use of predictive tools to narrow down which candidate molecules could be successfully developed as therapeutics, and developing novel protein-based scaffolds with superior properties to those already in use will be major areas of research and development in the coming decades. A decade from now it is likely that many antibody-based therapeutics based on different scaffolds will be approved for clinical use, with hundreds more in preclinical and clinical development.

ACKNOWLEDGMENTS

The authors would like to thank John Owens from the group Protein Interactions for discussions and help.

REFERENCES

1. Dillman RO. Cancer immunotherapy. Cancer Biother Radiopharm 2011;26(1): 1–64.
2. Kohler G, Milstein C. Continuous cultures of fused cells secreting antibody of predefined specificity. Nature 1975;256:495–7.
3. Carter PJ. Potent antibody therapeutics by design. Nat Rev Immunol 2006;6(5): 343–57.
4. Schrama D, Reisfeld RA, Becker JC. Antibody targeted drugs as cancer therapeutics. Nat Rev Drug Discov 2006;5(2):147–59.
5. Waldmann TA. Immunotherapy: past, present and future. Nat Med 2003;9(3): 269–77.
6. Casadevall A, Dadachova E, Pirofski LA. Passive antibody therapy for infectious diseases. Nat Rev Microbiol 2004;2(9):695–703.
7. Carter PJ. Introduction to current and future protein therapeutics: a protein engineering perspective. Exp Cell Res 2011;317(9):1261–9.
8. Dimitrov DS. Therapeutic antibodies, vaccines and antibodyomes. MAbs 2010; 2(3):347–56.
9. Walsh G. Biopharmaceutical benchmarks 2010. Nat Biotechnol 2010;28(9): 917–24.
10. Leader B, Baca QJ, Golan DE. Protein therapeutics: a summary and pharmacological classification. Nat Rev Drug Discov 2008;7(1):21–39.
11. Dimitrov DS, Marks JD. Therapeutic antibodies: current state and future trends—is a paradigm change coming soon? Methods Mol Biol 2009;525:1–27.
12. Ashkenazi A. Directing cancer cells to self-destruct with pro-apoptotic receptor agonists. Nat Rev Drug Discov 2008;7(12):1001–12.
13. Beck A, Reichert JM. Therapeutic Fc-fusion proteins and peptides as successful alternatives to antibodies. MAbs 2011;3(5):415–6.
14. Reichert JM. Antibody-based therapeutics to watch in 2011. MAbs 2011;3(1): 76–99.
15. Reichert JM. Metrics for antibody therapeutics development. MAbs 2010;2(6): 695–700.

16. Teicher BA, Chari RV. Antibody conjugate therapeutics: challenges and potential. Clin Cancer Res 2011;17(20):6389–97.
17. Pasquetto MV, Vecchia L, Covini D, et al. Targeted drug delivery using immunoconjugates: principles and applications. J Immunother 2011;34(9):611–28.
18. Ricart AD. Immunoconjugates against solid tumors: mind the gap. Clin Pharmacol Ther 2011;89(4):513–23.
19. Ricart AD. Antibody-drug conjugates of calicheamicin derivative: gemtuzumab ozogamicin and inotuzumab ozogamicin. Clin Cancer Res 2011;17(20):6417–27.
20. Grillo-Lopez AJ. Rituximab: an insider's historical perspective. Semin Oncol 2000;27(6 Suppl 12):9–16.
21. Maloney DG. Mechanism of action of rituximab. Anticancer Drugs 2001;12(Suppl 2):S1–4.
22. Byrd JC, Kitada S, Flinn I, et al. The mechanism of tumor cell clearance by rituximab in vivo in patients with B-cell chronic lymphocytic leukemia: evidence of caspase activation and apoptosis induction. Blood 2002;99(3):1038–43.
23. Hilchey SP, Hyrien O, Mosmann TR, et al. Rituximab immunotherapy results in the induction of a lymphoma idiotype-specific T-cell response in patients with follicular lymphoma: support for a "vaccinal effect" of rituximab. Blood 2009;113(16):3809–12.
24. Mathas S, Rickers A, Bommert K, et al. Anti-CD20- and B-cell receptor-mediated apoptosis: evidence for shared intracellular signaling pathways. Cancer Res 2000;60(24):7170–6.
25. Shan D, Ledbetter J, Press O. Signaling events involved in anti-CD20-induced apoptosis of malignant human B cells. Cancer Immunol Immunother 2000;48:673–83.
26. Dillman RO, Hendrix CS. Unique aspects of supportive care using monoclonal antibodies in cancer treatment. Support Cancer Ther 2003;1(1):38–48.
27. Allison M. PML problems loom for Rituxan. Nat Biotechnol 2010;28(2):105–6.
28. Paues J, Vrethem M. Fatal progressive multifocal leukoencephalopathy in a patient with non-Hodgkin lymphoma treated with rituximab. J Clin Virol 2010;48(4):291–3.
29. Coiffier B, Lepage E, Briere J, et al. CHOP chemotherapy plus rituximab compared with CHOP alone in elderly patients with diffuse large-B-cell lymphoma. N Engl J Med 2002;346(4):235–42.
30. Keating MJ, O'Brien S, Albitar M, et al. Early results of a chemoimmunotherapy regimen of fludarabine, cyclophosphamide, and rituximab as initial therapy for chronic lymphocytic leukemia. J Clin Oncol 2005;23(18):4079–88.
31. Harting R, Venogopal P, Gregory SA, et al. Efficacy and safety of rituximab combined with ESHAP chemotherapy for the treatment of relapsed/refractory aggressive B-cell non-Hodgkin lymphoma. Clin Lymphoma Myeloma 2007;7(6):406–12.
32. Fischer K, Cramer P, Busch R, et al. Bendamustine combined with rituximab in patients with relapsed and/or refractory chronic lymphocytic leukemia: a multicenter phase II trial of the German Chronic Lymphocytic Leukemia Study Group. J Clin Oncol 2011;29(26):3559–66.
33. Datta YH, Kampalath B, Binion DG. Rituximab-induced remission of a gastric MALT lymphoma. Leuk Lymphoma 2004;45(6):1297–9.
34. Chong EA, Svoboda J, Cherian S, et al. Regression of pulmonary MALT lymphoma after treatment with rituximab. Leuk Lymphoma 2005;46(9):1383–6.
35. Kluin-Nelemans HC, Doorduijn JK. Treatment of elderly patients with mantle cell lymphoma. Semin Hematol 2011;48(3):208–13.

36. Fenot M, Quereux G, Brocard A, et al. Rituximab for primary cutaneous diffuse large B-cell lymphoma-leg type. Eur J Dermatol 2010;20(6):753–7.
37. Bennett M, Schechter GP. Treatment of splenic marginal zone lymphoma: splenectomy versus rituximab. Semin Hematol 2010;47(2):143–7.
38. Dimopoulos MA, Kastritis E, Roussou M, et al. Rituximab-based treatments in Waldenstrom's macroglobulinemia. Clin Lymphoma Myeloma 2009;9(1):59–61.
39. Rai KR, Peterson BL, Appelbaum FR, et al. Fludarabine compared with chlorambucil as primary therapy for chronic lymphocytic leukemia. N Engl J Med 2000; 343(24):1750–7.
40. Flinn IW, Neuberg DS, Grever MR, et al. Phase III trial of fludarabine plus cyclophosphamide compared with fludarabine for patients with previously untreated chronic lymphocytic leukemia: US Intergroup Trial E2997. J Clin Oncol 2007; 25(7):793–8.
41. Robak T, Dmoszynska A, Solal-Céligny P, et al. Rituximab plus fludarabine and cyclophosphamide prolongs progression-free survival compared with fludarabine and cyclophosphamide alone in previously treated chronic lymphocytic leukemia. J Clin Oncol 2010;28(10):1756–65.
42. McLaughlin P. Rituximab chimeric anti-CD20 monoclonal antibody therapy for relapsed indolent lymphoma: half of patients respond to a four-dose treatment program. J Clin Oncol 1998;16:2825–33.
43. Huhn D, von Schilling C, Wilhelm M, et al. Rituximab therapy of patients with B-cell chronic lymphocytic leukemia. Blood 2001;98(5):1326–31.
44. Nabhan C, Kay NE. The emerging role of ofatumumab in the treatment of chronic lymphocytic leukemia. Clin Med Insights Oncol 2011;5:45–53.
45. Teeling JL, Mackus WJ, Wiegman LJ, et al. The biological activity of human CD20 monoclonal antibodies is linked to unique epitopes on CD20. J Immunol 2006;177(1):362–71.
46. Pawluczkowycz AW, Beurskens FJ, Beum PV, et al. Binding of submaximal C1q promotes complement-dependent cytotoxicity (CDC) of B cells opsonized with anti-CD20 mAbs ofatumumab (OFA) or rituximab (RTX): considerably higher levels of CDC are induced by OFA than by RTX. J Immunol 2009;183(1):749–58.
47. Li B, Zhao L, Guo H, et al. Characterization of a rituximab variant with potent antitumor activity against rituximab-resistant B-cell lymphoma. Blood 2009; 114(24):5007–15.
48. Coiffier B, Lepretre S, Pedersen LM, et al. Safety and efficacy of ofatumumab, a fully human monoclonal anti-CD20 antibody, in patients with relapsed or refractory B-cell chronic lymphocytic leukemia: a phase 1-2 study. Blood 2008;111(3):1094–100.
49. Keating MJ, Flinn I, Jain V, et al. Therapeutic role of alemtuzumab (Campath-1H) in patients who have failed fludarabine: results of a large international study. Blood 2002;99(10):3554–61.
50. Wierda WG, Kipps TJ, Mayer J, et al. Ofatumumab as single-agent CD20 immunotherapy in fludarabine-refractory chronic lymphocytic leukemia. J Clin Oncol 2010;28(10):1749–55.
51. Lemery SJ, Zhang J, Rothmann MD, et al. U.S. Food and Drug Administration approval: ofatumumab for the treatment of patients with chronic lymphocytic leukemia refractory to fludarabine and alemtuzumab. Clin Cancer Res 2010; 16(17):4331–8.
52. Wierda WG, Kipps TJ, Durig J, et al. Chemoimmunotherapy with O-FC in previously untreated patients with chronic lymphocytic leukemia. Blood 2011; 117(24):6450–8.

53. Haskova Z, Whitacre MN, Dede KA, et al. Combination therapy with ofatumumab and bendamustine in xenograft model of chronic lymphocytic leukaemia. Br J Haematol 2012;156(3):402–4.
54. Sondak VK, Flaherty LE. Targeted therapies: improved outcomes for patients with metastatic melanoma. Nat Rev Clin Oncol 2011;8(9):513–5.
55. Leach DR, Krummel MF, Allison JP. Enhancement of antitumor immunity by CTLA-4 blockade. Science 1996;271(5256):1734–6.
56. Peggs KS, Quezada SA, Allison JP. Cell intrinsic mechanisms of T-cell inhibition and application to cancer therapy. Immunol Rev 2008;224:141–65.
57. Tivol EA, Borriello F, Schweitzer AN, et al. Loss of CTLA-4 leads to massive lymphoproliferation and fatal multiorgan tissue destruction, revealing a critical negative regulatory role of CTLA-4. Immunity 1995;3(5):541–7.
58. Peggs KS, Quezada SA, Chambers CA, et al. Blockade of CTLA-4 on both effector and regulatory T cell compartments contributes to the antitumor activity of anti-CTLA-4 antibodies. J Exp Med 2009;206(8):1717–25.
59. Weber J. Review: anti-CTLA-4 antibody ipilimumab: case studies of clinical response and immune-related adverse events. Oncologist 2007;12(7):864–72.
60. Hodi FS. Improved survival with ipilimumab in patients with metastatic melanoma. N Engl J Med 2010;363:711–23.
61. Schwartzentruber DJ. gp100 peptide vaccine and interleukin-2 in patients with advanced melanoma. N Engl J Med 2011;364:2119–27.
62. Robert C, Thomas L, Bondarenko I, et al. Ipilimumab plus dacarbazine for previously untreated metastatic melanoma. N Engl J Med 2011;364(26):2517–26.
63. Di Giacomo AM, Biagioli M, Maio M. The emerging toxicity profiles of anti-CTLA-4 antibodies across clinical indications. Semin Oncol 2010;37(5):499–507.
64. Attia P, Phan GQ, Maker AV, et al. Autoimmunity correlates with tumor regression in patients with metastatic melanoma treated with anti-cytotoxic T-lymphocyte antigen-4. J Clin Oncol 2005;23(25):6043–53.
65. Sondak VK, Smalley KS, Kudchadkar R, et al. Ipilimumab. Nat Rev Drug Discov 2011;10(6):411–2.
66. Slamon DJ, Clark GM, Wong SG, et al. Human breast cancer: correlation of relapse and survival with amplification of the HER-2/neu oncogene. Science 1987;235(4785):177–82.
67. Pauletti G, Dandekar S, Rong H, et al. Assessment of methods for tissue-based detection of the HER-2/neu alteration in human breast cancer: a direct comparison of fluorescence in situ hybridization and immunohistochemistry. J Clin Oncol 2000;18(21):3651–64.
68. Dowsett M, Bartlett J, Ellis IO, et al. Correlation between immunohistochemistry (HercepTest) and fluorescence in situ hybridization (FISH) for HER-2 in 426 breast carcinomas from 37 centres. J Pathol 2003;199(4):418–23.
69. Perez EA, Suman VJ, Davidson NE, et al. HER2 testing by local, central, and reference laboratories in specimens from the North Central Cancer Treatment Group N9831 intergroup adjuvant trial. J Clin Oncol 2006;24(19):3032–8.
70. Yarden Y. The EGFR family and its ligands in human cancer. signalling mechanisms and therapeutic opportunities. Eur J Cancer 2001;37(Suppl 4):S3–8.
71. Cho HS, Mason K, Ramyar KX, et al. Structure of the extracellular region of HER2 alone and in complex with the Herceptin Fab. Nature 2003;421(6924):756–60.
72. Bashey A, Medina B, Corringham S, et al. CTLA4 blockade with ipilimumab to treat relapse of malignancy after allogeneic hematopoietic cell transplantation. Blood 2009;113(7):1581–8.

73. Yarden Y, Sliwkowski MX. Untangling the ErbB signalling network. Nat Rev Mol Cell Biol 2001;2(2):127–37.

74. Nagata Y, Lan KH, Zhou X, et al. PTEN activation contributes to tumor inhibition by trastuzumab, and loss of PTEN predicts trastuzumab resistance in patients. Cancer Cell 2004;6(2):117–27.

75. Junttila TT, Akita RW, Parsons K, et al. Ligand-independent HER2/HER3/PI3K complex is disrupted by trastuzumab and is effectively inhibited by the PI3K inhibitor GDC-0941. Cancer Cell 2009;15(5):429–40.

76. Sliwkowski MX, Lofgren JA, Lewis GD, et al. Nonclinical studies addressing the mechanism of action of trastuzumab (Herceptin). Semin Oncol 1999;26(4 Suppl 12):60–70.

77. Weiner LM, Adams GP. New approaches to antibody therapy. Oncogene 2000; 19(53):6144–51.

78. Gennari R, Menard S, Fagnoni F, et al. Pilot study of the mechanism of action of preoperative trastuzumab in patients with primary operable breast tumors over-expressing HER2. Clin Cancer Res 2004;10(17):5650–5.

79. Kumar R, Yarmand-Bagheri R. The role of HER2 in angiogenesis. Semin Oncol 2001;28(5 Suppl 16):27–32.

80. Hudis CA. Trastuzumab–mechanism of action and use in clinical practice. N Engl J Med 2007;357(1):39–51.

81. Slamon D. Use of chemotherapy plus a monoclonal antibody against HER2 for metastatic breast cancer that overexpresses HER2. N Engl J Med 2001;344: 783–92.

82. Esteva FJ, Valero V, Booser D, et al. Phase II study of weekly docetaxel and tras-tuzumab for patients with HER-2-overexpressing metastatic breast cancer. J Clin Oncol 2002;20(7):1800–8.

83. Burstein HJ, Harris LN, Marcom PK, et al. Trastuzumab and vinorelbine as first-line therapy for HER2-overexpressing metastatic breast cancer: multicenter phase II trial with clinical outcomes, analysis of serum tumor markers as predic-tive factors, and cardiac surveillance algorithm. J Clin Oncol 2003;21(15): 2889–95.

84. Chia S, Clemons M, Martin LA, et al. Pegylated liposomal doxorubicin and tras-tuzumab in HER-2 overexpressing metastatic breast cancer: a multicenter phase II trial. J Clin Oncol 2006;24(18):2773–8.

85. Costa RB, Kurra G, Greenberg L, et al. Efficacy and cardiac safety of adjuvant trastuzumab-based chemotherapy regimens for HER2-positive early breast cancer. Ann Oncol 2010;21(11):2153–60.

86. Baselga J, Perez EA, Pienkowski T, et al. Adjuvant trastuzumab: a milestone in the treatment of HER-2-positive early breast cancer. Oncologist 2006;11(Suppl 1):4–12.

87. Gianni L, Eiermann W, Semiglazov V, et al. Neoadjuvant chemotherapy with tras-tuzumab followed by adjuvant trastuzumab versus neoadjuvant chemotherapy alone, in patients with HER2-positive locally advanced breast cancer (the NOAH trial): a randomised controlled superiority trial with a parallel HER2-negative cohort. Lancet 2010;375(9712):377–84.

88. Jorgensen JT. Targeted HER2 treatment in advanced gastric cancer. Oncology 2010;78(1):26–33.

89. Kelly H, Kimmick G, Dees EC, et al. Response and cardiac toxicity of trastuzu-mab given in conjunction with weekly paclitaxel after doxorubicin/cyclophos-phamide. Clin Breast Cancer 2006;7(3):237–43.

90. Perez EA, Suman VJ, Rowland KM, et al. Two concurrent phase II trials of pacli-taxel/carboplatin/trastuzumab (weekly or every-3-week schedule) as first-line

therapy in women with HER2-overexpressing metastatic breast cancer: NCCTG study 983252. Clin Breast Cancer 2005;6(5):425–32.

91. Adams GP, Weiner LM. Monoclonal antibody therapy of cancer. Nat Biotechnol 2005;23(9):1147–57.
92. Banerjee S, Flores-Rozas H. Monoclonal antibodies for targeted therapy in colorectal cancer. Cancer Biol Ther 2010;9(8):563–71.
93. Folkman J. The role of angiogenesis in tumor growth. Semin Cancer Biol 1992; 3(2):65–71.
94. Eskens FA, Verweij J. The clinical toxicity profile of vascular endothelial growth factor (VEGF) and vascular endothelial growth factor receptor (VEGFR) targeting angiogenesis inhibitors; a review. Eur J Cancer 2006;42(18):3127–39.
95. Choueiri TK, Mayer EL, Je Y, et al. Congestive heart failure risk in patients with breast cancer treated with bevacizumab. J Clin Oncol 2011;29(6):632–8.
96. Nalluri SR, Chu D, Keresztes R, et al. Risk of venous thromboembolism with the angiogenesis inhibitor bevacizumab in cancer patients: a meta-analysis. JAMA 2008;300(19):2277–85.
97. Hurwitz HI, Saltz LB, Van Cutsem E, et al. Venous thromboembolic events with chemotherapy plus bevacizumab: a pooled analysis of patients in randomized phase II and III studies. J Clin Oncol 2011;29(13):1757–64.
98. Sandler AB, Schiller JH, Gray R, et al. Retrospective evaluation of the clinical and radiographic risk factors associated with severe pulmonary hemorrhage in first-line advanced, unresectable non-small-cell lung cancer treated with Carboplatin and Paclitaxel plus bevacizumab. J Clin Oncol 2009;27(9):1405–12.
99. Badgwell BD, Camp ER, Feig B, et al. Management of bevacizumab-associated bowel perforation: a case series and review of the literature. Ann Oncol 2008; 19(3):577–82.
100. Gordon MS, Margolin K, Talpaz M, et al. Phase I safety and pharmacokinetic study of recombinant human anti-vascular endothelial growth factor in patients with advanced cancer. J Clin Oncol 2001;19(3):843–50.
101. Yang JC, Haworth L, Sherry RM, et al. A randomized trial of bevacizumab, an anti-vascular endothelial growth factor antibody, for metastatic renal cancer. N Engl J Med 2003;349(5):427–34.
102. Hurwitz H, Fehrenbacher L, Novotny W, et al. Bevacizumab plus irinotecan, fluorouracil, and leucovorin for metastatic colorectal cancer. N Engl J Med 2004; 350:2335–42.
103. Fuchs CS, Marshall J, Mitchell E, et al. Randomized, controlled trial of irinotecan plus infusional, bolus, or oral fluoropyrimidines in first-line treatment of metastatic colorectal cancer: results from the BICC-C Study. J Clin Oncol 2007; 25(30):4779–86.
104. Fuchs CS, Marshall J, Barrueco J. Randomized, controlled trial of irinotecan plus infusional, bolus, or oral fluoropyrimidines in first-line treatment of metastatic colorectal cancer: updated results from the BICC-C study. J Clin Oncol 2008;26(4):689–90.
105. Hochster HS, Hart LL, Ramanathan RK, et al. Safety and efficacy of oxaliplatin and fluoropyrimidine regimens with or without bevacizumab as first-line treatment of metastatic colorectal cancer: results of the TREE Study. J Clin Oncol 2008;26(21):3523–9.
106. Vincenzi B, Santini D, Russo A, et al. Bevacizumab in association with de Gramont 5-fluorouracil/folinic acid in patients with oxaliplatin-, irinotecan-, and cetuximab-refractory colorectal cancer: a single-center phase 2 trial. Cancer 2009;115(20):4849–56.

107. Kabbinavar FF, Schulz J, McCleod M, et al. Addition of bevacizumab to bolus fluorouracil and leucovorin in first-line metastatic colorectal cancer: results of a randomized phase II trial. J Clin Oncol 2005;23(16):3697–705.
108. Allegra CJ, Yothers G, O'Connell MJ, et al. Phase III trial assessing bevacizumab in stages II and III carcinoma of the colon: results of NSABP protocol C-08. J Clin Oncol 2011;29(1):11–6.
109. de Gramont A, Van Cutsem E, Tabernero J, et al. AVANT: Results from a randomized, three-arm multinational phase III study to investigate bevacizumab with either XELOX or FOLFOX4 versus FOLFOX4 alone as adjuvant treatment for colon cancer. J Clin Oncol 2011;29(Suppl 4):[abstract: 362].
110. Sandler A, Gray R, Perry MC, et al. Paclitaxel-carboplatin alone or with bevacizumab for non-small-cell lung cancer. N Engl J Med 2006;355(24):2542–50.
111. Reck M, von Pawel J, Zatloukal P, et al. Overall survival with cisplatin-gemcitabine and bevacizumab or placebo as first-line therapy for nonsquamous non-small-cell lung cancer: results from a randomised phase III trial (AVAiL). Ann Oncol 2010;21(9):1804–9.
112. Patel JD, Hensing TA, Rademaker A, et al. Phase II study of pemetrexed and carboplatin plus bevacizumab with maintenance pemetrexed and bevacizumab as first-line therapy for nonsquamous non-small-cell lung cancer. J Clin Oncol 2009;27(20):3284–9.
113. Patel JD, Bonomi P, Socinski MA, et al. Treatment rationale and study design for the pointbreak study: a randomized, open-label phase III study of pemetrexed/carboplatin/bevacizumab followed by maintenance pemetrexed/bevacizumab versus paclitaxel/carboplatin/bevacizumab followed by maintenance bevacizumab in patients with stage IIIB or IV nonsquamous non-small-cell lung cancer. Clin Lung Cancer 2009;10(4):252–6.
114. Miller K, Wang M, Gralow J, et al. Paclitaxel plus bevacizumab versus paclitaxel alone for metastatic breast cancer. N Engl J Med 2007;357(26):2666–76.
115. Miles DW, Chan A, Dirix LY, et al. Phase III study of bevacizumab plus docetaxel compared with placebo plus docetaxel for the first-line treatment of human epidermal growth factor receptor 2-negative metastatic breast cancer. J Clin Oncol 2010;28(20):3239–47.
116. Robert NJ, Dieras V, Glaspy J, et al. RIBBON-1: randomized, double-blind, placebo-controlled, phase III trial of chemotherapy with or without bevacizumab for first-line treatment of human epidermal growth factor receptor 2-negative, locally recurrent or metastatic breast cancer. J Clin Oncol 2011;29(10):1252–60.
117. Escudier B, Pluzanska A, Koralewski P, et al. Bevacizumab plus interferon alfa-2a for treatment of metastatic renal cell carcinoma: a randomised, double-blind phase III trial. Lancet 2007;370(9605):2103–11.
118. Rini BI, Halabi S, Rosenberg JE, et al. Bevacizumab plus interferon alfa compared with interferon alfa monotherapy in patients with metastatic renal cell carcinoma: CALGB 90206. J Clin Oncol 2008;26(33):5422–8.
119. Escudier B, Bellmunt J, Negrier S, et al. Phase III trial of bevacizumab plus interferon alfa-2a in patients with metastatic renal cell carcinoma (AVOREN): final analysis of overall survival. J Clin Oncol 2010;28(13):2144–50.
120. Rini BI, Halabi S, Rosenberg J, et al. Bevacizumab plus interferon-alpha versus interferon-alpha monotherapy in patients with metastatic renal cell carcinoma: results of overall survival for CALGB 90206. J Clin Oncol 2009;27:18s.
121. Vredenburgh JJ, Desjardins A, Herndon JE 2nd, et al. Phase II trial of bevacizumab and irinotecan in recurrent malignant glioma. Clin Cancer Res 2007;13(4):1253–9.

122. Desjardins A, Reardon DA, Herndon JE 2nd, et al. Bevacizumab plus irinotecan in recurrent WHO grade 3 malignant gliomas. Clin Cancer Res 2008;14(21): 7068–73.

123. Friedman HS, Prados MD, Wen PY, et al. Bevacizumab alone and in combination with irinotecan in recurrent glioblastoma. J Clin Oncol 2009;27(28):4733–40.

124. Burger R, Brady MF, Bookman MA, et al. Phase III trial of bevacizumab (BEV) in the primary treatment of advanced epithelial ovarian cancer (EOC), primary peritoneal cancer (PPC), or fallopian tube cancer (FTC): a Gynecologic Oncology Group study. J Clin Oncol 2010;28(Suppl):18s: p. LBA1.

125. Kristensen G, Perren T, Qian W, et al. Result of interim analysis of overall survival in the GCIG ICON7 phase III randomized trial of bevacizumab in women with newly diagnosed ovarian cancer. J Clin Oncol 2011;29(Suppl):[abstract: LBA5006].

126. Siegel AB, Cohen EI, Ocean A, et al. Phase II trial evaluating the clinical and biologic effects of bevacizumab in unresectable hepatocellular carcinoma. J Clin Oncol 2008;26(18):2992–8.

127. Zhu AX, Blaszkowsky LS, Ryan DP, et al. Phase II study of gemcitabine and oxaliplatin in combination with bevacizumab in patients with advanced hepatocellular carcinoma. J Clin Oncol 2006;24(12):1898–903.

128. Xu L, Duda DG, di Tomaso E, et al. Direct evidence that bevacizumab, an anti-VEGF antibody, up-regulates SDF1alpha, CXCR4, CXCL6, and neuropilin 1 in tumors from patients with rectal cancer. Cancer Res 2009;69(20):7905–10.

129. Miles D, Harbeck N, Escudier B, et al. Disease course patterns after discontinuation of bevacizumab: pooled analysis of randomized phase III trials. J Clin Oncol 2011;29(1):83–8.

130. Kerr DJ, Young AM. Targeted therapies: bevacizumab—has it reached its final resting place? Nat Rev Clin Oncol 2011;8(4):195–6.

131. Ranpura V, Hapani S, Wu S. Treatment-related mortality with bevacizumab in cancer patients: a meta-analysis. JAMA 2011;305(5):487–94.

132. Mendelsohn J. Blockade of receptors for growth factors: an anticancer therapy—the fourth annual Joseph H. Burchenal American Association of Cancer Research Clinical Research Award Lecture. Clin Cancer Res 2000;6(3):747–53.

133. Chung KY, Shia J, Kemeny NE, et al. Cetuximab shows activity in colorectal cancer patients with tumors that do not express the epidermal growth factor receptor by immunohistochemistry. J Clin Oncol 2005;23(9):1803–10.

134. Lenz HJ, Van Cutsem E, Khambata-Ford S, et al. Multicenter phase II and translational study of cetuximab in metastatic colorectal carcinoma refractory to irinotecan, oxaliplatin, and fluoropyrimidines. J Clin Oncol 2006;24(30): 4914–21.

135. Tsuchihashi Z, Khambata-Ford S, Hanna N, et al. Responsiveness to cetuximab without mutations in EGFR. N Engl J Med 2005;353(2):208–9.

136. Allegra CJ, Jessup JM, Somerfield MR, et al. American Society of Clinical Oncology provisional clinical opinion: testing for KRAS gene mutations in patients with metastatic colorectal carcinoma to predict response to anti-epidermal growth factor receptor monoclonal antibody therapy. J Clin Oncol 2009;27(12):2091–6.

137. Jonker DJ, O'Callaghan CJ, Karapetis CS, et al. Cetuximab for the treatment of colorectal cancer. N Engl J Med 2007;357(20):2040–8.

138. Cunningham D, Humblet Y, Siena S, et al. Cetuximab monotherapy and cetuximab plus irinotecan in irinotecan-refractory metastatic colorectal cancer. N Engl J Med 2004;351(4):337–45.

139. Sobrero AF, Maurel J, Fehrenbacher L, et al. EPIC: phase III trial of cetuximab plus irinotecan after fluoropyrimidine and oxaliplatin failure in patients with metastatic colorectal cancer. J Clin Oncol 2008;26(14):2311–9.

140. Van Cutsem E, Kohne CH, Lang I, et al. Cetuximab plus irinotecan, fluorouracil, and leucovorin as first-line treatment for metastatic colorectal cancer: updated analysis of overall survival according to tumor KRAS and BRAF mutation status. J Clin Oncol 2011;29(15):2011–9.

141. Amado RG, Wolf M, Peeters M, et al. Wild-type KRAS is required for panitumumab efficacy in patients with metastatic colorectal cancer. J Clin Oncol 2008;26(10):1626–34.

142. Maughan TS, Adams RA, Smith CG, et al. Addition of cetuximab to oxaliplatin-based first-line combination chemotherapy for treatment of advanced colorectal cancer: results of the randomised phase 3 MRC COIN trial. Lancet 2011; 377(9783):2103–14.

143. Bonner JA, Harari PM, Giralt J, et al. Radiotherapy plus cetuximab for squamous-cell carcinoma of the head and neck. N Engl J Med 2006;354(6):567–78.

144. Bonner JA, Harari PM, Giralt J, et al. Radiotherapy plus cetuximab for locoregionally advanced head and neck cancer: 5-year survival data from a phase 3 randomised trial, and relation between cetuximab-induced rash and survival. Lancet Oncol 2010;11(1):21–8.

145. Vermorken JB, Herbst RS, Leon X, et al. Overview of the efficacy of cetuximab in recurrent and/or metastatic squamous cell carcinoma of the head and neck in patients who previously failed platinum-based therapies. Cancer 2008; 112(12):2710–9.

146. Pirker R, Pereira JR, Szczesna A, et al. Cetuximab plus chemotherapy in patients with advanced non-small-cell lung cancer (FLEX): an open-label randomised phase III trial. Lancet 2009;373(9674):1525–31.

147. Gatzemeier U, von Pawel J, Vynnychenko I, et al. First-cycle rash and survival in patients with advanced non-small-cell lung cancer receiving cetuximab in combination with first-line chemotherapy: a subgroup analysis of data from the FLEX phase 3 study. Lancet Oncol 2011;12(1):30–7.

148. Lynch TJ, Patel T, Dreisbach L, et al. Cetuximab and first-line taxane/carboplatin chemotherapy in advanced non-small-cell lung cancer: results of the randomized multicenter phase III trial BMS099. J Clin Oncol 2010;28(6):911–7.

149. Giusti RM, Shastri KA, Cohen MH, et al. FDA drug approval summary: panitumumab (Vectibix). Oncologist 2007;12(5):577–83.

150. Berlin J, Posey J, Tchekmedyian S, et al. Panitumumab with irinotecan/leucovorin/5-fluorouracil for first-line treatment of metastatic colorectal cancer. Clin Colorectal Cancer 2007;6(6):427–32.

151. Martinelli E, De Palma R, Orditura M, et al. Anti-epidermal growth factor receptor monoclonal antibodies in cancer therapy. Clin Exp Immunol 2009;158(1):1–9.

152. Hecht JR, Mitchell E, Neubauer MA, et al. Lack of correlation between epidermal growth factor receptor status and response to panitumumab monotherapy in metastatic colorectal cancer. Clin Cancer Res 2010;16(7):2205–13.

153. Peeters M, Siena S, Van Cutsem E, et al. Association of progression-free survival, overall survival, and patient-reported outcomes by skin toxicity and KRAS status in patients receiving panitumumab monotherapy. Cancer 2009; 115(7):1544–54.

154. Di Nicolantonio F, Martini M, Molinari F, et al. Wild-type BRAF is required for response to panitumumab or cetuximab in metastatic colorectal cancer. J Clin Oncol 2008;26(35):5705–12.

155. Van Cutsem E, Peeters M, Siena S, et al. Open-label phase III trial of panitumumab plus best supportive care compared with best supportive care alone in patients with chemotherapy-refractory metastatic colorectal cancer. J Clin Oncol 2007;25(13):1658–64.
156. Douillard JY, Siena S, Cassidy J, et al. Randomized, phase III trial of panitumumab with infusional fluorouracil, leucovorin, and oxaliplatin (FOLFOX4) versus FOLFOX4 alone as first-line treatment in patients with previously untreated metastatic colorectal cancer: the PRIME study. J Clin Oncol 2010;28(31):4697–705.
157. Peeters M, Price TJ, Cervantes A, et al. Randomized phase III study of panitumumab with fluorouracil, leucovorin, and irinotecan (FOLFIRI) compared with FOLFIRI alone as second-line treatment in patients with metastatic colorectal cancer. J Clin Oncol 2010;28(31):4706–13.
158. Chiarle R, Podda A, Prolla G, et al. CD30 in normal and neoplastic cells. Clin Immunol 1999;90(2):157–64.
159. Sureda A, Constans M, Iriondo A, et al. Prognostic factors affecting long-term outcome after stem cell transplantation in Hodgkin's lymphoma autografted after a first relapse. Ann Oncol 2005;16(4):625–33.
160. Younes A, Bartlett NL, Leonard JP, et al. Brentuximab vedotin (SGN-35) for relapsed CD30-positive lymphomas. N Engl J Med 2010;363(19):1812–21.
161. Chen R, Gopal A. Results of a pivotal phase 2 study of brentuximab vedontin (SGN-35) in patients with relapsed or refractory Hodgkin's lymphoma. Blood 2010;116:128–9.
162. Foyil KV, Kennedy DA, Grove LE, et al. Extended retreatment with brentuximab vedotin (SGN-35) maintains complete remission in patient with recurrent systemic anaplastic large-cell lymphoma. Leuk Lymphoma 2012;53(3):560–7.
163. Bartlett N, Grove L. Objective responses with brentuximab vedontin retreatment in CD30-positive hematologic malignancies: a case series. J Clin Oncol 2010; 28(Suppl 15):[abstract: 8062].
164. Katz J, Janik JE, Younes A. Brentuximab vedotin (SGN-35). Clin Cancer Res 2011;17(20):6428–36.
165. Aldinucci D, Gloghini A, Pinto A, et al. The classical Hodgkin's lymphoma microenvironment and its role in promoting tumour growth and immune escape. J Pathol 2010;221(3):248–63.
166. Lorusso PM, Weiss D, Guardino E, et al. Trastuzumab emtansine: a unique antibody-drug conjugate in development for human epidermal growth factor receptor 2-positive cancer. Clin Cancer Res 2011;17(20):6437–47.
167. Kaufman M, Rai KR. Alemtuzumab in the up-front setting. Ther Clin Risk Manag 2008;4(2):459–64.
168. Dyer MJ. The role of CAMPATH-1 antibodies in the treatment of lymphoid malignancies. Semin Oncol 1999;26(5 Suppl 14):52–7.
169. Dearden C. The role of alemtuzumab in the management of T-cell malignancies. Semin Oncol 2006;33(2 Suppl 5):S44–52.
170. Dearden CE, Matutes E. Alemtuzumab in T-cell lymphoproliferative disorders. Best Pract Res Clin Haematol 2006;19(4):795–810.
171. Kimby E. Management of advanced-stage peripheral T-cell lymphomas. Curr Hematol Malig Rep 2007;2(4):242–8.
172. Lundin J, Hagberg H, Repp R, et al. Phase 2 study of alemtuzumab (anti-CD52 monoclonal antibody) in patients with advanced mycosis fungoides/Sezary syndrome. Blood 2003;101(11):4267–72.
173. Ricci F, Tedeschi A, Morra E, et al. Fludarabine in the treatment of chronic lymphocytic leukemia: a review. Ther Clin Risk Manag 2009;5(1):187–207.

174. Montillo M, Tedeschi A, Petrizzi VB, et al. An open-label, pilot study of fludara-bine, cyclophosphamide, and alemtuzumab in relapsed/refractory patients with B-cell chronic lymphocytic leukemia. Blood 2011;118(15):4079–85.

175. Grever MR, Lucas DM, Dewald GW, et al. Comprehensive assessment of genetic and molecular features predicting outcome in patients with chronic lymphocytic leukemia: results from the US Intergroup Phase III Trial E2997. J Clin Oncol 2007;25(7):799–804.

176. Stilgenbauer S, Zenz T. Understanding and managing ultra high-risk chronic lympho-cytic leukemia. Hematology Am Soc Hematol Educ Program 2010;2010:481–8.

177. Fiegl M, Erdel M, Tinhofer I, et al. Clinical outcome of pretreated B-cell chronic lymphocytic leukemia following alemtuzumab therapy: a retrospective study on various cytogenetic risk categories. Ann Oncol 2010;21(12):2410–9.

178. Stilgenbauer S, Dohner H. Campath-1H-induced complete remission of chronic lymphocytic leukemia despite p53 gene mutation and resistance to chemo-therapy. N Engl J Med 2002;347(6):452–3.

179. Lozanski G, Heerema NA, Flinn IW, et al. Alemtuzumab is an effective therapy for chronic lymphocytic leukemia with p53 mutations and deletions. Blood 2004;103(9):3278–81.

180. Stilgenbauer S, Zenz T, Winkler D, et al. Subcutaneous alemtuzumab in fludarabine-refractory chronic lymphocytic leukemia: clinical results and prog-nostic marker analyses from the CLL2H study of the German Chronic Lympho-cytic Leukemia Study Group. J Clin Oncol 2009;27(24):3994–4001.

181. Faderl S, Thomas DA, O'Brien S, et al. Experience with alemtuzumab plus ritux-imab in patients with relapsed and refractory lymphoid malignancies. Blood 2003;101(9):3413–5.

182. Parikh SA, Keating MJ, O'Brien S, et al. Frontline chemoimmunotherapy with flu-darabine, cyclophosphamide, alemtuzumab, and rituximab for high-risk chronic lymphocytic leukemia. Blood 2011;118(8):2062–8.

183. Hainsworth JD, Vazquez ER, Spigel DR, et al. Combination therapy with fludar-abine and rituximab followed by alemtuzumab in the first-line treatment of patients with chronic lymphocytic leukemia or small lymphocytic lymphoma: a phase 2 trial of the Minnie Pearl Cancer Research Network. Cancer 2008; 112(6):1288–95.

184. Schweighofer CD, Ritgen M, Eichhorst BF, et al. Consolidation with alemtuzumab improves progression-free survival in patients with chronic lymphocytic leukaemia (CLL) in first remission: long-term follow-up of a randomized phase III trial of the German CLL Study Group (GCLLSG). Br J Haematol 2009;144(1):95–8.

185. Wierda WG, Kipps TJ, Keating MJ, et al. Self-administered, subcutaneous alem-tuzumab to treat residual disease in patients with chronic lymphocytic leukemia. Cancer 2011;117(1):116–24.

186. Lin TS, Donohue KA, Byrd JC, et al. Consolidation therapy with subcutaneous alemtuzumab after fludarabine and rituximab induction therapy for previously untreated chronic lymphocytic leukemia: final analysis of CALGB 10101. J Clin Oncol 2010;28(29):4500–6.

187. Kipps TJ. Genomic complexity in chronic lymphocytic leukemia. Blood 2008; 112(5):1550.

188. Döhner H, Stilgenbauer S, Benner A, et al. Genomic aberrations and survival in chronic lymphocytic leukemia. N Engl J Med 2000;343(26):1910–6.

189. Feng Y, Dimitrov DS. Monoclonal antibodies against components of the IGF system for cancer treatment. Curr Opin Drug Discov Devel 2008;11(2): 178–85.

190. Skerra A. Alternative non-antibody scaffolds for molecular recognition. Curr Opin Biotechnol 2007;18(4):295–304.
191. Chen W, Dimitrov DS. Human monoclonal antibodies and engineered antibody domains as HIV-1 entry inhibitors. Curr Opin HIV AIDS 2009;4(2):112–7.
192. Chen W, Zhu Z, Feng Y, et al. Construction of a large phage-displayed human antibody domain library with a scaffold based on a newly identified highly soluble, stable heavy chain variable domain. J Mol Biol 2008;382(3):779–89.
193. Dimitrov DS. Engineered CH2 domains (nanoantibodies). MAbs 2009;1(1):26–8.
194. Xiao X, Feng Y, Vu BK, et al. A large library based on a novel (CH2) scaffold: identification of HIV-1 inhibitors. Biochem Biophys Res Commun 2009;387(2): 387–92.
195. Gong R, Vu BK, Feng Y, et al. Engineered human antibody constant domains with increased stability. J Biol Chem 2009;284(21):14203–10.
196. Gong R, Wang Y, Feng Y, et al. Shortened engineered human antibody CH2 domains: increased stability and binding to the human neonatal receptor. J Biol Chem 2011;286(31):27288–93.
197. Descotes J, Gouraud A. Clinical immunotoxicity of therapeutic proteins. Expert Opin Drug Metab Toxicol 2008;4(12):1537–49.
198. Suntharalingam G, Perry MR, Ward S, et al. Cytokine storm in a phase 1 trial of the anti-CD28 monoclonal antibody TGN1412. N Engl J Med 2006;355(10): 1018–28.
199. Ewer SM, Ewer MS. Cardiotoxicity profile of trastuzumab. Drug Saf 2008;31(6): 459–67.
200. Chung CH. Managing premedications and the risk for reactions to infusional monoclonal antibody therapy. Oncologist 2008;13(6):725–32.
201. Winter MC, Hancock BW. Ten years of rituximab in NHL. Expert Opin Drug Saf 2009;8(2):223–35.
202. Pendley C, Schantz A, Wagner C. Immunogenicity of therapeutic monoclonal antibodies. Curr Opin Mol Ther 2003;5(2):172–9.
203. Schellekens H. How to predict and prevent the immunogenicity of therapeutic proteins. Biotechnol Annu Rev 2008;14:191–202.
204. Onda M. Reducing the immunogenicity of protein therapeutics. Curr Drug Targets 2009;10(2):131–9.
205. Baker MP, Jones TD. Identification and removal of immunogenicity in thera-peutic proteins. Curr Opin Drug Discov Devel 2007;10(2):219–27.
206. Stas P, Lasters I. Strategies for preclinical immunogenicity assessment of protein therapeutics. IDrugs 2009;12(3):169–73.
207. De Groot AS, McMurry J, Moise L. Prediction of immunogenicity: in silico para-digms, ex vivo and in vivo correlates. Curr Opin Pharmacol 2008;8(5):620–6.
208. Emi Aikawa N, de Carvalho JF, Artur Almeida Silva C, et al. Immunogenicity of anti-TNF-alpha agents in autoimmune diseases. Clin Rev Allergy Immunol 2010;38(2–3):82–9.
209. Hangartner L, Zinkernagel RM, Hengartner H. Antiviral antibody responses: the two extremes of a wide spectrum. Nat Rev Immunol 2006;6(3):231–43.
210. Dixit R, Coats S. Preclinical efficacy and safety models for mAbs: the challenge of developing effective model systems. IDrugs 2009;12(2):103–8.
211. Castillo J, Winer E, Quesenberry P. Newer monoclonal antibodies for hematolog-ical malignancies. Exp Hematol 2008;36(7):755–68.
212. Mariani G, Fasolo A, De Benedictis E, et al. Trastuzumab as adjuvant systemic therapy for HER2-positive breast cancer. Nat Clin Pract Oncol 2009;6(2): 93–104.

213. Bedard PL, Piccart-Gebhart MJ. Current paradigms for the use of HER2-targeted therapy in early-stage breast cancer. Clin Breast Cancer 2008; 8(Suppl 4):S157–65.
214. Hall PS, Cameron DA. Current perspective—trastuzumab. Eur J Cancer 2009; 45(1):12–8.
215. Cameron D, Casey M, Press M, et al. A phase III randomized comparison of lapatinib plus capecitabine versus capecitabine alone in women with advanced breast cancer that has progressed on trastuzumab: updated efficacy and biomarker analyses. Breast Cancer Res Treat 2008;112(3):533–43.
216. Norden AD, Drappatz J, Wen PY. Novel anti-angiogenic therapies for malignant gliomas. Lancet Neurol 2008;7(12):1152–60.
217. Sachdev JC, Jahanzeb M. Evolution of bevacizumab-based therapy in the management of breast cancer. Clin Breast Cancer 2008;8(5):402–10.
218. Patel DK. Clinical use of anti-epidermal growth factor receptor monoclonal antibodies in metastatic colorectal cancer. Pharmacotherapy 2008;28(11 Pt 2): 31S–41S.
219. Tassev DV, Cheung NK. Monoclonal antibody therapies for solid tumors. Expert Opin Biol Ther 2009;9(3):341–53.
220. Hopper-Borge EA, Churchill T, Paulose C, et al. Mechanisms of tumor resistance to EGFR-targeted therapies. Expert Opin Ther Targets 2009;13(3):339–62.
221. Presta LG. Molecular engineering and design of therapeutic antibodies. Curr Opin Immunol 2008;20(4):460–70.
222. Jefferis R. Glycosylation as a strategy to improve antibody-based therapeutics. Nat Rev Drug Discov 2009;8(3):226–34.
223. Labrijn AF, Aalberse RC, Schuurman J. When binding is enough: nonactivating antibody formats. Curr Opin Immunol 2008;20(4):479–85.
224. Kiewe P, Thiel E. Ertumaxomab: a trifunctional antibody for breast cancer treatment. Expert Opin Investig Drugs 2008;17(10):1553–8.
225. Weber J. Ipilimumab: controversies in its development, utility and autoimmune adverse events. Cancer Immunol Immunother 2009;58(5):823–30.
226. Yuan J, Gnjatic S, Li H, et al. CTLA-4 blockade enhances polyfunctional NY-ESO-1 specific T cell responses in metastatic melanoma patients with clinical benefit. Proc Natl Acad Sci U S A 2008;105(51):20410–5.
227. Bellail AC, Ling Q, Mulligan P, et al. TRAIL agonists on clinical trials for cancer therapy: the promises and the challenges. Rev Recent Clin Trials 2009;4(1): 34–41.
228. Feng Y, Xiao X, Zhu Z, et al. Identification and characterization of a novel agonistic anti-DR4 human monoclonal antibody. MAbs 2010;2(5):565–70.
229. Zhang MY, Shu Y, Phogat S, et al. Broadly cross-reactive HIV neutralizing human monoclonal antibody Fab selected by sequential antigen panning of a phage display library. J Immunol Methods 2003;283(1–2):17–25.
230. Choudhry V, Zhang MY, Sidorov IA, et al. Cross-reactive HIV-1 neutralizing monoclonal antibodies selected by screening of an immune human phage library against an envelope glycoprotein (gp140) isolated from a patient (R2) with broadly HIV-1 neutralizing antibodies. Virology 2007;363(1): 79–90.
231. Zhang MY, Dimitrov DS. Novel approaches for identification of broadly cross-reactive HIV-1 neutralizing human monoclonal antibodies and improvement of their potency. Curr Pharm Des 2007;13(2):203–12.
232. Liu H, Gaza-Bulseco G, Faldu D, et al. Heterogeneity of monoclonal antibodies. J Pharm Sci 2008;97(7):2426–47.

233. Birch JR, Racher AJ. Antibody production. Adv Drug Deliv Rev 2006;58(5–6): 671–85.
234. Zhou JX, Tressel T, Yang X, et al. Implementation of advanced technologies in commercial monoclonal antibody production. Biotechnol J 2008;3(9–10): 1185–200.

mTOR Signaling Pathway and mTOR Inhibitors in Cancer Therapy

Alejandro Gomez-Pinillos, MD, Anna C. Ferrari, MD*

KEYWORDS

- mTOR • Inhibitor • Rapalog • Cancer

KEY POINTS

- Mammalian target of rapamycin (mTOR) is a serine/threonine protein kinase. It is ubiquitously expressed in cells and is a therapeutic target for the cancer treatment arsenal.
- Despite the great responses obtained in tumors addicted to specific mutations or overactivation of key members of the mTOR pathway (HiF1α in RCC, cyclin D1 in MCL, or TSC in SEGA), mTOR inhibitors as single agents have modest activity.
- Dual PI3K/mTOR kinase inhibitors have been developed with the idea of overcoming resistance to the mTOR inhibition through preventing the activation of PI3K/Akt as a result of release negative feedback loops.

mTOR PATHWAY AND FUNCTION

Mammalian target of rapamycin (mTOR) is a serine/threonine protein kinase. It is ubiquitously expressed in cells and is a therapeutic target for the cancer treatment arsenal. The mTOR kinase was first identified during the study of the small molecule rapamycin (also known as sirolimus), a compound obtained from the bacterium *Streptomyces hygroscopicus* that was known to have antifungal properties.[1] However, the use of rapamycin as an antifungal agent was abandoned when potent immunosuppressive and antiproliferative properties were observed. The mTOR kinase is part of a pathway that integrates signals that govern protein biosynthesis, cell growth, and cell cycle progression (**Fig. 1**). mTOR protein is the catalytic subunit of two molecular complexes: mTORC1 and mTORC2. The rapamycin-sensitive mTOR complex 1

Anna C. Ferrari participates in advisory boards for Novartis; Dendreon Corporation; Janssen Pharmaceuticals, Inc.; OSI Pharmaceuticals, Inc.; Astellas Pharma US, Inc.; OrhtoBiotech; Bayer Corporation; Merck & Co., Inc.; Osuka; Natrogene; Amgen, Inc.; Oxford BioMedica; and Cougar Biotechnology/Johnson & Johnson, and is a recipient of a grant from Novartis.
Department of Medicine, NYU Cancer Institute, New York University School of Medicine, 160 East 34th Street, 8th Floor, New York, NY 10016, USA
* Corresponding author.
E-mail address: Anna.Ferrari@nyumc.org

Hematol Oncol Clin N Am 26 (2012) 483–505
doi:10.1016/j.hoc.2012.02.014
0889-8588/12/$ – see front matter © 2012 Elsevier Inc. All rights reserved.

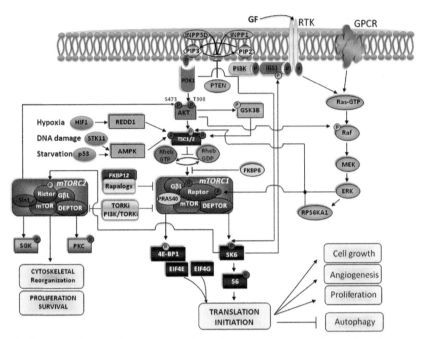

Fig. 1. Targeting the mTOR signaling pathway in cancer. mTOR inhibitors (rapalogs, mTOR kinase inhibitors, and dual PI3K/TORKi) are represented in the context of the mTOR pathway. Growth signaling factors and receptors activate the PI3K/Akt axis upstream to mTORC1. mTORC1 key driver downstream (SK6 and 4EBP1) integrates nutrient availability and cellular stress to regulate protein synthesis and induce cell growth, angiogenesis, and proliferation. Feedback loops within mTOR pathway are also represented. mTORC2 is inactivated by S6K1 through phosphorylating rictor. mTORC2 promotes survival by Akt phosphorylation. Crosstalk between PI3K/Akt/mTOR and Ras/Raf/MEK/ERK pathways are also represented. Green "P" circles represent inactivating phosphorylation; red "P" circles represent activating phosphorylation; the black spot represents a node shared by two molecules.

(mTORC1) contains mTOR, the regulatory-associated protein of mTOR (raptor), the proline-rich Akt substrate 40 (PRAS40), mLST8/G-protein β-subunit–like protein (GβL), and deptor.[2] mTORC1 stimulates protein synthesis through phosphorylating the ribosomal S6 kinase 1 (S6K1) and the eukaryotic translation initiation factor 4E-binding protein 1 (4EBP1). S6K1 activates the ribosomal protein S6 that stimulates the translation of mRNA with a 5′ oligopyrimidine tract. This class of mRNA represents up to 30% of the mRNA that encodes many of the components of the protein synthesis machinery, including ribosomal proteins, translation initiation, and elongation factors.[3–6] The phosphorylation of 4EBP1 (eIF-4E-binding protein) releases eIF4E, allowing the association of eIF4E with eIF4G to form the active eIF4F complex, a key component of the protein synthesis machinery that is particularly important for the translation of 5′ capped mRNA. The latter encodes relevant proteins for cell growth and cell cycle progression, such as growth factors (GFs), receptors, cyclins, c-myc, and signaling proteins.[6–8] Thus, the activation of mTORC1 in response to insulin, GFs, availability of nutrients, oxygen, and increased intracellular levels of energy (high ATP concentrations) promotes ribosome biogenesis, protein synthesis, and angiogenesis to support cell growth and proliferation. Rapamycin and rapamycin derivatives (rapalogs) bind to FK506 binding protein 12 (FKBP12), which interferes with mTORC1 and inhibits its activation.

The more recently discovered mTOR complex 2 (mTORC2) contains mTOR, the rapamycin-insensitive companion of mTOR (rictor), mLST8, deptor, and the stress-activated MAPK-interacting protein 1 (Sin1).[9] mTORC2 phosphorylates serum- and glucocorticoid-regulated kinase (SGK), protein kinase C (PKC), and also Akt at Ser 473, which in turn regulates cell cycle progression and survival.[10–12] mTORC2 has also been involved in the organization of the actin cytoskeleton.[13] Although mTORC2 has been described as the rapamycin-insensitive component of the mTOR pathway, prolonged treatment with rapamycin inhibited mTORC2 activity in PC3 xenografts and U937 lymphoma cells.[13–15]

As the biogenesis of proteins is the most energetically expensive process performed by the cell,[16] the activation of the protein synthesis machinery is tightly regulated and perfectly coupled to the availability of nutrients, oxygen, and GFs in the microenvironment. To optimize mTOR activation in response to these biologic conditions, the cell resorts to a coordinated interplay between positive and negative regulators of the molecules that participate in the mTOR pathway, and the activation of intrinsic feedback loops that modulate its function and impose a self-limiting control over its activation.

UPSTREAM REGULATORS OF mTOR

Under normal physiologic conditions, amino acids, glucose, oxygen availability, and GFs are the key signals to stimulate mTORC1 activity. The intake of nutrients combined with adequate supplies of oxygen increase intracellular transport of glucose, glycolysis, the mitochondrial Krebs cycle, and production of ATP. ATP prevents the inhibitory effect exerted by AMP-activated kinase (AMPK) on mTORC1. Then, mTORC1 activation by increased pools of intracellular energy couples the intake of glucose and amino acids to protein synthesis. Growth signaling factors also play an important role in the regulation of mTOR activity. Growth factors (eg, epidermal growth factor [EGF], transforming growth factor [TGF], vascular endothelial growth factor [VEGF], hepatocyte growth factor [HGF], platelet-derived growth factor [PDGF], insulin-like growth factor 1 [IGF-1]) stimulate cell growth and mTOR activation through binding to the external domain of transmembrane receptor tyrosine kinases (RTKs). The ligand-receptor interaction induces a conformational change in the RTK-ligand complex that causes the intracellular region of the receptor to become active, effecting transfer of phosphate groups from ATP to the tyrosine residues on the receptor itself. The autophosphorylation of an RTK activates its enzymatic activity and phosphorylates the next protein in the kinase cascade of the PI3K/Akt/mTOR pathway. For example, In the case of the IGF receptor (IGFR), on binding of the IGF-1, the insulin receptor phosphorylates substrates 1 and 2 (IRS1-2), which relay the activation downstream to PI3K, in turn activating Akt through phosphorylation on Thr 308. Phosphorylated Akt unleashes mTORC1 through inactivating phosphorylation of three negative regulators. One is the tuberous sclerosis 1 (TSC1)/TSC2 complex, which prevents phosphorylation and activation of mTORC1 through inhibiting the Ras homolog enriched in brain GTPase (Rheb).[17,18] The second is glycogen synthase kinase 3 beta (GSK3B), which inhibits mTORC1 through inducing AMPK-dependent activation of the TSC1/2 complex.[19] The third is PRAS40, which competes with Rheb-dependent phosphorylation of raptor in the mTORC1 complex.[20] Little is known about upstream regulators of mTORC2. However, because SGK and PKC are known to be regulated by GFs, regulation of mTORC2 has been thought to be modulated by the same GFs as mTORC1.

NEGATIVE REGULATORS

The negative regulators of mTOR are biologic conditions and molecules that modulate upstream stimulatory signals to prevent uncontrolled cellular energy expenditure through limiting the activation of mTOR. The more effective negative regulator signals of the mTOR pathway are nutrient deprivation (starvation), hypoxia, and negative regulators of the PI3K/Akt/mTOR signaling pathway. The latter include primarily the TSC1/2 complex and the phosphatase and tensin homolog (PTEN). Nutrient deprivation, chemical inhibition of glycolysis, or inhibition of mitochondrial respiration activate the serine/threonine kinase 11 (STK11) that induces the AMPK-mediated activation of TSC1/2, with the subsequent inhibition of mTORC1 activity.[21,22] Thus, through inhibiting mTORC1 activity, starvation prevents the biogenesis of lipids and proteins and promotes autophagy to optimize the use of limited energy supplies.[23-26] Other adverse conditions, such as DNA damage and hypoxia, also promote the inhibitory effect of TSC1/2 on mTORC1. DNA damage prevents mTORC1 activation through the p53-mediated activation of AMPK, whereas hypoxia induces the activation of HIF1α-responsive RTP801 (REDD1), which antagonizes the Akt-mediated inhibition of TSC1/2.[27-29]

Under normal physiologic conditions, the *PTEN* gene provides the paradigm for modulation of PI3K/Akt/mTOR signaling.[30,31] On activation of RTK through ligand-binding, PI3K is activated and converts phosphatidylinositol 4,5-bisphosphate (PIP2) into phosphatidylinositol 3,4,5-triphosphate (PIP3), which triggers Akt phosphorylation and mTORC1 activation. Thus, conversion of PIP23 to PIP3 is a critical rate-limiting step to modulate the PI3K/Akt-dependent activation of mTOR. PTEN regulates the conversion of PIP3 to PIP2; therefore, PTEN loss of function provides the basis for aberrant activation of Akt and mTOR signaling, as is frequently seen in cancer. In addition to PTEN, the inositol polyphosphate-5-phosphatase and the inositol polyphosphate phosphatase-like 1 are also involved in the restoration of PIP2 levels and modulation of the PI3K/Akt/mTOR pathway activation.[32,33]

Other negative regulators within the pathway are the FK506-binding protein 8 and PRAS40, which prevent Rheb from activating mTORC1.[17,18] Less is known about repression of mTORC2; however, in vitro and in vivo studies have shown that mTORC1 activation prevents mTORC2 activity in an S6K1-dependent way, as shown through direct inhibitory phosphorylation of rictor at Thr1135 in mTORC2-active cells.[34]

NEGATIVE FEEDBACK AND POSITIVE FEED-FORWARD LOOPS

Negative feedback and positive feed-forward loops are intrinsic mechanisms of self-control in the mTOR pathway that refrain or trigger its activation. For instance, activated S6K1 through mTORC1 phosphorylation blocks upstream overstimulation of the PI3K/Akt/mTOR through destabilizing IRS1-2 and uncoupling IGF-1 from the PI3K/Akt/mTOR cascade.[35-37] Negative feedback control is also exerted by mTORC1 through preventing the activation mTORC2.[34] In contrast, the 3-phosphoinositide–dependent protein kinase-1 (PDK1, known as PDPK1) can also directly activate S6K1 through Thr299 phosphorylation and prevent the uncoupling of IGF-1.[38] In addition, the degradation of GSK3B through Akt phosphorylation reinforces the activation of mTORC1 through destabilizing the TSC1/2 complex.[19]

CROSSTALK

The Ras/Raf/MEK/ERK pathway is also a key regulator of cell growth and metabolism, cell division, and survival. This pathway is activated by GFs, hormones, neurotransmitters, and chemokines that signal through RTK and G protein-coupled receptors. These extracellular stimuli only partially overlap with those that signal through the PI3K/Akt/mTOR pathway. The degree of activation of each pathway depends on the interplay between GF availability and the density and distribution of RTK within the cell. In addition, a dynamic interaction or crosstalk between the PI3K/Akt/mTOR and Raf/Raf/MEK/ERK pathways provides a balanced cellular response to growth signals. Thus, inhibition of these interactions may result in unpredictable responses.

Examples of inhibition through negative crosstalk between PI3K/Akt/mTOR and Raf/Raf/MEK/ERK pathways[37,39] are the inactivating phosphorylation of the *N*-terminus domain of Raf by Akt[40,41] and the inhibition of PI3K/Akt/mTOR signaling through blocking of the recruitment of PI3K to the intracellular domain of RTK in response to GFs by Erk.[42,43] An example of positive crosstalk is the enhanced PI3K/Akt/mTOR signaling in response to Ras/Raf/MEK/ERK activation that results in dissociation of the TSC1/2 complex, direct phosphorylation of raptor, and activation of mTORC1.[44,45] In addition, inhibition of Akt or MEK can lead to the activation of other pathways through releasing interactive cross-inhibition.

mTOR IN CANCER

Tumors harbor a great spectrum of molecular alterations that deregulate the mTOR pathway and support the increased metabolic demands required by high rates of cell growth and proliferation (**Table 1**). The spectrum of alterations observed in different tumor types include mutations of the PI3K/Akt/mTOR pathway members and regulators, mutations of *p53*, deregulation of RTK activation through overexpression or increased affinity/availability of ligands, and alteration in crosstalk signaling and angiogenesis. Although no mTOR-activating mutations have been described to date, activating mutations of RTKs, more frequently of the catalytic alpha subunit of phosphoinositide-3-kinase (PI3KCA), a critical upstream activator of the PI3K/Akt/mTOR pathway, have been linked to overactivation of mTOR in human cancer tissues.[46–48] Alternatively, inactivating mutations or deletions of suppressors is also a frequent mechanism of activation of the mTOR pathway. Most commonly, this involves the loss of PTEN function in tumor tissues,[49,50] which constitutively activates Akt and mTOR in tumor cells.[37] Heritable inactivating mutations of *TSC1/2*, *NF1*, and *STK11* are less frequently observed.[51] In the case of mantle cell lymphoma, mutations of *STK11* uncouple the critical negative feedback of nutrient deprivation from the mTOR pathway.[52] In addition, tumors that harbor *p53*-inactivating mutations uncouple mTORC1 inactivation from DNA damage, which sustains aberrant mTOR activation.[29]

In the absence of mutations, overactive PI3K/Akt/mTOR signaling can result from deregulated activation of different molecules that participate directly or indirectly in the pathway through feedback loops or crosstalk. RTK can be activated through increased binding affinity or availability of GFs.[47,48] Rheb can be aberrantly activated by gene amplification, suggesting it is a proto-oncogene in prostate cancer.[53] Alterations in the crosstalk between PI3/Akt/mTOR and the Ras/Raf/MEK/ERK pathways have also been described. Tumors that have overactive Erk sustain high mTORC1 activation in a PI3K-independent manner through dissociation of the TSC1/2 repressor complex that inhibits mTORC1. Dissociation of the TSC1/2 repressor by Erk is achieved through direct phosphorylation of TSC2 at Ser 664, resulting in release

Table 1
mTOR pathway alterations in human cancers

Gene	Mechanisms of Activation	Disease/Prevalence	Reference
EGFR	Overexpression	CRC (50%)	Yen et al,[129] 2010
	Mutation	NSCLC (55%–80%)	Lynch et al,[130] 2004
HER2	Mutation	BC (25%–30%)	Slamon et al,[131] 1989
		Ovarian (30%)	
IGFR	Autocrine IGFR-IGF-1 loop	AML (35%)	Chapuis et al,[132] 2010
	Overexpression	RCC (80%)	Schips et al,[133] 2004
c-MET	Overexpression	RCC (100%)	Pisters et al,[134] 1997
		PC (80%–100%)	Pisters et al,[135] 1995
PDGFR	Mutation	GIST (35% in KIT-negative)	Heinrich et al,[136] 2003
	Overexpression	BC (39%)	Carvalho et al,[137] 2005
VEGFR	Overexpression	CRC (52%)	Hashim et al,[138] 2010
	Autocrine loop	GBM (100%)	Steiner et al,[139] 2004
PTEN	Mutation	CRPC (20%–30%)	Suzuki et al,[140] 1998
	Deletion	CRPC (30%)	Yoshimoto et al,[141] 2007
	Lost expression	CRPC (80%)	Bertram et al,[112] 2006
PIK3CA	Mutation	BC (25%)	Bachman et al,[142] 2004
	Mutation	CRC (20%–30%)	Frattini et al,[143] 2005
	Mutation	Glioblastoma (27%)	Samuels et al,[144] 2004
	Amplification	PC (50%)	Edwards et al,[145] 2003
VHL	Mutation	RCC (60%–80% in sporadic RCC)	Gallou et al,[146] 1999
Ras	Overexpression	CRC (42%)	Karapetis et al,[147] 2008
		Pancreas cancer (85%)	Laghi et al,[148] 2002

Abbreviations: AML, acute myeloid leukemia; BC, breast cancer; c-MET, hepatocyte growth factor receptor; CRC, colorectal cancer; CRPC, castration-resistant prostate cancer; EGFR, epidermal growth factor receptor; GBM, glioblastoma multiforme; GIST, gastrointestinal stromal tumor; HER2, human epidermal growth factor receptor 2; IGF-1, insulin-like growth factor 1; IGFR, insulin-like growth factor 1 receptor; NSCLC, non–small cell lung cancer; PC, prostate cancer; PDGFR, platelet-derived growth factor receptor; PIK3CA, phosphoinositide-3-kinase, catalytic, alpha polypeptide; PTEN, phosphatase and tensin homolog; Ras, rat sarcoma viral oncogene homolog; RCC, renal cell carcinoma; VEGFR, vascular endothelial growth factor receptor; VHL, von Hippel-Lindau tumor suppressor.

of TORC1,[45] and through phosphorylation and activation of the TSC1/2 inhibitor ribosomal protein S6 kinase polypeptide 1 (RPS6KA1, also denominated RSK1).[54]

Another mechanism of activation of the mTOR pathway in cancer is aberrant HIF1α activation. Under normal conditions, induction of HIF1α by hypoxia inhibits mTOR activation and stimulates the VEGF-VEGFR1-PAI1 angiogenic pathway, which is turned off as hypoxia subsides. In renal cell carcinoma (RCC), high levels of HIF1α transcriptional activity and increased angiogenesis are seen in the presence of adequate oxygen levels as a result of inactivating mutations of the Von Hippel-Lindau tumor suppressor gene (VHL) that prevent HIF1α degradation. Concurrently, HIF1α stimulation of glucose uptake (GLUT1, GLUT3) and glycolysis (PKM2, LDHA, ENO1)[55] increases the nutrient availability and sustains high levels of PI3K/Akt/mTOR pathway activity. Thus, mTOR became a prime target for therapeutic inhibition in RCC, and this has proven to be an effective approach to controlling advanced metastatic disease.

Tumor cells can turn on an extensive, complex, and redundant network of proteins that support uncontrolled growth and survival, which is a major reason why specific inhibitors have limited success in killing human cancer cells and why resistance to therapy can develop rapidly.[37,39]

mTOR PATHWAY INHIBITORS IN CANCER

The inhibition of the mTOR signaling pathway by rapamycin was discovered in the early 1990s. Although the mechanism of rapamycin action (Rapamune) as an anti-cancer agent has not been completely elucidated, rapamycin binds to FKBP12, and the rapamycin-FKBP12 complex binds to mTORC1 to prevent phosphorylation of the mTORC1 effectors 4EBP1 and S6K1. Therefore, the inhibition of the mTOR pathway prevents protein synthesis and cell proliferation, arresting the cells in the G1 phase of the cell cycle.

In the past 10 years, several agents have been designed to target the mTOR pathway. Temsirolimus, everolimus, and ridaforolimus are rapalogs that share the same mechanism of action but differ in pharmacokinetic properties because of different substitutions at position C-40 of rapamycin.[56] Currently, temsirolimus and everolimus are approved for the treatment of metastatic RCC. More recently, everolimus has also been approved for treatment of subependimal giant cell astrocytoma and neuroendocrine tumors of the pancreas. Many other mTOR pathway inhibitors are being studied in clinical trials.

mTOR INHIBITORS APPROVED BY FDA FOR TREATMENT OF CANCER
Renal Cell Carcinoma

In the United States 58,240 new cases of RCC were diagnosed in 2010, and 2.3% of cancer deaths are attributed to RCC.[57] Most renal epithelial tumors are clear cell carcinomas, of which 80% show VHL loss of heterozygosity with inactivating mutations of the remaining allele. Despite complete surgical resection of localized tumors, 30% of patients experience recurrence with distant metastasis.[58] Metastatic RCC is highly resistant to standard chemotherapy but sensitive to the immune-modulatory cytokines interleukin 2 and interferon (IFN)-alfa 2a[59]; the inhibitors of angiogenesis sunitinib (Sutent),[60] sorafenib (Nevaxar),[61] and bevacizumab (Avastin) in combination with IFN-alpha 2a[62]; and, two mTOR inhibitors, temsirolimus and everolimus, which were approved by the U.S. Food and Drug Administration (FDA) in 2007 and 2010, respectively.

Temsirolimus (Torisel) is a prodrug of rapamycin and the first mTOR inhibitor approved for increasing survival of patients with previously untreated metastatic RCC with poor prognostic features as defined by the Memorial Sloan-Kettering Cancer Center (MSKCC) prognostic model.[63] A randomized phase II trial of temsirolimus at three doses (25, 75, and 250 mg) conducted in 111 patients with heavily pretreated metastatic RCC had shown a clinical benefit (objective and minor response plus stable disease) in 51% cases.[64] Overall, the median time to progression was 6 months and the median overall survival was 15 months. Neither toxicity nor efficacy was influenced by temsirolimus dose levels, and because the intravenous infusion of 25 mg once weekly dose was the optimal biologic dose, it was selected for further clinical development.

The Global Advanced Renal-Cell Carcinoma (ARCC) multicenter phase III trial randomized 626 treatment-naive patients with advanced/stage IV RCC with poor prognosis to receive either weekly temsirolimus at 25 mg (TEM) or 3 million IU of subcutaneous IFN (with an increase to 18 million IU) or the combination of both temsirolimus at 15 mg plus IFN (TEM-IFN).[65] Treatment groups, stratified by nephrectomy status and region, were well balanced. Clear cell RCC was the most common histologic type (80%) and nephrectomy was performed in 66% of cases. The primary end point was overall survival, and to reach statistical significance, a 40% improvement in either one of the temsirolimus-containing regimens was necessary over IFN. Overall survival was significantly longer in the TEM-only group than in the IFN-only group (10.9 vs 7.3 months; hazard ratio [HR], 0.73; 95% CI, 0.58–0.92; $P = .008$). The TEM-IFN combination did not significantly improved overall survival compared with IFN and had more toxicity (8.4 vs 7.3 months; HR, 0.93; 95% CI, 0.76–1.20; $P = .7$). The median progression-free survival according to RECIST criteria was 5.5, 4.7, and 3.1 months, respectively, for TEM, TEM-IFN, and IFN. The objective response rates were not significantly different among the three groups, 8.6%, 8.1%, and 4.8%, respectively. By contrast, the proportion of patients with a durable (>6 months) clinical benefit (objective response rate plus stable disease) was significantly higher in TEM and TEM-IFN compared with IFN (32.1%, 28.1%, and 15.5%; $P<.001$ and $P = .002$, respectively).

Asthenia was the most common adverse effect (60%) in patients receiving IFN alone or in combination. Temsirolimus-containing regimens showed a higher incidence of mild to moderate rash, peripheral edema, stomatitis, hyperglycemia, hyperlipidemia, and hypercholesterolemia. Grade 3/4 adverse events occurred in 67% of patients in the TEM arm, compared with 87% in the TEM-IFN arm ($P = .02$) and 78% in the IFN arm ($P = .02$). Grade 3/4 asthenia was reported in 11% of patients in the TEM arm, 28% in the TEM-IFN arm ($P<.001$), and 26% in the IFN arm ($P<.001$). TEM-IFN showed higher rates of grade 3/4 neutropenia and thrombocytopenia compared with TEM (15% and 9% vs 3% and 1%, respectively). Based on these findings, weekly temsirolimus at 25 mg was approved for first-line treatment of metastatic, poor-prognosis RCC. Responses were observed in all histologic subtypes, including sarcomatoid variants. The differences in efficacy among temsirolimus-containing regimens were attributed to lower mean dose-intensity of temsirolimus in the TEM-IFN arm (10.9 mg/wk) versus the TEM arm (23.1 mg).

Everolimus (RAD001) is the first oral mTOR inhibitor to reach the oncology clinic. Unlike temsirolimus, everolimus is not a prodrug of rapamycin and is taken daily by mouth in a 10-mg tablet.

The Renal Cell Cancer Treatment with Oral RAD001 Given Daily (RECORD-I) double-blind, placebo-controlled, multicenter phase III trial enrolled 410 patients with poor-prognosis RCC (MSKCC model) that progressed within 6 months of stopping treatment with either sunitinib, sorafenib, or both agents.[66] All patients had the clear cell histologic type of RCC and were randomized in a 2:1 ratio to everolimus at 10 mg daily or placebo until disease progression. On progression, patients randomized to placebo were able to receive open-label everolimus. The study was powered to detect a 50% improvement in the primary end point of progression-free survival and two interim analyses were planned. Median progression-free survival of patients in the everolimus group was significantly longer than placebo (4.9 vs 1.9 months; HR, 0.33; 95% CI, 0.25–0.43; $P<.001$).[67] The probability of remaining progression-free for at least 10 months was 25% in the everolimus group compared with less than 2% in the placebo. However, the overall survival in months was not significantly different because of the crossover effect (14.8 vs 14.4 months, respectively; $P = .177$). Objective response rate according to RECIST was observed in fewer than 2% of patients on everolimus. As expected, the incidence of adverse effects was higher in the everolimus group: mild to moderate stomatitis in 40%, rash in 25%, fatigue in 20%, and asthenia in 18%. Severe grade 3/4 adverse events were in the everolimus group were lymphopenia (14%), hyperglycemia (12%), anemia

(9%), hyperphosphatemia (4%), stomatitis (3%), noninfectious pneumonitis (3%), and hypercholesterolemia (3%). Dose reduction from 10 to 5 mg was required in 39% of the patients and 13% of the total discontinued everolimus because of lung disorder or fatigue. Everolimus was approved by the FDA for increasing progression-free survival of patients with advanced RCC progressing after treatment with sunitinib or sorafenib.

Pancreatic Neuroendocrine Tumors

Pancreatic neuroendocrine tumors (PNET) represents 1.3% of all pancreatic cancer and according to the Centers for Disease Control and Prevention, approximately 1000 cases are diagnosed annually in the United States. However, although rare, its incidence is rising because of improvements in diagnostic methods.[68,69] Everolimus and sunitinib, were recently FDA-approved for the treatment of metastatic or unresectable PNET.

The RAD001 in Advanced Neuroendocrine Tumors, third trial (RADIANT-3), a multicenter, double-blind, and placebo-controlled phase III study of everolimus at 10 mg daily was conducted in 410 patients with metastatic unresectable PNET.[70] Patients were stratified by previous treatment and World Health Organization performance status and those randomized to placebo were allowed to crossover to everolimus at progression. The study was powered to detect a 50% improvement in the primary end point of progression-free survival. More than 90% of the patients had metastases and 24% had gastrinoma, VIPoma, insulinoma, or somatostatinoma. The median progression-free survival was significantly longer in the everolimus group (11 vs 4.6 months; HR, 0.34; 95% CI, 0.26–0.44; $P<.001$)[70]; the probability of remaining progression-free at least 18 months was 34% in the everolimus group and 9% in placebo. The objective response rate was not significantly different (5% in everolimus and 2% in placebo), indicating that the observed clinical benefit was primarily because of stabilization of the disease and that the lack of overall survival benefit was confounded by the high rate of patients on placebo who crossed over to everolimus at progression (73%). Most common adverse events associated with everolimus were stomatitis (52.9%), rash (48.5%), diarrhea (34.3%), and fatigue (32.4%). Grade 3 or 4 anemia (5.9%), hyperglycemia (5.9%), stomatitis (4.9%), and noninfectious pneumonitis (2%) events were rare but more frequent in the everolimus group.

The RADIANT-2 phase III trial randomized 429 patients with neuroendocrine tumors involving multiple sites and carcinoid syndrome to long-acting release (LAR) octreotide at 30 mg intramuscularly every 28 days in combination with either everolimus at 10 mg daily or placebo.[71] Everolimus plus octreotide increased the median progression-free survival to 16.4 compared with 11.3 months for placebo. However, the HR fell short of the prespecified boundary of statistical significance (HR, 0.77; 95% CI, 0.59–1.00; one-sided, $P = .026$).

Subependymal Giant-Cell Astrocytomas in Tuberous Sclerosis

The tuberous sclerosis (TS) complex is a rare multisystem autosomal dominant disorder (1 in 6000 live births)[72] that causes nonmalignant tumors to grow in the brain and on other vital organs. Subependymal giant-cell astrocytomas (SEGA) are slow-growing tumors that present in up to 20% of TS cases and typically arise from the foramen of Monro, blocking the circulation of the cerebrospinal fluid and leading to hydrocephalus. Current standard is surgical resection, which is not always possible.

A single-arm, open-label phase I/II trial conducted at the Cincinnati Children's Hospital Medical Center enrolled 28 patients with SEGA to receive everolimus at 3 mg per square meter of body surface area.[73] The primary end point of tumor reduction equal or higher than 30% was reached in 21 (75%) patients. The largest phase III study in TS that was presented at the International TSC Research Conference 2011 showed that 35% of patients treated with everolimus had a 50% or greater reduction in SEGA volume, whereas no responses were observed in placebo. On October 2010, the FDA approved everolimus for the treatment of SEGA in patients with TS who were not candidates for surgical intervention.

mTOR INHIBITORS IN OTHER MALIGNANCIES
Hematologic Malignancies

Activation of the PI3K/Akt/mTOR pathway in non-Hodgkin's lymphomas (NHL), Waldenström's macroglobulinemia (WM), chronic lymphocytic leukemia (CLL), and acute leukemias provided the basis for testing rapalogs in these settings.[74–76] **Table 2** summarizes the results of rapalogs in hematologic malignancies. Mantle cell lymphoma (MCL) represents an ideal target for mTOR inhibitors because the t(11;14) translocation induces overexpression of cyclin D1 messenger RNA,[77] which is regulated by mTOR.

Two trials of single-agent temsirolimus in heavily pretreated patients with relapsed MCL showed a small benefit. One was a single-arm trial of temsirolimus at 250 mg weekly for six cycles in 34 patients with refractory MCL.[78] Results showed 13 (38%) responders, 12 of whom (35%) experienced a partial response and 1 (3%) a complete response. The median time to progression was 6 months. Grade 3/4 hematologic toxicity was observed in 75% and 11% of the patients, respectively. A subsequent study by the same group of investigators treated 29 patients with MCL with a tenfold lower dose of temsirolimus (25 mg weekly).[79] Objective responses were experienced in 11 (41%) patients, among whom 10 (37%) experienced a partial response and 1 (3.7%) a complete response. The median time to progression was 6 months and the grade 3 and 4 hematologic toxicity decreased to 50% and 4% of the patients, respectively.

The subsequent phase III trial randomized 162 patients with relapsed MCL after a median of three to four prior chemotherapy schedules to receive either two dose levels of temsirolimus monotherapy (175 mg weekly for 3 weeks followed by either 75 or 25 mg weekly) or investigator's choice of therapy.[80] The primary efficacy end point was median progression-free survival, which reached 4.8, 3.4, and 1.9 months, respectively, for the 175/75-mg and 175/25-mg temsirolimus and investigator's-choice groups. The 175/75-mg dose level of temsirolimus had significantly better median progression-free survival than the investigator's choice (HR, 0.44; $P = .0009$ for the 175/75-mg group vs HR, 0.65; $P = .0618$ for the 175/25-mg group), but the median overall survival was not significantly different between high- or low-dose temsirolimus-containing regimens and the investigator's choice (11.1, 8.8, and 9.5 months, respectively). Grade 3/4 thrombocytopenia (52%–59%), anemia (11%–20%), neutropenia (15%–22%), and asthenia (13%–19%) were frequent. These results established temsirolimus as a new therapeutic option for relapsed/refractory MCL and led to its inclusion in the NCCN Clinical Practice Guidelines in Oncology for NHL.[81]

A multicenter phase II trial of temsirolimus at 25 mg that included 89 patients with relapsed/refractory non-MCL NHL B-cell lymphomas (MCL excluded) and indolent lymphomas[82] showed a 28.1% response rate, with 12.5% complete responses in diffuse large B-cell lymphomas (DLBCLs); a 53.8% response rate with 25.65% complete response in follicular lymphomas (FLs); and a 11% response rate with no complete response in CLL. The median progression-free survival was 2.6 months for DLBCL and 12.7 months for FL.

Table 2
Trials of rapalogs in hematologic malignancies

Author	Phase	Agent/Dose	Disease	n	RR	Survival
Witzig et al,[78] 2005	2	Temsirolimus, 250 mg weekly	MCL	34	38%	6.5 mo (mTTP)
Ansell et al,[79] 2008	2	Temsirolimus, 25 mg weekly	MCL	29	41%	6 mo (mTTP)
Hess et al,[80] 2009	3	Temsirolimus, 175 mg/wk × 3 wk +75 or 25 mg weekly	MCL	108	22%	4.8 mo (mPFS)
Smith et al,[82] 2010	2	Temsirolimus, 25 mg weekly	NHL (MCL excluded)	89	DLBCL, 28.1% FL, 55.5% CLL, 11%	2.6 DLBCL 12.7 FL (mTTP mo)
Tobinai et al,[84] 2010	1	Everolimus, 5–10 mg daily	NHL	13	30%	NR
Witzig et al,[85] 2011	2	Everolimus, 10 mg daily	NHL	77	DLBCL, 30% MCL, 32% FL, 38%	5.7 mo (duration of response)
Ghobrial et al,[86] 2010	2	Everolimus, 10 mg daily	WM	50	70%	mPFS not reached
Zent et al,[149] 2010	2	Everolimus, 10 mg daily	CLL	22	18%	NR
Rizzieri et al,[83] 2008	2	Ridaforolimus, 12.5 mg daily × 5 d	Multiple malignancies	55	MCL, 33% Agn.M.met 15%	NR

Abbreviations: Agn.M.met, agnogenic myeloid metaplasia; CLL, chronic lymphocytic leukemia; DLBCL, diffuse large B-cell lymphoma; FL, follicular lymphoma; MCL, mantle cell lymphoma; mPFS, median progression-free survival; mTTP, median time to progression; NHL, non-Hodgkin's lymphoma; NR, not reported; RR, response rate; WM, Waldenström's macroglobulinemia.

Ridaforolimus, also known as deforolimus (ARIAD in collaboration with Merck), is a nonprodrug rapamycin analog studied in a phase II trial of 55 patients with relapsed/refractory disease with different hematologic malignancies (acute leukemia, agnogenic myeloid metaplasia, and MCL).[83] At a dose of 12.5 mg intravenous daily for 5 days every 2 weeks on a 4-week cycle, ridaforolimus showed partial response in 2 of 7 patients with agnogenic myeloid metaplasia and 3 of 9 patients with MCL but no activity in acute leukemias. The most common mild and transient adverse effects were stomatitis, fatigue, nausea, and thrombocytopenia.

Everolimus has also been tested in NHL, WM, and CLL. A small phase I trial of everolimus at 5 and 10 mg daily showed no dose-limiting toxicities in 13 patients with NHL (5 FL, 2 DLBCL, 2 MCL, and 4 T-cell NHL lymphomas) and, similar to other rapalogs, a response rate of 30%.[84] A subsequent phase II trial conducted at the Mayo Clinic and Dana-Farber Cancer Institute enrolled 77 patients with aggressive NHL who were heavily pretreated to receive everolimus at 10 mg/d.[85] The overall response rate was 30%, with 25% (n = 20) experiencing a partial response and 4% (n = 3) a complete response; stable disease was observed in 23% (n = 18). The overall response rate by NHL type was 30% (14/47) in DLBCL, 32% (6/19) in MCL, and 38% (3/8) in grade 3 FL. Median duration of response was 5.7 months, and grade 3/4 thrombocytopenia, neutropenia, and anemia were observed in 38%, 18%, and 14% of patients, respectively. A phase II trial of everolimus 10 mg/d in 50 previously treated patients with WM showed an overall response rate of 70%, with 42% experiencing a partial response and 28% a minimal response.[86] Estimated progression-free survival rates at 6 and 12 months were 75% and 62%, respectively. A phase II study of everolimus at 10 mg in 22 patients with recurrent/refractory CLL showed an 18% (4/22) partial response rate and a median decrease of 75% in the size of lymphadenopathies in 8 (36%) patients. The response rate described in this study is similar to that reported with temsirolimus.

For more information, the Schatz[87] review is strongly recommended.

Sarcoma

Small phase I trials with temsirolimus and ridaforolimus showed encouraging responses in patients with heavily pretreated soft tissue sarcomas (STS). A phase II trial of temsirolimus at 25 mg weekly in 41 patients with advanced STS who had no prior chemotherapy for metastatic disease showed limited activity (two partial responses, median time to progression of 2 months).[88] Results of a larger phase II trial of ridaforolimus given at 12.5 mg intravenously for 5 days every 2 weeks in 212 patients with STS or bone sarcoma, with no restrictions on prior chemotherapy, showed 49 patients with stable disease and 5 with partial responses.[89] Based on these results, a double-blind phase III trial of ridaforolimus randomized 711 patients with metastatic sarcoma (stratified STS vs bone sarcoma; first- vs second-/third-line prior chemotherapy) to placebo or ridaforolimus at 40 mg orally for 5 days a week as maintenance therapy after experiencing stable disease or better response to prior chemotherapy. Ridaforolimus significantly improved the medial progression-free survival from 14.6 weeks to 17.7 weeks (HR, 0.69; P = .0001) in all prespecified strata. The safety profile was similar to other rapalogs. Follow-up for overall survival is ongoing.[90]

Breast Cancer

Preclinical breast cancer models indicate that activation of the PI3K/Akt/mTOR pathway through growth factor signaling confers resistance to hormonal manipulations through interfering with estrogen receptor antagonists,[91,92] and that mTOR inhibition restores hormonal response.[93]

A randomized phase II trial of letrozole alone or in combination with two schedules of temsirolimus (temsirolimus, 10 mg daily, or temsirolimus, 30 mg intermittent) conducted in 90 patients with metastatic breast cancer showed a higher progression-free survival rate at 1 year in the combination arms compared with letrozole alone (daily TEM, 69%; intermittent TEM, 62%; letrozole, 48%).[94] However, the subsequent phase III trial of intermittent TEM combined with letrozole in metastatic breast cancer was stopped after the interim analysis of 992 of 1236 patients showed no benefit in median progression-free survival.[95]

Two everolimus schedules (10 mg orally daily vs 70 mg orally weekly) were studied in a randomized phase II trial in metastatic breast cancer. The combined complete and partial response in the daily schedule was 12% versus 0% in the weekly dosing.[96] Thus, everolimus regimen of 10 mg orally daily was selected for further development. The results of the randomized phase III trial of everolimus at 10 mg plus examestane versus examestane alone in postmenopausal women with estrogen receptor–positive, HER2-negative metastatic breast cancer resistant to aromatase inhibitors (BOLERO-2) was recently presented at the 2011 European Multidisciplinary Cancer Congress in Stockholm, Sweden. The interim analysis through central assessment of 724 patients showed a significant improvement in the medial progression-free survival favoring the combination (10.6 vs 4.1 months; HR, 0.36; $P<.0001$).

Similar approaches combining everolimus with hormonal manipulation have been tested in the neoadjuvant setting of breast cancer.[97]

Lung Cancer

Rapalogs have shown very limited activity as single agents in phase II trials of small cell lung cancer (SCLC). Temsirolimus at 25 mg and 250 mg daily in either patients experiencing response or stable disease after induction with platinum-etoposide showed a median progression-free survival ranging from 1.9 to 2.5 months.[98] Everolimus at 10 mg orally daily in 40 pretreated patients showed 1 (3%) with a partial response and 8 (23%) with stable disease, with a median progression-free survival of 1.3 months.[99]

In patients with stage IIIb–IV non–small cell lung cancer (NSCLC) previously treated with platinums, everolimus at 10 mg daily showed modest activity (overall disease control rate, 47.1%; median progression-free survival, 2.6 months).[100]

Gastric Cancer

The rationale to use rapalogs in gastric cancer is supported by studies of patient-derived samples of gastric cancer showing phosphorylated mTOR.[101] In addition, mTOR activation was correlated with tumor progression and poor survival.[102,103]

In a multicenter phase II trial of everolimus at 10 mg/d conducted in 53 patients with pathologically confirmed advanced gastric cancer refractory to any of the first-line treatments (5-fluorouracil [5FU] and derivatives, taxanes, irinotecan, or platinums) showed stable disease in 56% of cases, with a median progression-free survival of 2.7 months.[104] Adverse events were similar to other trials, including mild to moderate stomatitis (74%), anorexia (53%), fatigue (51%), rash (45%), and nausea (32%). A second phase II trial of everolimus at 10 mg/d in 54 patients with advanced gastric cancer refractory to both fluoropyrimidine and platinum showed stable disease in 35% of the patients and 2 partial responses. The median progression-free survival (primary end point) was 1.7 months.[105] Grade 3/4 toxicity included anemia (9.4%), thrombocytopenia (9.4%), hepatic dysfunction (11.3%), one case of interstitial pneumonitis, and one case of diffuse alveolar hemorrhage.

Endometrial Cancer

PTEN loss and PI3K/Akt/mTOR activation have been observed in 40% to 60% of endometrial cancers, suggesting that this pathway is important in the pathogenesis of this disease.[106,107]

A single-arm phase II trial of everolimus at 10 mg daily conducted in 35 patients with progressive or recurrent endometrioid endometrial carcinoma refractory to chemotherapy showed stable disease according to RECIST in 12 of 28 (43%) and 6 of 28 (21%) evaluable patients at 8 and 20 weeks, respectively.[108] Up to 50% of patients required dose reduction. Grade 3/4 toxicities were lymphopenia (29%), fatigue (23%), nausea (11%), and elevated glucose (9%). A randomized multicenter phase II trial of temsirolimus at 25 mg intravenously weekly in 60 patients with chemotherapy-naïve/refractory endometrial carcinoma of multiple histology types showed that 14% experienced a partial response (median duration, 5.1 months) and 69% had stable disease (median duration, 9.7 months) in the chemotherapy-naïve group versus 4% experienced a partial response (median duration, 4.9 months) and 48% had stable disease (median duration, 3.8 months) in the chemotherapy-refractory group.[109] The most common adverse effects were fatigue, rash, nausea, and anemia; grade 3/4 toxicities were fatigue in seven patients, diarrhea in five, and pneumonitis in five.

Prostate Cancer

Loss of PTEN and activation of the PI3/Akt/mTOR pathway is a frequent and well-established mechanism of prostate cancer progression[110–112] that by crosstalk induction of ligand-independent activation of the androgen receptor supports the development of resistance to androgen deprivation therapy.[113,114] In turn, although androgen receptor upregulates mTOR activity by increasing the androgen receptor–dependent transcription of nutrient transporters,[115] the inhibition of mTOR with rapamycin increases androgen receptor mRNA and transcriptional activity.[116,117] Therefore, inhibiting both pathways would be essential to achieve complete responses.

A randomized phase II trial of everolimus and bicalutamide versus bicalutamide alone in metastatic castration-resistant prostate cancer (CRPC) is testing the effect on prostate-specific antigen (PSA) response.[118] The same approach is being studied in the randomized phase II trial of ridaforolimus-bicalutamide versus bicalutamide alone for treating CRPC (ClinicalTrials.gov identifier: NCT00777959). In line with inhibiting mTOR through blocking Akt, the phase II trial ECOG 2809 is testing MK-2206 in combination with bicalutamide (Casodex) as an approach to avoiding androgen deprivation in men with recurrent, nonmetastatic, noncastrate prostate cancer at high risk for progression after primary therapy (ClinicalTrials.gov identifier: NCT01251861).

Several clinical trials are testing the effect of rapalogs in other malignancies; however, it is apparent that their activity as monotherapy remains limited.

NEW STRATEGIES TO IMPLEMENT THE EFFECT OF mTOR INHIBITORS IN CANCER

Despite of the great responses obtained in tumors addicted to specific mutations or overactivation of key members of the mTOR pathway (HiF1α in RCC, cyclin D1 in MCL, or TSC in SEGA), mTOR inhibitors as single agents have modest activity. The transient and partial inhibition of 4EBP1, the increased phosphorylation of Akt through the loss of negative feedback loops, and the activation of alternative oncogenic pathways through crosstalk support the notion that rapalogs may be more effective in combination with other targeted agents or to enhance activity of hormones and chemotherapy. Clinical trials in a variety of solid tumors and hematologic malignancies are testing these approaches. Two phase I trials evaluating the combination of everolimus and trastuzumab (Herceptin) have shown activity in patients with breast cancer that progresses after trastuzumab-based therapies.[119,120] Everolimus-gefitinib (Iressa) in recurrent glioblastoma multiforme showed partial response in 14% of cases and stable disease in 36%,[121] and the same combination is in phase II in NSCLC.[122] Everolimus combined with IGF1R inhibitors is in phase I in sarcomas.[123] Randomized phase II trial of temsirolimus-bevacizumab as first-line treatment for advanced RCC compared with standard sunitinib or IFN-bevacizumab has shown increased toxicity with no survival benefit.[124] Temsirolimus in combination with bortezomib (Velcade) or rituximab (Rituxan) is in phase II studies in refractory multiple myeloma and MCL, respectively.[125,126]

Another approach has been to design small-molecule inhibitors with a broader spectrum of activity in the PI3K/Akt/mTOR pathway. Early clinical trials are in progress with inhibitors of the kinase-dependent function of both mTORC1 and mTORC2, including WYE354 and WYE132, AZD805, OSI-027, and INK128.

Dual PI3K/mTOR kinase inhibitors have also been developed with the idea of overcoming resistance to the mTOR inhibition through preventing the activation of PI3K/Akt as a result of release negative feedback loops. Preclinical testing indicated these agents have significant activity alone and in combination with antiandrogens and chemotherapy in several solid tumors.[127,128] Agents in early clinical trials are GDC-0980, GSK2126458, NVP-BEZ235, PF-04691502, and XL765.

REFERENCES

1. Vezina C, Kudelski A, Sehgal SN. Rapamycin (AY-22,989), a new antifungal antibiotic. I. Taxonomy of the producing streptomycete and isolation of the active principle. J Antibiot (Tokyo) 1975;28(10):721–6.
2. Foster KG, Acosta-Jaquez HA, Romeo Y, et al. Regulation of mTOR complex 1 (mTORC1) by raptor Ser863 and multisite phosphorylation. J Biol Chem 2010; 285(1):80–94.
3. Tang H, Hornstein E, Stolovich M, et al. Amino acid-induced translation of TOP mRNAs is fully dependent on phosphatidylinositol 3-kinase-mediated signaling, is partially inhibited by rapamycin, and is independent of S6K1 and rpS6 phosphorylation. Mol Cell Biol 2001;21(24):8671–83.
4. Raught B, Gingras AC, Sonenberg N. The target of rapamycin (TOR) proteins. Proc Natl Acad Sci U S A 2001;98(13):7037–44.
5. Jefferies HB, Fumagalli S, Dennis PB, et al. Rapamycin suppresses 5'TOP mRNA translation through inhibition of p70s6k. EMBO J 1997;16(12):3693–704.
6. Martin KA, Blenis J. Coordinate regulation of translation by the PI 3-kinase and mTOR pathways. Adv Cancer Res 2002;86:1–39.
7. West MJ, Stoneley M, Willis AE. Translational induction of the c-myc oncogene via activation of the FRAP/TOR signalling pathway. Oncogene 1998;17(6): 769–80.
8. Gingras AC, Raught B, Sonenberg N. Regulation of translation initiation by FRAP/mTOR. Genes Dev 2001;15(7):807–26.
9. Sarbassov DD, Ali SM, Kim DH, et al. Rictor, a novel binding partner of mTOR, defines a rapamycin-insensitive and raptor-independent pathway that regulates the cytoskeleton. Curr Biol 2004;14(14):1296–302.

10. Garcia-Martinez JM, Alessi DR. mTOR complex 2 (mTORC2) controls hydrophobic motif phosphorylation and activation of serum- and glucocorticoid-induced protein kinase 1 (SGK1). Biochem J 2008;416(3):375–85.

11. Facchinetti V, Ouyang WM, Wei H, et al. The mammalian target of rapamycin complex 2 controls folding and stability of Akt and protein kinase C. EMBO J 2008;27(14):1932–43.

12. Sarbassov DD, Guertin DA, Ali SM, et al. Phosphorylation and regulation of Akt/PKB by the rictor-mTOR complex. Science 2005;307(5712):1098–101.

13. Jacinto E, Loewith R, Schmidt A, et al. Mammalian TOR complex 2 controls the actin cytoskeleton and is rapamycin insensitive. Nat Cell Biol 2004;6(11):1122–8.

14. Sarbassov DD, Ali SM, Sengupta S, et al. Prolonged rapamycin treatment inhibits mTORC2 assembly and Akt/PKB. Mol Cell 2006;22(2):159–68.

15. Zeng Z, Sarbassov dos D, Samudio IJ, et al. Rapamycin derivatives reduce mTORC2 signaling and inhibit AKT activation in AML. Blood 2007;109(8):3509–12.

16. Schmidt EV. The role of c-myc in cellular growth control. Oncogene 1999;18(19):2988–96.

17. Zhang Y, Gao X, Saucedo LJ, et al. Rheb is a direct target of the tuberous sclerosis tumour suppressor proteins. Nat Cell Biol 2003;5(6):578–81.

18. Saucedo LJ, Gao X, Chiarelli DA, et al. Rheb promotes cell growth as a component of the insulin/TOR signalling network. Nat Cell Biol 2003;5(6):566–71.

19. Inoki K, Ouyang H, Zhu T, et al. TSC2 integrates Wnt and energy signals via a coordinated phosphorylation by AMPK and GSK3 to regulate cell growth. Cell 2006;126(5):955–68.

20. Guertin DA, Sabatini DM. Defining the role of mTOR in cancer. Cancer Cell 2007;12(1):9–22.

21. Shaw RJ, Bardeesy N, Manning BD, et al. The LKB1 tumor suppressor negatively regulates mTOR signaling. Cancer Cell 2004;6(1):91–9.

22. Shackelford DB, Shaw RJ. The LKB1-AMPK pathway: metabolism and growth control in tumour suppression. Nat Rev Cancer 2009;9(8):563–75.

23. Kim DH, Sarbassov DD, Ali SM, et al. mTOR interacts with raptor to form a nutrient-sensitive complex that signals to the cell growth machinery. Cell 2002;110(2):163–75.

24. Dennis PB, Jaeschke A, Saitoh M, et al. Mammalian TOR: a homeostatic ATP sensor. Science 2001;294(5544):1102–5.

25. Shamji AF, Nghiem P, Schreiber SL. Integration of growth factor and nutrient signaling: implications for cancer biology. Mol Cell 2003;12(2):271–80.

26. Jung CH, Ro SH, Cao J, et al. mTOR regulation of autophagy. FEBS lett 2010;584(7):1287–95.

27. Feng Z, Zhang H, Levine AJ, et al. The coordinate regulation of the p53 and mTOR pathways in cells. Proc Natl Acad Sci U S A 2005;102(23):8204–9.

28. Brugarolas J, Lei K, Hurley RL, et al. Regulation of mTOR function in response to hypoxia by REDD1 and the TSC1/TSC2 tumor suppressor complex. Genes Dev 2004;18(23):2893–904.

29. Jones RG, Thompson CB. Tumor suppressors and cell metabolism: a recipe for cancer growth. Genes Dev 2009;23(5):537–48.

30. Carracedo A, Pandolfi PP. The PTEN-PI3K pathway: of feedbacks and cross-talks. Oncogene 2008;27(41):5527–41.

31. Pandolfi PP. P-TEN exciting years: from the cytosol to the nucleus and back to keep cancer at bay. Oncogene 2008;27(41):5386.

32. Sharrard RM, Maitland NJ. Regulation of protein kinase B activity by PTEN and SHIP2 in human prostate-derived cell lines. Cell Signal 2007;19(1): 129–38.
33. Prasad NK, Tandon M, Badve S, et al. Phosphoinositol phosphatase SHIP2 promotes cancer development and metastasis coupled with alterations in EGF receptor turnover. Carcinogenesis 2008;29(1):25–34.
34. Julien LA, Carriere A, Moreau J, et al. mTORC1-activated S6K1 phosphorylates Rictor on threonine 1135 and regulates mTORC2 signaling. Mol Cell Biol 2010; 30(4):908–21.
35. Dibble CC, Asara JM, Manning BD. Characterization of Rictor phosphorylation sites reveals direct regulation of mTOR complex 2 by S6K1. Mol Cell Biol 2009;29(21):5657–70.
36. Harrington LS, Findlay GM, Gray A, et al. The TSC1-2 tumor suppressor controls insulin-PI3K signaling via regulation of IRS proteins. J Cell Biol 2004;166(2): 213–23.
37. Carracedo A, Ma L, Teruya-Feldstein J, et al. Inhibition of mTORC1 leads to MAPK pathway activation through a PI3K-dependent feedback loop in human cancer. J Clin Invest 2008;118(9):3065–74.
38. Pullen N, Dennis PB, Andjelkovic M, et al. Phosphorylation and activation of p70s6k by PDK1. Science 1998;279(5351):707–10.
39. Kinkade CW, Castillo-Martin M, Puzio-Kuter A, et al. Targeting AKT/mTOR and ERK MAPK signaling inhibits hormone-refractory prostate cancer in a preclinical mouse model. J Clin Invest 2008;118(9):3051–64.
40. Zimmermann S, Moelling K. Phosphorylation and regulation of Raf by Akt (protein kinase B). Science 1999;286(5445):1741–4.
41. Guan KL, Figueroa C, Brtva TR, et al. Negative regulation of the serine/threonine kinase B-Raf by Akt. J Biol Chem 2000;275(35):27354–9.
42. Yu CF, Liu ZX, Cantley LG. ERK negatively regulates the epidermal growth factor-mediated interaction of Gab1 and the phosphatidylinositol 3-kinase. J Biol Chem 2002;277(22):19382–8.
43. Lehr S, Kotzka J, Avci H, et al. Identification of major ERK-related phosphorylation sites in Gab1. Biochemistry 2004;43(38):12133–40.
44. Roux PP, Blenis J. ERK and p38 MAPK-activated protein kinases: a family of protein kinases with diverse biological functions. Microbiol Mol Biol Rev 2004; 68(2):320–44.
45. Ma L, Chen Z, Erdjument-Bromage H, et al. Phosphorylation and functional inactivation of TSC2 by Erk implications for tuberous sclerosis and cancer pathogenesis. Cell 2005;121(2):179–93.
46. Huang CH, Mandelker D, Schmidt-Kittler O, et al. The structure of a human p110alpha/p85alpha complex elucidates the effects of oncogenic PI3Kalpha mutations. Science 2007;318(5857):1744–8.
47. Gschwind A, Fischer OM, Ullrich A. The discovery of receptor tyrosine kinases: targets for cancer therapy. Nat Rev Cancer 2004;4(5):361–70.
48. Chiang GG, Abraham RT. Targeting the mTOR signaling network in cancer. Trends Mol Med 2007;13(10):433–42.
49. Keniry M, Parsons R. The role of PTEN signaling perturbations in cancer and in targeted therapy. Oncogene 2008;27(41):5477–85.
50. Bonneau D, Longy M. Mutations of the human PTEN gene. Hum Mutat 2000; 16(2):109–22.
51. Faivre S, Kroemer G, Raymond E. Current development of mTOR inhibitors as anticancer agents. Nat Rev Drug Discov 2006;5(8):671–88.

52. Drakos E, Atsaves V, Li J, et al. Stabilization and activation of p53 downregulates mTOR signaling through AMPK in mantle cell lymphoma. Leukemia 2009;23(4): 784–90.

53. Nardella C, Chen Z, Salmena L, et al. Aberrant Rheb-mediated mTORC1 activation and Pten haploinsufficiency are cooperative oncogenic events. Genes Dev 2008;22(16):2172–7.

54. Roux PP, Ballif BA, Anjum R, et al. Tumor-promoting phorbol esters and activated Ras inactivate the tuberous sclerosis tumor suppressor complex via p90 ribosomal S6 kinase. Proc Natl Acad Sci U S A 2004;101(37):13489–94.

55. Zagorska A, Dulak J. HIF-1: the knowns and unknowns of hypoxia sensing. Acta Biochim Pol 2004;51(3):563–85.

56. Ballou LM, Lin RZ. Rapamycin and mTOR kinase inhibitors. J Chem Biol 2008; 1(1–4):27–36.

57. Jemal A, Siegel R, Xu J, et al. Cancer statistics, 2010. CA Cancer J Clin 2010; 60(5):277–300.

58. Motzer RJ, Agarwal N, Beard C, et al. Kidney cancer. J Natl Compr Canc Netw 2011;9(9):960–77.

59. McDermott DF, Regan MM, Clark JI, et al. Randomized phase III trial of high-dose interleukin-2 versus subcutaneous interleukin-2 and interferon in patients with metastatic renal cell carcinoma. J Clin Oncol 2005;23(1):133–41.

60. Motzer RJ, Hutson TE, Tomczak P, et al. Overall survival and updated results for sunitinib compared with interferon alfa in patients with metastatic renal cell carcinoma. J Clin Oncol 2009;27(22):3584–90.

61. Escudier B, Eisen T, Stadler WM, et al. Sorafenib for treatment of renal cell carcinoma: final efficacy and safety results of the phase III treatment approaches in renal cancer global evaluation trial. J Clin Oncol 2009;27(20):3312–8.

62. Escudier B, Bellmunt J, Negrier S, et al. Phase III trial of bevacizumab plus interferon alfa-2a in patients with metastatic renal cell carcinoma (AVOREN): final analysis of overall survival. J Clin Oncol 2010;28(13):2144–50.

63. Motzer RJ, Mazumdar M, Bacik J, et al. Survival and prognostic stratification of 670 patients with advanced renal cell carcinoma. J Clin Oncol 1999;17(8): 2530–40.

64. Atkins MB, Hidalgo M, Stadler WM, et al. Randomized phase II study of multiple dose levels of CCI-779, a novel mammalian target of rapamycin kinase inhibitor, in patients with advanced refractory renal cell carcinoma. J Clin Oncol 2004; 22(5):909–18.

65. Hudes G, Carducci M, Tomczak P, et al. Temsirolimus, interferon alfa, or both for advanced renal-cell carcinoma. N Engl J Med 2007;356(22):2271–81.

66. Motzer RJ, Escudier B, Oudard S, et al. Efficacy of everolimus in advanced renal cell carcinoma: a double-blind, randomised, placebo-controlled phase III trial. Lancet 2008;372(9637):449–56.

67. Kay A, Motzer R, Figlin R, et al. Updated data from a phase III randomized trial of everolimus (RAD001) versus PBO in metastatic renal cell carcinoma (mRCC) [abstract 278]. Presented at the American Society of Clinical Oncology 2009 Genitourinary Cancers Symposium. Orlando (FL), February 26–28, 2009.

68. Yao JC, Hassan M, Phan A, et al. One hundred years after "carcinoid": epidemiology of and prognostic factors for neuroendocrine tumors in 35,825 cases in the United States. J Clin Oncol 2008;26(18):3063–72.

69. Zhou J, Enewold L, Stojadinovic A, et al. Incidence rates of exocrine and endocrine pancreatic cancers in the United States. Cancer Causes Control 2010; 21(6):853–61.

70. Yao JC, Shah MH, Ito T, et al. Everolimus for advanced pancreatic neuroendocrine tumors. N Engl J Med 2011;364(6):514–23.

71. Pavel ME, Hainsworth JD, Baudin E, et al. Everolimus plus octreotide long-acting repeatable for the treatment of advanced neuroendocrine tumours associated with carcinoid syndrome (RADIANT-2): a randomised, placebo-controlled, phase 3 study. Lancet 2011;378(9808):2005–12.

72. Krueger DA, Franz DN. Current management of tuberous sclerosis complex. Paediatr Drugs 2008;10(5):299–313.

73. Krueger DA, Care MM, Holland K, et al. Everolimus for subependymal giant-cell astrocytomas in tuberous sclerosis. N Engl J Med 2010;363(19):1801–11.

74. Sakai A, Thieblemont C, Wellmann A, et al. PTEN gene alterations in lymphoid neoplasms. Blood 1998;92(9):3410–5.

75. Zheng B, Fiumara P, Li YV, et al. MEK/ERK pathway is aberrantly active in Hodgkin disease: a signaling pathway shared by CD30, CD40, and RANK that regulates cell proliferation and survival. Blood 2003;102(3):1019–27.

76. Isaacson TV, Smith LB, Tripp S, et al. Expression of mTOR pathway proteins in malignant lymphoma. Lab Invest 2007;87:246a.

77. Bertoni F, Zucca E, Cotter FE. Molecular basis of mantle cell lymphoma. Br J Haematol 2004;124(2):130–40.

78. Witzig TE, Geyer SM, Ghobrial I, et al. Phase II trial of single-agent temsirolimus (CCI-779) for relapsed mantle cell lymphoma. J Clin Oncol 2005;23(23):5347–56.

79. Ansell SM, Inwards DJ, Rowland KM Jr, et al. Low-dose, single-agent temsirolimus for relapsed mantle cell lymphoma: a phase 2 trial in the North Central Cancer Treatment Group. Cancer 2008;113(3):508–14.

80. Hess G, Herbrecht R, Romaguera J, et al. Phase III study to evaluate temsirolimus compared with investigator's choice therapy for the treatment of relapsed or refractory mantle cell lymphoma. J Clin Oncol 2009;27(23):3822–9.

81. Zelenetz AD, Abramson JS, Advani RH, et al. NCCN Clinical Practice Guidelines in Oncology: non-Hodgkin's lymphomas. J Natl Compr Canc Netw 2010;8(3):288–334.

82. Smith SM, van Besien K, Karrison T, et al. Temsirolimus has activity in non-mantle cell non-Hodgkin's lymphoma subtypes: the University of Chicago phase II consortium. J Clin Oncol 2010;28(31):4740–6.

83. Rizzieri DA, Feldman E, Dipersio JF, et al. A phase 2 clinical trial of deforolimus (AP23573, MK-8669), a novel mammalian target of rapamycin inhibitor, in patients with relapsed or refractory hematologic malignancies. Clin Cancer Res 2008;14(9):2756–62.

84. Tobinai K, Ogura M, Maruyama D, et al. Phase I study of the oral mammalian target of rapamycin inhibitor everolimus (RAD001) in Japanese patients with relapsed or refractory non-Hodgkin lymphoma. Int J Hematol 2010;92(4):563–70.

85. Witzig TE, Reeder CB, LaPlant BR, et al. A phase II trial of the oral mTOR inhibitor everolimus in relapsed aggressive lymphoma. Leukemia 2011;25(2):341–7.

86. Ghobrial IM, Gertz M, Laplant B, et al. Phase II trial of the oral mammalian target of rapamycin inhibitor everolimus in relapsed or refractory Waldenstrom macroglobulinemia. J Clin Oncol 2010;28(8):1408–14.

87. Schatz JH. Targeting the PI3K/AKT/mTOR pathway in non-Hodgkin's lymphoma: results, biology, and development strategies. Curr Oncol Rep 2011;13(5):398–406.

88. Okuno S, Bailey H, Mahoney MR, et al. A phase 2 study of temsirolimus (CCI-779) in patients with soft tissue sarcomas: a study of the Mayo phase 2 consortium (P2C). Cancer 2011;117(15):3468–75.

89. Chawla SP, Tolcher AW, Staddon AP, et al. Updated results of a phase II trial of AP23573, a novel mTOR inhibitor, in patients (pts) with advanced soft tissue or bone sarcomas. J Clin Oncol 2006;24(Suppl):[abstract: 9505].

90. Chawla SP, Blay J, Ray-Coquard IL, et al. Results of the phase III, placebo-controlled trial (SUCCEED) evaluating the mTOR inhibitor ridaforolimus (R) as maintenance therapy in advanced sarcoma patients (pts) following clinical benefit from prior standard cytotoxic chemotherapy (CT). J Clin Oncol 2011; 29(Suppl):[abstract: 10005].

91. Kurokawa H, Lenferink AE, Simpson JF, et al. Inhibition of HER2/neu (erbB-2) and mitogen-activated protein kinases enhances tamoxifen action against HER2-overexpressing, tamoxifen-resistant breast cancer cells. Cancer Res 2000;60(20):5887–94.

92. Kurokawa H, Arteaga CL. ErbB (HER) receptors can abrogate antiestrogen action in human breast cancer by multiple signaling mechanisms. Clin Cancer Res 2003;9(1 Pt 2):511S–5S.

93. deGraffenried LA, Friedrichs WE, Russell DH, et al. Inhibition of mTOR activity restores tamoxifen response in breast cancer cells with aberrant Akt Activity. Clin Cancer Res 2004;10(23):8059–67.

94. Carpenter JT, Roche H, Campone M, et al. Randomized 3-arm, phase 2 study of temsirolimus (CCI-779) in combination with letrozole in postmenopausal women with locally advanced or metastatic breast cancer. J Clin Oncol 2005;23(Suppl): [abstract: 564].

95. Chow LW, SunY, Jassem J, et al. Phase 3 study of temsirolimus with letrozole or letrozole alone in postmenopausal women with locally advanced or metastatic breast cancer [abstract 6091]. 2006 Annual San Antonio Breast cancer Symposium. San Antonio (TX), December 14–17, 2006.

96. Ellard SL, Clemons M, Gelmon KA, et al. Randomized phase II study comparing two schedules of everolimus in patients with recurrent/metastatic breast cancer: NCIC Clinical Trials Group IND.163. J Clin Oncol 2009;27(27): 4536–41.

97. Baselga J, Semiglazov V, van Dam P, et al. Phase II randomized study of neoadjuvant everolimus plus letrozole compared with placebo plus letrozole in patients with estrogen receptor-positive breast cancer. J Clin Oncol 2009; 27(16):2630–7.

98. Pandya KJ, Dahlberg S, Hidalgo M, et al. A randomized, phase II trial of two dose levels of temsirolimus (CCI-779) in patients with extensive-stage small-cell lung cancer who have responding or stable disease after induction chemotherapy: a trial of the Eastern Cooperative Oncology Group (E1500). J Thorac Oncol 2007;2(11):1036–41.

99. Tarhini A, Kotsakis A, Gooding W, et al. Phase II study of everolimus (RAD001) in previously treated small cell lung cancer. Clin Cancer Res 2010;16(23): 5900–7.

100. Soria JC, Shepherd FA, Douillard JY, et al. Efficacy of everolimus (RAD001) in patients with advanced NSCLC previously treated with chemotherapy alone or with chemotherapy and EGFR inhibitors. Ann Oncol 2009;20(10):1674–81.

101. Lang SA, Gaumann A, Koehl GE, et al. Mammalian target of rapamycin is activated in human gastric cancer and serves as a target for therapy in an experimental model. Int J Cancer 2007;120(8):1803–10.

102. Yu G, Wang J, Chen Y, et al. Overexpression of phosphorylated mammalian target of rapamycin predicts lymph node metastasis and prognosis of chinese patients with gastric cancer. Clin Cancer Res 2009;15(5):1821–9.

103. An JY, Kim KM, Choi MG, et al. Prognostic role of p-mTOR expression in cancer tissues and metastatic lymph nodes in pT2b gastric cancer. Int J Cancer 2010; 126(12):2904–13.

104. Doi T, Muro K, Boku N, et al. Multicenter phase II study of everolimus in patients with previously treated metastatic gastric cancer. J Clin Oncol 2010;28(11): 1904–10.

105. Yoon D, Park Y, Lee H, et al. Phase II study of everolimus in patients with advanced gastric cancer refractory to chemotherapy including fluoropyrimidine and platinum. J Clin Oncol 2011;29(Suppl 4):[abstract: 93].

106. Slomovitz BM, Wu W, Broaddus RR, et al. mTOR inhibition is a rational target for the treatment of endometrial cancer. J Clin Oncol 2004;22(Suppl):[abstract: 5076].

107. Salvesen HB, Carter SL, Mannelqvist M, et al. Integrated genomic profiling of endometrial carcinoma associates aggressive tumors with indicators of PI3 kinase activation. Proc Natl Acad Sci U S A 2009;106(12):4834–9.

108. Slomovitz BM, Lu KH, Johnston T, et al. A phase 2 study of the oral mammalian target of rapamycin inhibitor, everolimus, in patients with recurrent endometrial carcinoma. Cancer 2010;116(23):5415–9.

109. Oza AM, Elit L, Tsao MS, et al. Phase II study of temsirolimus in women with recurrent or metastatic endometrial cancer: a trial of the NCIC Clinical Trials Group. J Clin Oncol 2011;29(24):3278–85.

110. Mulholland DJ, Dedhar S, Wu H, et al. PTEN and GSK3beta: key regulators of progression to androgen-independent prostate cancer. Oncogene 2006;25(3): 329–37.

111. Sircar K, Yoshimoto M, Monzon FA, et al. PTEN genomic deletion is associated with p-Akt and AR signalling in poorer outcome, hormone refractory prostate cancer. J Pathol 2009;218(4):505–13.

112. Bertram J, Peacock JW, Fazli L, et al. Loss of PTEN is associated with progression to androgen independence. Prostate 2006;66(9):895–902.

113. Lin HK, Hu YC, Lee DK, et al. Regulation of androgen receptor signaling by PTEN (phosphatase and tensin homolog deleted on chromosome 10) tumor suppressor through distinct mechanisms in prostate cancer cells. Mol Endocrinol 2004;18(10):2409–23.

114. Pienta KJ, Bradley D. Mechanisms underlying the development of androgen-independent prostate cancer. Clin Cancer Res 2006;12(6):1665–71.

115. Xu Y, Chen SY, Ross KN, et al. Androgens induce prostate cancer cell proliferation through mammalian target of rapamycin activation and post-transcriptional increases in cyclin D proteins. Cancer Res 2006;66(15):7783–92.

116. Cinar B, De Benedetti A, Freeman MR. Post-transcriptional regulation of the androgen receptor by Mammalian target of rapamycin. Cancer Res 2005; 65(7):2547–53.

117. Wang Y, Mikhailova M, Bose S. Regulation of androgen receptor transcriptional activity by rapamycin in prostate cancer cell proliferation and survival. Oncogene 2008;27(56):7106–17.

118. Pan C, Ghosh P, Lara P Jr, et al. Encouraging activity of bicalutamide and everolimus in castration-resistant prostate cancer (CRPC): Early results from a phase II clinical trial. J Clin Oncol 2011;29(Suppl 7):[abstract: 157].

119. André F, Hurvitz SA, Vittori L, et al. Multicenter phase I clinical trial of daily and weekly RAD001 in combination with weekly paclitaxel and trastuzumab in

patients with HER2-overexpressing metastatic breast cancer with prior resistance to trastuzumab. J Clin Oncol 2008;26(Suppl):[abstract: 1003].

120. Morrow PK, Wulf GM, Ensor J, et al. Phase I/II study of trastuzumab in combination with everolimus (RAD001) in patients with HER2-overexpressing metastatic breast cancer who progressed on trastuzumab-based therapy. J Clin Oncol 2011;29(23):3126–32.

121. Kreisl TN, Lassman AB, Mischel PS, et al. A pilot study of everolimus and gefitinib in the treatment of recurrent glioblastoma (GBM). J Neurooncol 2009;92(1): 99–105.

122. Milton DT, Riely GJ, Azzoli CG, et al. Phase 1 trial of everolimus and gefitinib in patients with advanced nonsmall-cell lung cancer. Cancer 2007;110(3): 599–605.

123. Quek R, Wang Q, Morgan JA, et al. Combination mTOR and IGF-1R inhibition: phase I trial of everolimus and figitumumab in patients with advanced sarcomas and other solid tumors. Clin Cancer Res 2011;17(4):871–9.

124. Negrier S, Gravis G, Perol D, et al. Temsirolimus and bevacizumab, or sunitinib, or interferon alfa and bevacizumab for patients with advanced renal cell carcinoma (TORAVA): a randomised phase 2 trial. Lancet Oncol 2011;12(7): 673–80.

125. Ghobrial IM, Weller E, Vij R, et al. Weekly bortezomib in combination with temsirolimus in relapsed or relapsed and refractory multiple myeloma: a multicentre, phase 1/2, open-label, dose-escalation study. Lancet Oncol 2011;12(3):263–72.

126. Ansell SM, Tang H, Kurtin PJ, et al. Temsirolimus and rituximab in patients with relapsed or refractory mantle cell lymphoma: a phase 2 study. Lancet Oncol 2011;12(4):361–8.

127. Gomez-Pinillos A, Liu X, Ferrari AC. Targeted combinatorial therapy of androgen receptor in androgen-independent prostate cancer cells. J Clin Oncol 2011; 29(Suppl 7):[abstract: 29].

128. Dubrovska A, Elliott J, Salamone RJ, et al. Combination therapy targeting both tumor-initiating and differentiated cell populations in prostate carcinoma. Clin Cancer Res 2010;16(23):5692–702.

129. Yen LC, Uen YH, Wu DC, et al. Activating KRAS mutations and overexpression of epidermal growth factor receptor as independent predictors in metastatic colorectal cancer patients treated with cetuximab. Ann Surg 2010;251(2): 254–60.

130. Lynch TJ, Bell DW, Sordella R, et al. Activating mutations in the epidermal growth factor receptor underlying responsiveness of non-small-cell lung cancer to gefitinib. N Engl J Med 2004;350(21):2129–39.

131. Slamon DJ, Godolphin W, Jones LA, et al. Studies of the HER-2/neu proto-oncogene in human breast and ovarian cancer. Science 1989;244(4905):707–12.

132. Chapuis N, Tamburini J, Cornillet-Lefebvre P, et al. Autocrine IGF-1/IGF-1R signaling is responsible for constitutive PI3K/Akt activation in acute myeloid leukemia: therapeutic value of neutralizing anti-IGF-1R antibody. Haematologica 2010;95(3):415–23.

133. Schips L, Zigeuner R, Ratschek M, et al. Analysis of insulin-like growth factors and insulin-like growth factor I receptor expression in renal cell carcinoma. Am J Clin Pathol 2004;122(6):931–7.

134. Pisters LL, el-Naggar AK, Luo W, et al. C-met proto-oncogene expression in benign and malignant human renal tissues. J Urol 1997;158(3 Pt 1):724–8.

135. Pisters LL, Troncoso P, Zhau HE, et al. c-met proto-oncogene expression in benign and malignant human prostate tissues. J Urol 1995;154(1):293–8.

136. Heinrich MC, Corless CL, Duensing A, et al. PDGFRA activating mutations in gastrointestinal stromal tumors. Science 2003;299(5607):708–10.
137. Carvalho I, Milanezi F, Martins A, et al. Overexpression of platelet-derived growth factor receptor alpha in breast cancer is associated with tumour progression. Breast Cancer Res 2005;7(5):R788–95.
138. Hashim AF, Al-Janabi AA, Mahdi LH, et al. Vascular endothelial growth factor (VEGF) receptor expression correlates with histologic grade and stage of colorectal cancer. Libyan J Med 2010;5.
139. Steiner HH, Karcher S, Mueller MM, et al. Autocrine pathways of the vascular endothelial growth factor (VEGF) in glioblastoma multiforme: clinical relevance of radiation-induced increase of VEGF levels. J Neurooncol 2004;66(1–2): 129–38.
140. Suzuki H, Freije D, Nusskern DR, et al. Interfocal heterogeneity of PTEN/MMAC1 gene alterations in multiple metastatic prostate cancer tissues. Cancer Res 1998;58(2):204–9.
141. Yoshimoto M, Cunha IW, Coudry RA, et al. FISH analysis of 107 prostate cancers shows that PTEN genomic deletion is associated with poor clinical outcome. Br J Cancer 2007;97(5):678–85.
142. Bachman KE, Argani P, Samuels Y, et al. The PIK3CA gene is mutated with high frequency in human breast cancers. Cancer Biol Ther 2004;3(8):772–5.
143. Frattini M, Signoroni S, Pilotti S, et al. Phosphatase protein homologue to tensin expression and phosphatidylinositol-3 phosphate kinase mutations in colorectal cancer. Cancer Res 2005;65(23):11227.
144. Samuels Y, Wang Z, Bardelli A, et al. High frequency of mutations of the PIK3CA gene in human cancers. Science 2004;304(5670):554.
145. Edwards J, Krishna NS, Witton CJ, et al. Gene amplifications associated with the development of hormone-resistant prostate cancer. Clin Cancer Res 2003;9(14): 5271–81.
146. Gallou C, Joly D, Mejean A, et al. Mutations of the VHL gene in sporadic renal cell carcinoma: definition of a risk factor for VHL patients to develop an RCC. Hum Mutat 1999;13(6):464–75.
147. Karapetis CS, Khambata-Ford S, Jonker DJ, et al. K-ras mutations and benefit from cetuximab in advanced colorectal cancer. N Engl J Med 2008;359(17): 1757–65.
148. Laghi L, Orbetegli O, Bianchi P, et al. Common occurrence of multiple K-RAS mutations in pancreatic cancers with associated precursor lesions and in biliary cancers. Oncogene 2002;21(27):4301–6.
149. Zent CS, LaPlant BR, Johnston PB, et al. The treatment of recurrent/refractory chronic lymphocytic leukemia/small lymphocytic lymphoma (CLL) with everolimus results in clinical responses and mobilization of CLL cells into the circulation. Cancer 2010;116(9):2201–7.

Topoisomerase 1 Inhibitors and Cancer Therapy

Julia Moukharskaya, MD, Claire Verschraegen, MD*

KEYWORDS

- Topoisomerase 1 • Ovarian cancer • Irinotecan • Topotecan

KEY POINTS

- Topoisomerase 1 inhibitors cure human cancer xenografts in animal models, more so than most other chemotherapy agents. However, their activity in patients with cancer is modest.
- Ongoing research is studying the optimal analogs that could reproduce animal data in the cancer population.
- This article analyzes the clinical research with topoisomerase 1 inhibitors in ovarian cancer.

The first type I topoisomerase (Top1) inhibitors were found in the wood bark of *Camptotheca acuminata*, an oriental tree, the powder or injectable extracts of which have been used in traditional Chinese medicine.[1] The class was named camptothecin (CPT) for the basic CPT compound (**Fig. 1**). Clinical studies of this group of drugs were initiated in the 1970s, and in the 1980s the Top1 enzyme was identified as the cellular target of CPT.[2,3]

Topoisomerases relax the DNA supercoiling and perform catalytic functions during replication and transcription.[4] There are two classes of topoisomerases. Type I enzymes cleave one strand of DNA and type II cleave both strands. Six topoisomerase genes have been identified in mammalian somatic cells within these two classes. Type IA enzymes consist of Top3 α and Top3 β; type IB consist of Top1 and Top1mt (mitochondrial); and type IIA consist of Top2 α and Top2 β. CPT is an inhibitor of Top1. Top1 cleaves the DNA phosphodiester backbone, nicking one strand of the DNA duplex and forming a Top1-DNA reversible cleavage complex by covalent bonding of a tyrosine residue. Single-strand breaks induced by Top1 help untangle excessive DNA supercoils during DNA replication and transcription (**Fig. 2**).[5,6] Top1 is essential for survival.

Department of Medicine, Vermont Cancer Center, 89 Beaumont Avenue, Given 214, Burlington, VT 05405, USA
* Corresponding author.
E-mail address: Claire.Verschraegen@vtmednet.org

Hematol Oncol Clin N Am 26 (2012) 507–525
doi:10.1016/j.hoc.2012.03.002
0889-8588/12/$ – see front matter © 2012 Elsevier Inc. All rights reserved.

1: R = H, Camptothecin (Lactone)   **3: R = H, Camptothecin (Carboxylate)**

Fig. 1. Camptothecin lactone – carboxylate equilibrium.

Mouse embryos lacking Top1 die before the tenth cell division. There are no known wild Top1 mutants. The only mutants detected were in vitro manipulations of cell lines.[7] However, compared with Top1 found in normal tissues, a significant increase of the enzyme was detected in surgical specimens of colon adenocarcinoma; several types of non-Hodgkin's lymphoma; specimens of leukemia; carcinoma of the stomach, breast, and lung; and malignant melanoma.[8]

Top1 inhibitors work by stabilizing the Top1 cleavage complexes, leading to DNA damage, because the DNA cannot repair itself.[9,10] The cytotoxicity of Top1 inhibitors is caused by the paralyzing of Top1 cleavage complexes (where CPT interferes with the Top1/DNA complex by binding to Top1) rather than by the inhibition of Top1 catalytic activity (see **Fig. 2**).[11] Because malignant cells often contain greater amounts of Top1 than normal cells, they should be more sensitive to the toxic effects of the CPT. Binding of CPT to the DNA-topoisomerase complex is reversible and dependent on the chemical structure of CPT. For maximal inhibitory activity, the cleavage complex needs to be maintained.[12] In an acidic milieu, CPT is in lactone form, and in more basic milieu, the equilibrium shifts toward a carboxylate form (see **Fig. 1**). The lactone form is the active form of the drug and the carboxylate form lacks the ability to stabilize the cleavage complex.[13,14] At the physiologic pH of the human serum, the equilibrium between lactone and carboxylate is in favor of the latter, with the area under the curve (AUC) of the lactone form being below 16%.[15] Additionally, most semisynthetic analogs are poorly water soluble. Two analogs designed to be soluble, irinotecan (CPT-11)[16] and topotecan (NSC 609699),[17] were then synthesized and are currently widely used in clinical practice.

Despite the proved anticancer activity of irinotecan and topotecan, there are major limitations. First, these CPTs are not very active as single agent, with a 10% to 15% response rate in specific cancer indications. They are certainly not curative, despite the potential for inhibiting one of the most crucial enzymes of DNA replication. Both

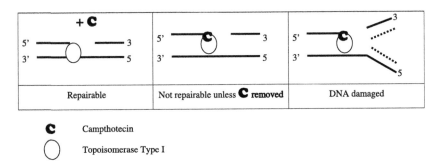

| Repairable | Not repairable unless **C** removed | DNA damaged |

C   Campthotecin

⬭   Topoisomerase Type I

Ⓒ   Cleavage complex

Fig. 2. Mechanism of camptothecin action.

drugs are inactivated within minutes at physiologic pH by lactone ring opening.[5] The E ring–opened carboxylate form has less than 10% potency of the lactone form. Second, the intracellular concentration is reduced by the efflux pumps, although these drugs freely enter the cells by passive diffusion.[18] To overcome these limitations, new CPT derivatives have been developed. In animal models, some of the new analogs are proved more active than irinotecan or topotecan, and a few are even curative of xenograft models instead of simply delaying tumor growth, which is usually the most common observation of anticancer agent activity in animal models. However, when tested in clinical studies none of these newer compounds is better than irinotecan or topotecan. Therefore, we hypothesize that there is either a specific human pharmacodynamics issue that is not understood, or a species response that prevents the replication of animal data in humans. Human blood stabilities of several CPT analogs indicated that serum albumin plays a dual role in the CPT pharmacokinetics. In the case of water-insoluble CPTs, human albumin acts as a sink for carboxylate drug form, binding the carboxylate species and thereby shifting the lactone-carboxylate equilibrium to the right, thus decreasing the potential activity of such CPTs. In the cases of water-soluble CPTs (topotecan, CPT-11), no such preferential binding of the carboxylate drug form by human serum albumin was observed. This might only in part explain the differences seen between human and mouse observed antitumor activity.[19,20]

IRINOTECAN
Activity and Metabolism

Irinotecan is chemically unique because of the presence of a bulky side chain on the core five-ring structure, which has to be cleaved for the drug to become pharmacologically active (**Fig. 3**). The active metabolite of irinotecan is SN-38. As with all CPTs, the carboxylate form is inactive and the lactone ring is the active form, accounting for approximately 60% to 70% of total plasma SN-38 after the end of irinotecan infusion.[21] The conversion of the lactone into the carboxylate form of irinotecan is rapid, with a mean half-life of the lactone form of 9.5 minutes.[22] The volume of distribution of irinotecan at steady state is large, suggesting extensive tissue distribution, and remains unchanged with increasing doses.[23]

The conversion of irinotecan to SN-38 is an enzyme-catalyzed reaction and liver carboxylesterases (CE; CE-1 and CE-2) are most likely responsible for this conversion. CE-2 plays the most important role in patients with cancer.[21] Because tumors have higher concentrations of CE enzymes compared with normal tissue, the activation of this enzyme may account for the irinotecan activity being higher in specific types of tumors compared with normal tissue.[24] SN-38 itself is further metabolized in human liver by uridine diphosphate glycoronosyltranferase 1A1 (UGT1A1) to an inactive compound, SN-38G (see **Fig. 1**). SN-38G concentrations are proportional to the dose of irinotecan, suggesting that hepatic glucuronidation is not saturated in the dose range studied, up to 600 mg/m^2.[21,25] Unlike hepatocytes, other cells in the body have no way of detoxifying SN-38 through glucuronidation, thus contributing to its high toxicity. The activity of UGT1A1 varies among different individuals. For example, in patients with Crigler-Najjar type I syndrome, UGT1A1 activity is totally lacking.[21] The UGT1A1*28 (a 7-TA repeat sequence in the promoter region) genotype is a significant risk factor for severe toxicity by irinotecan, with odds ratio of 7.23.[26] In 2005, the Food and Drug Administration recommended that treatment with irinotecan be altered for individuals with the UGT1A1*28 allele. Because the positive predictive value of the test is only 0.5 and no clear recommendation for dose reduction exists,

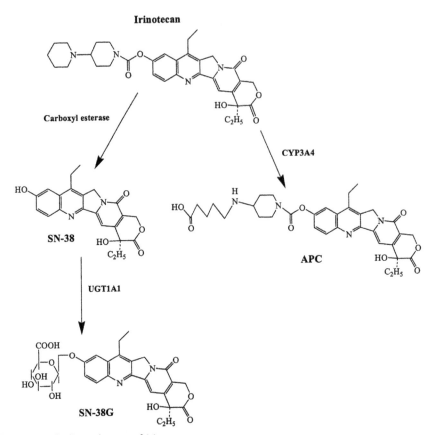

Fig. 3. Metabolic pathways of irinotecan.

it is not practical to use UGT1A1 genotyping.[27] A meta-analysis of nine studies including a total of 821 patients revealed a dose relationship between irinotecan and risk of hematologic toxic effects in patients with the *UGT1A1*28* genotype.[28] Thus, genotype-based decisions should be performed if higher doses of irinotecan (>250 mg/m^2) are administered, but at low doses the risk of increased toxicity is not defined by this genotype. CYP3A also metabolizes irinotecan into carbonyloxycamp-tothecin (APC), a metabolite with little cytotoxic activity (see **Fig. 3**). CYP3A pathway is inhibited by many drugs[21] (eg, ketoconazole, loperamide, and ondansetron), thus influencing the concentration of circulating irinotecan. Irinotecan is excreted by the kidney (11%–20%) and the liver (25%–50%). The excretion occurs in the first 24 hours after infusion, with almost complete excretion within 48 hours.[21] When SN-38G is excreted through the bile into the intestines several bacteria, including *Escherichia coli*, *Bacteroides* spp, and *Clostridium perfringens*, can convert the compound back to the active metabolite SN-38 by producing the enzyme β-glucuronidase,[29] poten-tially leading to late-onset intestinal toxicity (diarrhea). Diarrhea, one of the most common side effects of irinotecan, is associated with SN-38 exposure within the intes-tinal lumen. Myelosuppression, the second most common side effect of irinotecan, is related to plasma SN-38 exposure.[30]

Administration and Adverse Events

Irinotecan is administered intravenously over 90 minutes with a premedication consisting of atropine 0.25 mg subcutaneously or intravenously to prevent acute cholinergic reactions and a steroid with a serotonin 5-HT3 receptor antagonist to prevent emesis. The patient must be warned about the risk of diarrhea and instructed to take loperamide, 2 mg orally, after each liquid stools. If the diarrhea cannot be controlled within 24 hours, patients must return for intravenous hydration. Prolonged infusion might theoretically improve the efficacy by maintaining inhibition of the cleavage complex, but is not used clinically (**Table 1**).[31]

The newest use of irinotecan is for first-line pancreatic cancer in combination with oxaliplatin, 5-fluorouracil, and folinic acid (FOLFIRINOX). In the randomized study of this regimen compared with gemcitabine, the median overall survival of patients with chemotherapy-naive metastatic pancreatic cancer was 11.1 months compared with 6.8 months in the control group (hazard ratio for death, 0.57; 95% confidence interval, 0.45–0.73; $P<.001$). Median progression-free survival was doubled (hazard ratio for disease progression, 0.47; 95% confidence interval, 0.37–0.59; $P<.001$), and objective response rate was tripled ($P<.001$). The FOLFIRINOX was more toxic, but length of adequate quality of life was doubled.[40]

TOPOTECAN

Topotecan was synthesized in the 1980s as a hydrosoluble semisynthetic derivative of CPT, with a cytotoxic activity similar to the parent compound but a better toxicity profile. Topotecan is a 10-hydroxy camptothecin with a positively charged dimethylaminomethyl group at position 9.[41]

Activity and Metabolism

Topotecan, contrarily to irinotecan, is only metabolized to a minor extent. Topotecan undergoes a CYP3A catalyzed metabolism whereby N-desmethyl topotecan, a slightly less active agent, is irreversibly formed.[42] Only low levels of this metabolite have been found in plasma. Both compounds exist in an active lactone and inactive carboxylate form (see **Fig. 1**), but at equilibrium, a minor amount of total topotecan is present in the lactone form. Topotecan and N-desmethyl topotecan may undergo further metabolism to an UGT-mediated glucuronide product, but this transformation is reversible.[43] The kidneys are the most important route of excretion of the drug; hence, renal failure affects the clearance of the drug.

Topotecan has a high volume of distribution, indicating a good tissue penetration. Furthermore, topotecan has a good penetration in cerebrospinal fluid: about 1 hour after the administration, more than 50% of active drug is present in the cerebrospinal fluid. The elimination from cerebrospinal fluid follows a timing curve equivalent to that of elimination from plasma.[44,45] The fact that the blood–brain barrier is permeable to topotecan led to a series of studies where topotecan was used in patients with brain metastases with or without whole-brain radiation, with short-lasting objective response rates ranging from less than 10% to approximately 50% in patients with various solid tumors.[46]

Topotecan can be used in oral and intravenous formulations, which demonstrated similar efficacy in relapsed small-cell lung cancer.[47]

Administration and Adverse Events

Topotecan is administered as a 30-minute infusion every day for 5 days, every 3 weeks. Unfortunately, this schedule of administration is not very practical, and

Table 1
Current clinical use of irinotecan

Tumor Type	Indications	Food and Drug Administration Approval/ Strength of Recommendation[a]	References
Metastatic colorectal cancer	First-line therapy, in combination with 5-fluorouracil and folinic acid	Yes	32
	Second-line therapy, single agent after initial 5-fluorouracil-based therapy	Yes	33,34
Carcinoma of esophagus	Nonsurgical	No/Class IIA	35
Extensive stage small-cell lung cancer	First-line treatment, in combination with cisplatin	No/Class IIA	36
Acute lymphoid leukemia	Refractory	No/Class IIB	37
Acute myeloid leukemia	Refractory	No/Class IIB	37
Carcinoma of cervix	Refractory	No/Class IIB	38
Extensive stage small-cell lung cancer	First-line treatment, in combination with carboplatin	No/Class IIB	39
Gastric cancer	Refractory	No/Class IIB	37
Malignant glioma of brain	Recurrent or progressive disease	No/Class IIB	37
Metastatic breast cancer	Refractory	No/Class IIB	37
Non-Hodgkin's lymphoma	Refractory	No/Class IIB	37
Non-small cell lung cancer	Refractory	No/Class IIB	37
Ovarian cancer	Platinum-refractory or platinum-resistant	No/Class IIB	37
Pancreatic cancer	First-line therapy, in combination with oxaliplatin, 5-fluorouracil, and folinic acid	No/Class IIA	40

[a] Micromedex 2.0. Strength of recommendation definitions. In Edition 2011. Ann Arbor (MI): Thomson Reuters; 2011.

alternate schedules are being explored, such as 3 consecutive days or weekly in ovarian and recurrent small-cell lung cancer.[48–50]

The hematopoietic system is the most susceptible organ. Neutropenia, thrombocytopenia, and anemia are the most significant treatment-related toxicity. Gastrointestinal toxicity mainly manifests as nausea. No significant toxic effects have been observed in other organs, such as heart, lungs, liver, kidneys, bladder, and central nervous system (**Table 2**).[51]

CURRENT QUESTIONS AND FUTURE DIRECTIONS

Despite the widespread clinical uses of irinotecan and topotecan, many questions remain. An interesting hypothesis was the modulation of topoisomerase activities with various inhibitors of Top1 and Top2. Preclinical models suggest synergy when Top1 and Top2 inhibitors are given sequentially, but not simultaneously. Alternating the sequences of these inhibitors has been tried, with mitigated success. In a phase I study of 19 patients with previously treated ovarian or peritoneal carcinoma, sequential oral topotecan at 0.8 $mg/m^2/d$ for 5 days then oral etoposide at 50 $mg/m^2/d$ for another 5 days were administered as the starting dose. Dose escalation consisted of daily schedule intensification, but the adverse events were too pronounced. The main dose-limiting toxicity was neutropenia.[58] This trial and other alternating regimen studies reported a 20% to 30% activity in patients with ovarian cancer, without prolongation of disease-free progression.

Thus, improvements in CPT pharmacodynamics effects and anticancer effectiveness are needed. Reversal of drug resistance and reduction of toxicity would also be clinically beneficial. Therefore, new formulations and new analogs are being tested to achieve these goals.

New Formulations

To reduce toxicity, improve bioavailability, increase drug solubility, and enhance targeting to Top1, changes in formulation are being tested (**Fig. 4**). Several conjugates have entered clinical trials (**Table 3**).

CRLX101

For CRLX101 (formerly named IT-101), a cyclodextrin–polyethylene glycol (PEG) copolymer CPT conjugate (Cerulean Pharma, Cambridge, MA) is linked to a hydrophilic cyclodextrin-based linear polymer through ester bonds (see **Fig. 4**). This polymer conjugates with high molecular weights (3400 kDa) have shown significant antitumor effects against human colon carcinoma xenografts and irinotecan-resistant tumors. At equivalent doses, plasma concentrations and AUC are approximately 100-fold higher for CRLX10 than for CPT. The plasma half-life ranges from 17 to 20 hours and is significantly longer than that of CPT alone (1.3 hours). Tumor concentrations of active CPT released from the CRLX10 are about 160-fold higher when administered as a polymer conjugate than as CPT alone.[59] CRLX10 is currently tested in refractory non–small cell lung cancer (NCT01380769).

MAG-CPT

MAG-PT is a soluble N-(2-hydroxypropyl) methacrylamide (HPMA)-CPT conjugate (mureletecan; Pharmacia and Upjohn, Milan, Italy). HPMA copolymers are synthesized and covalently linked to CPT at the α-hydroxyl group through a Gly-Phe-Leu-Gly spacer. Active CPT is then released by elastase and cysteine-proteases. Although hydrolysis in plasma is minimal, retention of the conjugate in tumor leads to greater

Table 2
Current clinical use of topotecan

Tumor Type	Indications	Food and Drug Administration Approval/Strength of Recommendation[a]	References
Carcinoma of cervix	Stage IVB, recurrent, or persistent, in combination with cisplatin	Yes	52
Carcinoma of cervix	Advanced, recurrent, or persistent; as monotherapy in patients not amenable to curative treatment with surgery or radiotherapy	No/Class IIB	54
Ovarian cancer	Metastatic after failure of initial or subsequent chemotherapy	Yes	51
Small-cell carcinoma of lung	After failure of first-line therapy	Yes	53
Chronic myelomonocytic leukemia	Refractory	No/Class IIB	55
Myelodysplastic syndrome	Refractory	No/Class IIB	55
Nephroblastoma	Refractory	No/Class IIB	56
Non–small cell lung cancer	Refractory	No/Class IIB	57

[a] Micromedex 2.0. Strength of recommendation definitions. In Edition 2011. Ann Arbor (MI): Thomson Reuters; 2011.

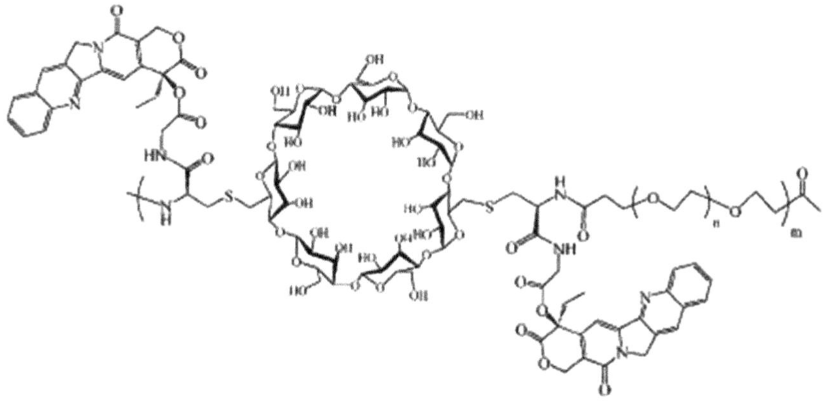

Fig. 4. Structure of IT-101, a conjugate between CPT and a linear cyclodextrin-based polymer. (*From* Schluep T, Hwang J, Cheng J, et al. Preclinical efficacy of the camptothecin-polymer conjugate IT-101 in multiple cancer models. Clin Cancer Res 2006;12:1607; with permission.)

than 90% tumor inhibition with no toxic deaths.[60] There are currently no ongoing clinical trials.

CT-2106

Another conjugate is CT-2106, a poly (L-glutamic acid) CPT conjugate (Cell Therapeutics, Seattle, WA). The linkage stabilizes the active lactone form of CPT and enhances aqueous solubility.[61] There might also be an improved retention effect in tumors. In a phase I study, CT-2106 was administered weekly in 26 patients. The dose-limiting toxicities are thrombocytopenia and fatigue. The maximum tolerated dose is 25 mg/m^2/wk given every 3 of 4 weeks. The pharmacokinetics profile showed a polyexponential decline with similar terminal half-life for conjugated and unconjugated CPT.[64] The drug was also combined with infusional 5-fluorouracil–folinic acid as second line in patients with metastatic colorectal cancer.

Pegamotecan

Pegamotecan, or CPT-di-20-O-ester of PEG (40-kDa) glycine (Gly), a pegylated CPT (also named EZ-246, PEG-beta-CPT, PEG-CPT, or Prothecan; Enzon, Piscataway, NY), was selected among various compounds for its biologic properties. Various amino acid spacers that conjugate CPT with PEG CPT were tested for antitumor activity, rates of hydrolysis, and in vivo efficacy.[65] These included PEG-CPT, PEG-Gly-CPT, PEG-sarcosine-CPT, and PEG-alanine-CPT.[66] The selected compound for phase I studies was PEG-Gly-CPT. It was administered as a 1-hour intravenous infusion every 3 weeks to 37 patients at different dose levels. The recommended dose for

Table 3
CPT conjugates

Name	CPT	Carrier	Linker	References
CRLX101	CPT	Cyclodextrin	Ester bonds	59
MAG-CPT	CPT	N-(2-hydroxypropyl) methacrylamide	Gly-Phe-Leu-Gly spacer	60
CT-2106	CPT	Poly-L-glutamic acid		61
Pegamotecan	CPT	Polyethylene glycol	Gly spacer	62
NKTR-102	Irinotecan	Polyethylene glycol		63

phase II studies is 7000 mg/m^2 as a 1-hour intravenous infusion every 3 weeks. Side effects include myelosuppression, cystitis, nausea, vomiting, and diarrhea. Free CPT accumulated slowly in plasma, with maximal plasma concentrations achieved at 23 ± 12.3 hours; the mean half-life of free CPT was thus prolonged to 77.46 ± 36.77 hours, accounting for a slow release of CPT from the conjugate.[62] In a phase II study of gastric cancer, some activity was observed.[67]

NKTR-102

NKTR-102, an irinotecan polymer conjugate (Nektar Therapeutics, Huntsville, AL, USA), has a reduced peak concentration and a continuous concentration profile with broad antitumor activity. In a phase II trial, patients with platinum-resistant or -refractory ovarian cancer were treated with NKTR-102 at 145 mg/m^2 every 2 or 3 weeks after a two-stage Simon design. Of 71 randomized patients, Response Evaluation Criteria In Solid Tumors (RECIST) responses were noted in 27% and 22% for the 2- and 3-week schedules, respectively. The progression-free survival was 4.4 months. Most common adverse events were diarrhea, dehydration, hypokalemia, fatigue, nausea, and neutropenia. The every-3-week regimen of NKTR-102 is better tolerated. The observed response rate is at the higher range of expected responses for a heavily pretreated population, but progression-free survival is not improved over any other chemotherapy regimen.[63] NKTR-102 is now tested in phase III trial for patients with refractory breast cancer, against physician choice (NCT01492101), and in a randomized phase II trial for second-line colon cancer against irinotecan for patients with KRAS-mutant, metastatic colorectal cancer (NCT00856375).

Reversal of Resistance

ATP-binding cassette subfamily G member 2 (ABCG2) is a protein encoded by the ABCG2 gene. It is a member of ATP-binding cassette transporters and is also called "breast cancer resistance protein" (BCRP). This protein functions as a transporter that might play a role in multidrug resistance to chemotherapeutic agents including anthracyclin and CPT analogs. It plays protective roles in blocking absorption at the apical membrane of the intestine, and at the blood–testis barrier, the blood–brain barrier, and the membranes of hematopoietic progenitor and other stem cells. The intestinal activity is important in the metabolism and enterohepatic cycling of irinotecan. Mao and Unadkat[68] provide a detailed review. Inhibitors of the BCRP transporter have been shown to reverse resistance to topotecan and SN-38 in vitro.[69] To determine the lowest effective dose of elacridar, a BCRP inhibitor, patients were randomized to receive various oral doses of elacridar along with topotecan. The recommended oral dose of topotecan was 2 mg plus 100 mg elacridar.[70] To date, BCRP inhibitors remain experimental.

Another way to revert resistance to chemotherapy is to block repair pathways. Poly(ADP-ribose) polymerases (PARPs) are repair proteins. They constitute a large family of 18 proteins, encoded by different genes but with a conserved catalytic domain. The catalytic activity of PARP-1 and PARP-2 is immediately stimulated by DNA strand breaks.[71] PARP-1 efficiently detects the presence of a single strand break, which leads to a posttranslational modification of histones H1 and H2B leading to chromatin structure relaxation and increased DNA accessibility. Activation of PARP-1 triggers the recruitment of XRCC1, which coordinates the repair process in less than 15 seconds in living cells by stimulating the base excision repair pathway.[72] Inhibitors of PARP are now in clinical trials, with various results. The combination of PARP inhibition with ABT-888 and irinotecan is being tested in one clinical trial for patients with metastatic or unresectable cancer (NCT00576654). In preclinical studies, although PARP inhibition increases the cytotoxicity of irinotecan, it prevents irinotecan-induced intestinal damage.[73,74]

Whether these strategies will be useful to improve the therapeutic index of CPTs remains to be seen.

New CPT Analogs

Some new CPT analogs have improved solubility, better clinical tolerability, and can be administered orally. All derivatives contain at least a pentacyclic ring system of CPT and an intact α-hydroxylactone group in the E ring (**Fig. 5**), which are required for the in vitro and in vivo activity of CPTs.[75] In general, modifications of the A and B ring have been shown to be well tolerated and in many cases enhanced the potency of CPT. Structure-activity relationship studies suggest that substitutions at positions 7, 9, or 10 of most CPT derivatives enhance their antitumor activity, but at positions 5 or 11 usually lead to activity decrease.[76]

Belotecan

Belotecan (Camptobell or CKD602) is a new CPT with a water-solubilizing group introduced at position 7 of the ring B of CPT (see **Fig. 5**). In preclinical studies it demonstrated good water solubility, and higher than CPT Top1-inhibiting activity.[77] Several phase II studies have been conducted demonstrating activity of belotecan in combination with carboplatin in recurrent ovarian cancer, and with cisplatin in extensive small-cell cancer.[77–79] Belotecan is approved in South Korea for treatment of ovarian and small-cell lung cancer.

Gimatecan

Gimatecan (7-t-butoxyiminomethyl-campthotecin) can also be administered orally and is mainly present in plasma as the lactone form (>85%).[80] Gimatecan is efficient in forming stable complexes with DNA and Top1 resulting in a higher number of DNA strand breaks than topotecan and SN38 under the same conditions.[81] Unlike topotecan and SN38 it is not a substrate to efflux pumps.[18] The half-life of gimatecan is 77 ± 29.6 hours, with an AUC raising threefold to sixfold after multiple dosing.[80] The efficacy has been evaluated in a phase II clinical trial, where gimatecan was active in patients with recurrent epithelial ovarian, fallopian tube, or peritoneal cancer, previously treated with platinum and taxanes.[82]

Lurtotecan

Lurtotecan is a water-soluble 7-(4-methylpiperazinomethylene) substituted ethylenedioxy CPT analog (also called GI147211, GG211, GW211, or NX 211). Compared with topotecan, lurtotecan was found to be approximately three times more potent in the cleavage complex assay and three to five times more potent in tumor cell cytotoxicity assays in vitro.[83] Lurtotecan (GI147211, GG211, or GW211) has been administered orally and intravenously, and in a liposomal formulation (NX 211). The liposomal formulation of lurtotecan was compared with the unencapsulated lurtotecan in preclinical models and produced a 1000-fold greater AUC of total lurtotecan and a half-life 5-fold longer. Furthermore, the therapeutic index of single-dose NX 211 in preclinical models was three- to 14-fold greater than that of lurtotecan or topotecan.[84] In clinical study, NX 211 demonstrated some activity in advanced ovarian cancer comparable with that of other Top1 inhibitors, but it is still uncertain whether it has any advantage over topotecan. The dose-limiting side effects of intravenous lurtotecan are neutropenia and thrombocytopenia.[85] The bioavailability of the oral formulation is not very high and showed a large interpatient variation of 11% ± 5% in one of the studies.[86]

Name	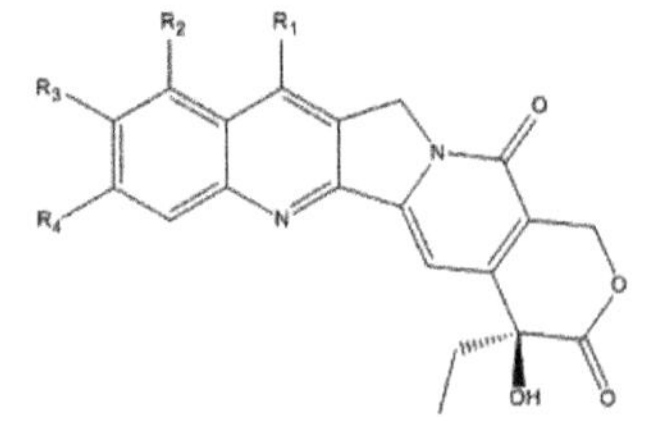			

	R_1 or C7	R_2 or C9	R_3 or C10	R_4 or C11
Camptothecin	H	H	H	H
Topotecan	H	CH₂NH(CH₃)₂	OH	H
Irinotecan	C₂H₅	H	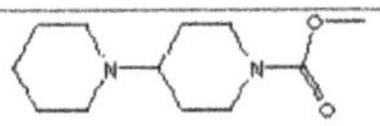 [piperidino-piperidino carbonyloxy group]	H
SN-38	C₂H₅	H	OH	H
Rubitecan	H	NO₂	H	H
Lurtotecan	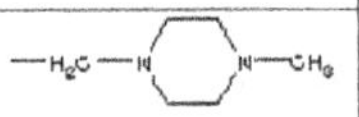 —H₂C—N⌉⌈N—CH₉	H	—OCH₂CH₂O—	H
Belotecan	(CH₂)₂NHCH(CH₃)₂	H	H	H
Silatecan (& Germanium) Analogs	7-t-butyldimethylsilyl CH2CH2Si(CH3)3	H	OH	H
Exatecan	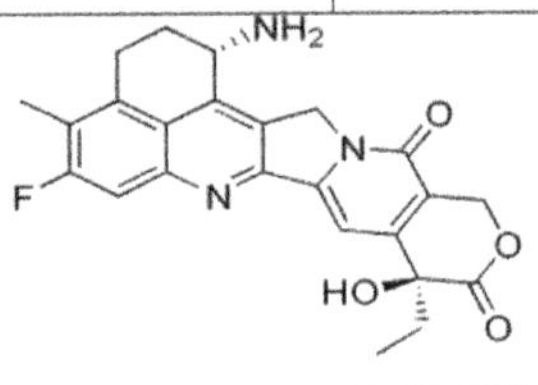 [structure with NH₂, F]		H	H
Homocampto thecin	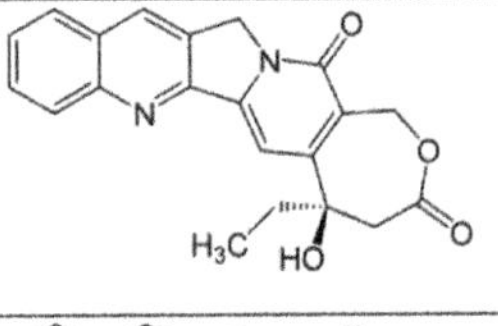 [structure]		H	H
Diflomotecan	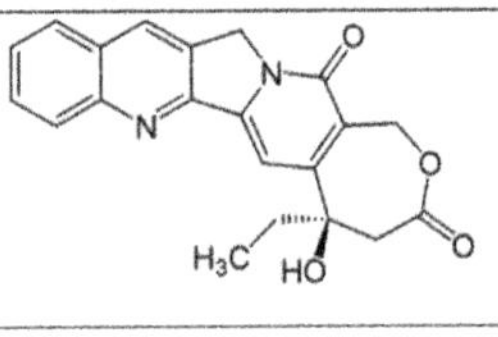 [structure]		F	F

Fig. 5. Chemical structures of camptothecin and analogs that are currently undergoing clinical trials. For examples, irinotecan is a CPT derivative with substitution of the (4-[1-piperidino]-1-piperidino carbonyloxy) group at position 10 of the A ring with an ethyl group at position 7 of the B ring, and topotecan is a 10 hydroxy camptothecin with a positively charged dimethyl-aminomethyl group at position 9. (*Data from* Mi Z, Malak H, Burke TG. Reduced albumin binding promotes the stability and activity of topotecan in human blood. Biochemistry 1995;34:13722–8.)

Rubitecan

Rubitecan (Orathecin) is another water-insoluble CPT analog, which exists in equilibrium as 9-nitro-CPT and 9-amino-CPT, a metabolite that is thought to be active, although it failed to be active when tested in clinical trials.[87] 9-Nitro-CPT has demonstrated significant antitumor activity in vitro and in vivo in human tumor xenograft models, but in clinic was found to be modestly effective against pancreatic cancer and possibly ovarian cancer.[88–90] Administration in patients with pancreatic cancer was associated with mild toxicity, mainly hematologic and gastrointestinal side effects.[87] Rubitecan is an orally available CPT analog that also has potential for delivery transdermally or by inhalation.[15] Because of marginal activity, clinical development has been halted.

Silatecans

Silatecans have a Si or Ge atom in the radical chain in R1 position. They have been tested in early clinical trials but did not show increased benefit over commercially available CPT.[91–93]

More recently, interest greatly increased in hexacyclic derivatives of CPT having an additional six-membered F ring. Several compounds have been synthesized and display an enhanced stability and increased Top1 inhibition and in vitro antitumor activities.[94,95] Another modification of the CPT lactone ring was studied, leading to the synthesis of a synthetic hepta cyclic E-ring, retaining anti-Top1 activity. This family is called homocamptothecin.[96,97]

Exatecan

Exatecan (4-methyl-5-fluoro substituted hexacyclic CPT analog) is water-soluble with significant in vitro antitumor activity.[98] At present, there are no oral formulations of exatecan, but an intravenous formulation demonstrated some clinical activity in pancreatic cancer[99] and metastatic breast carcinoma.[100] In addition, exatecan is not a substrate for the multidrug transporter P-glycoprotein and retains activity against cell lines with P-glycoprotein expression, which may be an advantage against other Top1 inhibitors.[101]

Homocamptothecin and diflomotecan

The stability of homocamptothecin and diflomotecan (heptacyclic E-ring modified analogs) is higher compared with "natural" six-membered α-hydroxylactone ring CPT derivatives, and Top1 cleavable complexes formed in the presence of synthetic E-ring modified analogs are also more stable.[102] Diflomotecan has been tested in clinical trials.[103]

NON-CPT TOP1 INHIBITORS

New Top1 inhibitors of different chemical natures are being explored. Although not a topic for this article, a few are mentioned for completeness. Edotecarin is a derivative of NB-506, an indolocarbazole antitumor agent. This novel inhibitor of Top1 induces single-strand DNA cleavage more effectively than NB-506 or CPT and at different DNA sequences.[104] However, in clinical trials the efficacy of edotecarin was not superior to currently available agents. Indenoisoquinolones, dibenzo naphthyridines, and aromathecins are still in the early stages of clinical development.[105–108]

SUMMARY

Top1 inhibitors belong to a group of drugs that target the Top1 enzyme leading to the stabilization of covalent complexes of DNA strands and Top1, prolonging the cleavage of DNA thereby inducing cell death. Only two Top1 inhibitors, irinotecan and topotecan, are approved by the Food and Drug Administration for use in clinical practice. Belotecan is approved in South Korea. No new analogs demonstrated superior activity in clinical settings, despite promising in vitro and in vivo activity. Newer analogs are still being developed. It is remarkable that such potent inhibitors in the experimental settings are not more active against cancers in the clinical setting. It seems that this class of agent undergoes potent inactivation by diverse mechanisms after administration and that sufficient inhibitory concentrations do not adequately penetrate cancer cells in humans. Innate resistance to CPT has not been demonstrated outside of laboratory systems. Therefore, the problem must either be early inhibition of CPT by mechanisms other than albumin sinking, because new analogs less adsorbed by human albumin are not clinically superior, or inability for CPT to reach the cancer cell targets in vivo. It is hoped that future research will solve this pharmacokinetics mystery.

REFERENCES

1. Wall ME, Wani MC. Camptothecin and taxol: discovery to clinic. Thirteenth Bruce F. Cain Memorial Award Lecture. Cancer Res 1995;55:753–60.
2. Wang JC. Interaction between DNA and an *Escherichia coli* protein omega. J Mol Biol 1971;55:523–33.
3. Hsiang YH, Hertzberg R, Hecht S, et al. Camptothecin induces protein-linked DNA breaks via mammalian DNA topoisomerase I. J Biol Chem 1985;260: 14873–8.
4. Liu LF, Wang JC. Supercoiling of the DNA template during transcription. Proc Natl Acad Sci U S A 1987;84:7024–7.
5. Pommier Y, Leo E, Zhang H, et al. DNA topoisomerases and their poisoning by anticancer and antibacterial drugs. Chem Biol 2010;17:421–33.
6. Pommier Y. DNA topoisomerase I inhibitors: chemistry, biology, and interfacial inhibition. Chem Rev 2009;109:2894–902.
7. Miao ZH, Player A, Shankavaram U, et al. Nonclassic functions of human topoisomerase I: genome-wide and pharmacologic analyses. Cancer Res 2007;67: 8752–61.
8. Potmesil M. Camptothecins: from bench research to hospital wards. Cancer Res 1994;54:1431–9.
9. Hsiang YH, Lihou MG, Liu LF. Arrest of replication forks by drug-stabilized topoisomerase I-DNA cleavable complexes as a mechanism of cell killing by camptothecin. Cancer Res 1989;49:5077–82.
10. Stewart L, Redinbo MR, Qiu X, et al. A model for the mechanism of human topoisomerase I. Science 1998;279:1534–41.
11. Pommier Y, Pourquier P, Fan Y, et al. Mechanism of action of eukaryotic DNA topoisomerase I and drugs targeted to the enzyme. Biochim Biophys Acta 1998;1400:83–105.
12. Lin CP, Ban Y, Lyu YL, et al. A ubiquitin-proteasome pathway for the repair of topoisomerase I-DNA covalent complexes. J Biol Chem 2008;283:21074–83.
13. Jaxel C, Kohn KW, Wani MC, et al. Structure-activity study of the actions of camptothecin derivatives on mammalian topoisomerase I: evidence for a specific receptor site and a relation to antitumor activity. Cancer Res 1989;49:1465–9.
14. Fukada M. Action of camptothecin and its derivatives on deoxyribonucleic acid. Biochem Pharmacol 1985;34:1225–30.
15. Glaberman U, Rabinowitz I, Verschraegen CF. Alternative administration of camptothecin analogues. Expert Opin Drug Deliv 2005;2:323–33.

16. Sawada S, Yokokura T, Miyasaka T. Synthesis of CPT-11 (irinotecan hydrochloride trihydrate). Ann N Y Acad Sci 1996;803:13–28.
17. Du W. Towards new anticancer drugs: a decade of advances in synthesis of camptothecins and related alkaloids. Tetrahedron 2003;59:8649–87.
18. Teicher BA. Next generation topoisomerase I inhibitors: rationale and biomarker strategies. Biochem Pharmacol 2008;75:1262–71.
19. Mi Z, Burke T. Differential interactions of camptothecin lactone and carboxylate forms with human blood components. Biochemistry 1994;33:10325–36.
20. Mi Z, Malak H, Burke TG. Reduced albumin binding promotes the stability and activity of topotecan in human blood. Biochemistry 1995;34:13722–8.
21. Mathijssen RH, van Alphen RJ, Verweij J, et al. Clinical pharmacokinetics and metabolism of irinotecan (CPT-11). Clin Cancer Res 2001;7:2182–94.
22. Rivory LP, Chatelut E, Canal P, et al. Kinetics of the in vivo interconversion of the carboxylate and lactone forms of irinotecan (CPT-11) and of its metabolite SN-38 in patients. Cancer Res 1994;54:6330–3.
23. Slatter JG, Schaaf LJ, Sams JP, et al. Pharmacokinetics, metabolism, and excretion of irinotecan (CPT-11) following I.V. infusion of [(14)C]CPT-11 in cancer patients. Drug Metab Dispos 2000;28:423–33.
24. Guichard S, Terret C, Hennebelle I, et al. CPT-11 converting carboxylesterase and topoisomerase activities in tumour and normal colon and liver tissues. Br J Cancer 1999;80:364–70.
25. Rivory LP, Haaz MC, Canal P, et al. Pharmacokinetic interrelationships of irinotecan (CPT-11) and its three major plasma metabolites in patients enrolled in phase I/II trials. Clin Cancer Res 1997;3:1261–6.
26. Ando Y, Saka H, Ando M, et al. Polymorphisms of UDP-glucuronosyltransferase gene and irinotecan toxicity: a pharmacogenetic analysis. Cancer Res 2000;60:6921–6.
27. Lee SY, McLeod HL. Pharmacogenetic tests in cancer chemotherapy: what physicians should know for clinical application. J Pathol 2011;223:15–27.
28. Hoskins JM, Goldberg RM, Qu P, et al. UGT1A1*28 genotype and irinotecan-induced neutropenia: dose matters. J Natl Cancer Inst 2007;99:1290–5.
29. Sperker B, Backman JT, Kroemer HK. The role of beta-glucuronidase in drug disposition and drug targeting in humans. Clin Pharmacokinet 1997;33:18–31.
30. Ratain MJ, Innocenti F. Individualizing dosing of irinotecan. Clin Cancer Res 2010;16:371–2.
31. Gerrits CJ, de Jonge MJ, Schellens JH, et al. Topoisomerase I inhibitors: the relevance of prolonged exposure for present clinical development. Br J Cancer 1997;76:952–62.
32. Saltz LB, Cox JV, Blanke C, et al. Irinotecan plus fluorouracil and leucovorin for metastatic colorectal cancer. Irinotecan Study Group. N Engl J Med 2000;343:905–14.
33. Cunningham D, Pyrhonen S, James RD, et al. Randomised trial of irinotecan plus supportive care versus supportive care alone after fluorouracil failure for patients with metastatic colorectal cancer. Lancet 1998;352:1413–8.
34. Rougier P, Van Cutsem E, Bajetta E, et al. Randomised trial of irinotecan versus fluorouracil by continuous infusion after fluorouracil failure in patients with metastatic colorectal cancer. Lancet 1998;352:1407–12.
35. Muhr-Wilkenshoff F, Hinkelbein W, Ohnesorge I, et al. A pilot study of irinotecan (CPT-11) as single-agent therapy in patients with locally advanced or metastatic esophageal carcinoma. Int J Colorectal Dis 2003;18:330–4.

36. Lara PN Jr, Natale R, Crowley J, et al. Phase III trial of irinotecan/cisplatin compared with etoposide/cisplatin in extensive-stage small-cell lung cancer: clinical and pharmacogenomic results from SWOG S0124. J Clin Oncol 2009; 27:2530–5.

37. Rosen LS. Irinotecan in lymphoma, leukemia, and breast, pancreatic, ovarian, and small-cell lung cancers. Oncology (Williston Park) 1998;12:103–9.

38. Verschraegen CF. Irinotecan for the treatment of cervical cancer. Oncology (Williston Park) 2002;16:32–4.

39. Schmittel A, Fischer von Weikersthal L, Sebastian M, et al. A randomized phase II trial of irinotecan plus carboplatin versus etoposide plus carboplatin treatment in patients with extended disease small-cell lung cancer. Ann Oncol 2006;17:663–7.

40. Conroy T, Desseigne F, Ychou M, et al. FOLFIRINOX versus gemcitabine for metastatic pancreatic cancer. N Engl J Med 2011;364:1817–25.

41. Underberg WJ, Goossen RM, Smith BR, et al. Equilibrium kinetics of the new experimental anti-tumour compound SK&F 104864-A in aqueous solution. J Pharm Biomed Anal 1990;8:681–3.

42. Mathijssen RH, Loos WJ, Verweij J, et al. Pharmacology of topoisomerase I inhibitors irinotecan (CPT-11) and topotecan. Curr Cancer Drug Targets 2002;2:103–23.

43. Rosing H, Herben VM, van Gortel-van Zomeren DM, et al. Isolation and structural confirmation of N-desmethyl topotecan, a metabolite of topotecan. Cancer Chemother Pharmacol 1997;39:498–504.

44. Blaney S, Heideman R, Cole D, et al. A phase I study of intrathecal topotecan. Proc Am Assoc Canc Res 1998;39:A2198.

45. Wong ET, Berkenblit A. The role of topotecan in the treatment of brain metastases. Oncologist 2004;9:68–79.

46. Neuhaus T, Ko Y, Muller RP, et al. A phase III trial of topotecan and whole brain radiation therapy for patients with CNS-metastases due to lung cancer. Br J Cancer 2009;100:291–7.

47. Riemsma R, Simons JP, Bashir Z, et al. Systematic review of topotecan (Hycamtin) in relapsed small cell lung cancer. BMC Cancer 2010;10:436.

48. Eckardt JR. Emerging role of weekly topotecan in recurrent small cell lung cancer. Oncologist 2004;9(Suppl 6):25–32.

49. Markman M. Can weekly topotecan substitute for a multi-day regimen in the treatment of ovarian cancer? Sadly, 10 years later the answer remains unknown. Gynecol Oncol 2011;122:213–4.

50. Sehouli J, Stengel D, Harter P, et al. Topotecan weekly versus conventional 5-day schedule in patients with platinum-resistant ovarian cancer: a randomized multicenter phase II trial of the North-Eastern German Society of Gynecological Oncology Ovarian Cancer Study Group. J Clin Oncol 2011;29:242–8.

51. Kudelka AP, Tresukosol D, Edwards CL, et al. Phase II study of intravenous topotecan as a 5-day infusion for refractory epithelial ovarian carcinoma. J Clin Oncol 1996;14:1552–7.

52. Long HJ III, Bundy BN, Grendys EC Jr, et al. Randomized phase III trial of cisplatin with or without topotecan in carcinoma of the uterine cervix: a Gynecologic Oncology Group study. J Clin Oncol 2005;23:4626–33.

53. Sorensen M, Jensen PB, Herrstedt J, et al. A dose escalating study of topotecan preceding cisplatin in previously untreated patients with small-cell lung cancer. Ann Oncol 2000;11:829–35.

54. Muderspach LI, Blessing JA, Levenback C, et al. A phase II study of topotecan in patients with squamous cell carcinoma of the cervix: a gynecologic oncology group study. Gynecol Oncol 2001;81:213–5.

55. Beran M, Estey E, O'Brien SM, et al. Results of topotecan single-agent therapy in patients with myelodysplastic syndromes and chronic myelomonocytic leukemia. Leuk Lymphoma 1998;31:521–31.
56. Metzger ML, Stewart CF, Freeman BB III, et al. Topotecan is active against Wilms' tumor: results of a multi-institutional phase II study. J Clin Oncol 2007;25:3130–6.
57. Weitz JJ, Marschke RF Jr, Sloan JA, et al. A randomized phase II trial of two schedules of topotecan for the treatment of advanced stage non-small cell lung cancer. Lung Cancer 2000;28:157–62.
58. Rose PG, Markman M, Bell JG, et al. Sequential prolonged oral topotecan and pro-longed oral etoposide as second-line therapy in ovarian or peritoneal carcinoma: a phase I Gynecologic Oncology Group study. Gynecol Oncol 2006;102:236–9.
59. Schluep T, Cheng J, Khin KT, et al. Pharmacokinetics and biodistribution of the camptothecin-polymer conjugate IT-101 in rats and tumor-bearing mice. Cancer Chemother Pharmacol 2006;57:654–62.
60. Caiolfa VR, Zamai M, Fiorino A, et al. Polymer-bound camptothecin: initial bio-distribution and antitumour activity studies. J Control Release 2000;65:105–19.
61. Li C, Wallace S. Polymer-drug conjugates: recent development in clinical oncology. Adv Drug Deliv Rev 2008;60:886–98.
62. Rowinsky EK, Rizzo J, Ochoa L, et al. A phase I and pharmacokinetic study of pegylated camptothecin as a 1-hour infusion every 3 weeks in patients with advanced solid malignancies. J Clin Oncol 2003;21:148–57.
63. Vergote I, Micha J, Pippitt C Jr, et al. Phase II study of NKTR-102 in women with platinum-resistant/refractory ovarian cancer. J Clin Oncol 2010;28:A5013.
64. Homsi J, Simon GR, Garrett CR, et al. Phase I trial of poly-L-glutamate campto-thecin (CT-2106) administered weekly in patients with advanced solid malignan-cies. Clin Cancer Res 2007;13:5855–61.
65. Conover CD, Greenwald RB, Pendri A, et al. Camptothecin delivery systems: the utility of amino acid spacers for the conjugation of camptothecin with polyeth-ylene glycol to create prodrugs. Anticancer Drug Des 1999;14:499–506.
66. Ying V, Haverstick K, Page RL, et al. Efficacy of camptothecin and polymer-conjugated camptothecin in tumor spheroids and solid tumors. J Biomater Sci Polym Ed 2007;18:1283–99.
67. Scott LC, Yao JC, Benson AB III, et al. A phase II study of pegylated-camptothecin (pegamotecan) in the treatment of locally advanced and metastatic gastric and gastro-oesophageal junction adenocarcinoma. Cancer Chemother Pharmacol 2009;63:363–70.
68. Mao Q, Unadkat JD. Role of the breast cancer resistance protein (ABCG2) in drug transport. AAPS J 2005;7:E118–33.
69. Houghton PJ, Germain GS, Harwood FC, et al. Imatinib mesylate is a potent inhibitor of the ABCG2 (BCRP) transporter and reverses resistance to topotecan and SN-38 in vitro. Cancer Res 2004;64:2333–7.
70. Schellens JH, Kuppens I, Jewell R, et al. Phase I and pharmacological study of oral topotecan and the BCRP and P-gp inhibitor elacridar. J Clin Oncol 2004;22: 14S(Suppl): [Abstract: 2003].
71. Ame JC, Spenlehauer C, de Murcia G. The PARP superfamily. Bioessays 2004; 26:882–93.
72. Okano S, Lan L, Tomkinson AE, et al. Translocation of XRCC1 and DNA ligase IIIalpha from centrosomes to chromosomes in response to DNA damage in mitotic human cells. Nucleic Acids Res 2005;33:422–9.
73. Chalmers AJ. The potential role and application of PARP inhibitors in cancer treatment. Br Med Bull 2009;89:23–40.

74. Tentori L, Leonetti C, Scarsella M, et al. Inhibition of poly(ADP-ribose) polymerase prevents irinotecan-induced intestinal damage and enhances irinotecan/temozolomide efficacy against colon carcinoma. FASEB J 2006;20: 1709–11.

75. Verschraegen CF, Kudelka AP, Kavanagh JJ. Topoisomerase-I inhibitors in gynaecologic tumours. Ann Acad Med Singapore 1998;27:683–7.

76. Basili S, Moro S. Novel camptothecin derivatives as topoisomerase I inhibitors. Expert Opin Ther Pat 2009;19:555–74.

77. Choi CH, Lee YY, Song TJ, et al. Phase II study of belotecan, a camptothecin analogue, in combination with carboplatin for the treatment of recurrent ovarian cancer. Cancer 2011;117:2104–11.

78. Lee DH, Kim SW, Suh C, et al. Multicenter phase 2 study of belotecan, a new camptothecin analog, and cisplatin for chemotherapy-naive patients with extensive-disease small cell lung cancer. Cancer 2010;116:132–6.

79. Hong J, Jung M, Kim YJ, et al. Phase II study of combined belotecan and cisplatin as first-line chemotherapy in patients with extensive disease of small cell lung cancer. Cancer Chemother Pharmacol 2012;69(1):215–20.

80. Frapolli R, Zucchetti M, Sessa C, et al. Clinical pharmacokinetics of the new oral camptothecin gimatecan: the inter-patient variability is related to alpha1-acid glycoprotein plasma levels. Eur J Cancer 2010;46:505–16.

81. Di Francesco AM, Riccardi A, Barone G, et al. The novel lipophilic camptothecin analogue gimatecan is very active in vitro in human neuroblastoma: a comparative study with SN38 and topotecan. Biochem Pharmacol 2005;70:1125–36.

82. Pecorelli S, Ray-Coquard I, Tredan O, et al. Phase II of oral gimatecan in patients with recurrent epithelial ovarian, fallopian tube or peritoneal cancer, previously treated with platinum and taxanes. Ann Oncol 2010;21:759–65.

83. Ulukan H, Swaan PW. Camptothecins: a review of their chemotherapeutic potential. Drugs 2002;62:2039–57.

84. Emerson DL, Bendele R, Brown E, et al. Antitumor efficacy, pharmacokinetics, and biodistribution of NX 211: a low-clearance liposomal formulation of lurtotecan. Clin Cancer Res 2000;6:2903–12.

85. Dark GG, Calvert AH, Grimshaw R, et al. Randomized trial of two intravenous schedules of the topoisomerase I inhibitor liposomal lurtotecan in women with relapsed epithelial ovarian cancer: a trial of the national cancer institute of Canada Clinical Trials group. J Clin Oncol 2005;23:1859–66.

86. Gerrits CJ, Schellens JH, Creemers GJ, et al. The bioavailability of oral GI147211 (GG211), a new topoisomerase I inhibitor. Br J Cancer 1997;76:946–51.

87. Verschraegen CF, Gupta E, Loyer E, et al. A phase II clinical and pharmacological study of oral 9-nitrocamptothecin in patients with refractory epithelial ovarian, tubal or peritoneal cancer. Anticancer Drugs 1999;10(4):375–83.

88. Verschraegen CF, Natelson EA, Giovanella BC, et al. A phase I clinical and pharmacological study of oral 9-nitrocamptothecin, a novel water-insoluble topoisomerase I inhibitor. Anticancer Drugs 1998;9:36–44.

89. Miller KD, Soule SE, Haney LG, et al. A phase II study of 9-nitro-camptothecin in patients with previously treated metastatic breast cancer. Invest New Drugs 2004;22(1):69–73.

90. Burris HA III, Rivkin S, Reynolds R, et al. Phase II trial of oral rubitecan in previously treated pancreatic cancer patients. Oncologist 2005;10:183–90.

91. Arnold SM, Rinehart JJ, Tsakalozou E, et al. A phase I study of 7-t-butyldimethylsilyl-10-hydroxycamptothecin in adult patients with refractory or metastatic solid malignancies. Clin Cancer Res 2010;16:673–80.

92. Miller AA, Herndon JE II, Gu L, et al. Phase II trial of karenitecin in patients with relapsed or refractory non-small cell lung cancer (CALGB 30004). Lung Cancer 2005;48:399–407.
93. Daud A, Valkov N, Centeno B, et al. Phase II trial of karenitecin in patients with malignant melanoma: clinical and translational study. Clin Cancer Res 2005;11: 3009–16.
94. Jew S, Kim HJ, Kim MG, et al. Synthesis and in vitro cytotoxicity of hexacyclic camptothecin analogues. Bioorg Med Chem Lett 1999;9:3203–6.
95. Sugimori M, Ejima A, Ohsuki S, et al. Synthesis and antitumor activity of ring A- and F-modified hexacyclic camptothecin analogues. J Med Chem 1998;41: 2308–18.
96. Bailly C, Lansiaux A, Dassonneville L, et al. Homocamptothecin, an E-ring-modified camptothecin analogue, generates new topoisomerase I-mediated DNA breaks. Biochemistry 1999;38:15556–63.
97. Lesueur-Ginot L, Demarquay D, Kiss R, et al. Homocamptothecin, an E-ring modified camptothecin with enhanced lactone stability, retains topoisomerase I-targeted activity and antitumor properties. Cancer Res 1999;59:2939–43.
98. Royce ME, Hoff PM, Dumas P, et al. Phase I and pharmacokinetic study of exatecan mesylate (DX-8951f): a novel camptothecin analog. J Clin Oncol 2001; 19:1493–500.
99. Abou-Alfa GK, Letourneau R, Harker G, et al. Randomized phase III study of exatecan and gemcitabine compared with gemcitabine alone in untreated advanced pancreatic cancer. J Clin Oncol 2006;24:4441–7.
100. Esteva FJ, Rivera E, Cristofanilli M, et al. A Phase II study of intravenous exatecan mesylate (DX-8951f) administered daily for 5 days every 3 weeks to patients with metastatic breast carcinoma. Cancer 2003;98:900–7.
101. Ishii M, Iwahana M, Mitsui I, et al. Growth inhibitory effect of a new camptothecin analog, DX-8951f, on various drug-resistant sublines including BCRP-mediated camptothecin derivative-resistant variants derived from the human lung cancer cell line PC-6. Anticancer Drugs 2000;11:353–62.
102. Miao Z, Zhang J, You L, et al. Phosphate ester derivatives of homocamptothecin: synthesis, solution stabilities and antitumor activities. Bioorg Med Chem 2010;18:3140–6.
103. Kroep JR, Gelderblom H. Diflomotecan, a promising homocamptothecin for cancer therapy. Expert Opin Investig Drugs 2009;18:69–75.
104. Hurwitz HI, Cohen RB, McGovren JP, et al. A phase I study of the safety and pharmacokinetics of edotecarin (J-107088), a novel topoisomerase I inhibitor, in patients with advanced solid tumors. Cancer Chemother Pharmacol 2007; 59:139–47.
105. Sunami S, Nishimura T, Nishimura I, et al. Synthesis and biological activities of topoisomerase I inhibitors, 6-arylmethylamino analogues of edotecarin. J Med Chem 2009;52:3225–37.
106. Cinelli MA, Morrell A, Dexheimer TS, et al. Design, synthesis, and biological evaluation of 14-substituted aromathecins as topoisomerase I inhibitors. J Med Chem 2008;51:4609–19.
107. Kurtzberg LS, Roth S, Krumbholz R, et al. Genz-644282, a novel non-camptothecin topoisomerase I inhibitor for cancer treatment. Clin Cancer Res 2011;17:2777–87.
108. Ruchelman AL, Singh SK, Ray A, et al. 5H-Dibenzo[c, h]1,6-naphthyridin-6-ones: novel topoisomerase I-targeting anticancer agents with potent cytotoxic activity. Bioorg Med Chem 2003;11:2061–73.

Targeting the Insulin Growth Factor Receptor 1

Fernanda I. Arnaldez, MD*, Lee J. Helman, MD

KEYWORDS

• IGF1R • IGF1 • IGF2 • Insulin • Kinase • Cancer

KEY POINTS

- The insulin growth factor (IGF) axis is a tightly controlled endocrine system that regulates cell growth and development.
- Alterations of this system have been found in neoplasias, including increased expression of ligands and receptors, loss of heterozygosity of the IGF2 locus, and increased IGF1 receptor (IGF1R) gene copy number.
- The IGF1 network is an attractive candidate for targeted therapy, including receptor blockade with monoclonal antibodies and small molecule inhibitors of receptor downstream signaling.
- Determining the most effective ways to combine IGF1R-targeted therapy with either cytotoxic chemotherapy or other targeted agents as well as identification of predictive biomarkers for patient selection are key future challenges.

Insulin growth factors (IGFs) were initially described as humoral mediators of growth hormone (GH) action.[1] This signaling network is involved in regulation of human development, energy balance, and cell growth.[2,3] In addition to its well-characterized role in glucose, protein, and lipid metabolism,[4] the complex nature of this hormonal axis continues to attract the attention of scientists and physicians, given the growing body of evidence that supports its critical role in cancer biology.[2,5] Unlike other trophic factors involved in neoplastic development, IGFs exert endocrine, paracrine, and autocrine effects. The components of this cellular network are summarized in **Table 1**.

In humans, both the insulin and the IGF receptors are composed of 2 globular extracellular alpha subunits that are each linked to a beta subunit and to each other by disulfide bonds. The tyrosine kinase activity resides in the beta subunit.[6] There are also hybrid receptors composed of half an insulin receptor and half an IGF receptor (IRαβ linked to IGF1Rαβ) (**Fig. 1**).[7,8] Binding of IGF2 to the IGF2/mannose-6-phosphate receptor (IGF2/M6P-R) triggers internalization and degradation of the

Disclosures: The authors have nothing to disclose.
Pediatric Oncology Branch, Center for Cancer Research, National Cancer Institute, National Institutes of Health, Building 10 CRC Room 1-3816, Bethesda, MD 20892, USA
* Corresponding author. Molecular Oncology Section, Pediatric Oncology Branch, NCI, 9000 Rockville Pike, Building 10/Room 1W-3816, Bethesda, MD 20892.
E-mail address: arnaldezf@mail.nih.gov

Hematol Oncol Clin N Am 26 (2012) 527–542
doi:10.1016/j.hoc.2012.01.004
0889-8588/12/$ – see front matter Published by Elsevier Inc.

Table 1
Components of the IGF axis and relevant features

IGF1	Binds IGF1R and hybrid receptors
IGF2	Binds IGF1R, IGF2R, IR-A, and hybrid receptors
Insulin	Binds IR-A, IR-B, and IGF1R
IGF1R	Binds IGF1 and IGF2 with high affinity and insulin with low affinity
IGF2/mannose-6-phosphate receptor	Binds IGF2, lacks intracellular signaling
IR-A	Lacks exon 11 (splice variant), binds insulin and IGF2 with high affinity
IR-B	Contains exon 11 (splice variant), binds insulin with high affinity
IGF1R/IR-A	Hybrid receptor
IGF1R/IR-B	Hybrid receptor
IGFBP 1–6 (IGFBP1-6)	Binds IGF1 and IGF2, forming tertiary complexes with IGFALS and prolonging the half-life of growth factors
IGFBP 7–8 (IGFBP7-8)	Binds IGF1 with low affinity
IGFALS	85-kDa protein, member of leucine-rich repeats superfamily; prolongs half-life of IGFBP-3/5 and IGF1 binary complexes

Abbreviations: IGF1R, IGF1 receptor; IGFALS, IGF acid-labile subunit; IGFBP, IGF binding protein; IR-A, insulin receptor A; IR-B, insulin receptor B.

ligand, without eliciting downstream signaling. Thus, the IGF2/M6P-R is considered a tumor suppressor[9,10] because it functions as a scavenger that reduces IGF2 availability to bind IGF1 receptor (IGF1R).[11–13]

Binding of IGF1 to the alpha subunit of IGF1R triggers a conformational change that causes activation of the catalytic domain in the intracellular beta subunit causing tyrosine autophosphorylation and transphosphorylation (Y1131, Y1135, and Y1136) that enhances its tyrosine kinase activity.[14] These events lead to recruitment of adaptor proteins such as IRS, CRK, and SHC. Downstream signaling is mostly channeled through the MAPK/Ras-Raf-Erk pathway, the phosphatidylinositol-3-kinase/AKT/mammalian target of rapamycin (PI3K/AKT/mTOR) pathway, and the Jak/STAT pathway. Ultimately, activation of IGF1R results in increased cell proliferation and decreased apoptosis.[5,15–17]

The central regulation of the IGF system resides in the hypothalamus. Various stimuli lead to growth hormone–releasing hormone or somatostatin secretion.[18,19] These peptides regulate the secretion of GH by the anterior pituitary gland. Binding of GH to its receptor in the liver results in stimulation of IGF1 synthesis and secretion. In addition, insulin can indirectly increase IGF1 production in part by upregulating GH receptors.[3,20,21] Cancer cells, however, can secrete significant quantities of IGF1 in a paracrine or autocrine manner, independently of GH regulation.[22] Thus, the IGF1 axis signals in a hormone-dependent manner to regulate physiologic growth and in a hormone-independent manner in the context of neoplasia.

Individuals with supraphysiologic levels of GH (acromegaly) seem to have an increased risk for cancer development, possibly via an IGF1-mediated mechanism.[3,23] Conversely, patients with Laron syndrome (IGF1 deficiency and insensitivity to GH) seem to have a lower cancer risk than their relatives.[24,25]

The influence of circulating IGF1 has been documented in mouse models of tumor development.[26] However, there is a clear distinction between murine and human IGF axis. Although mice present high IGF1 and almost undetectable IGF2 levels

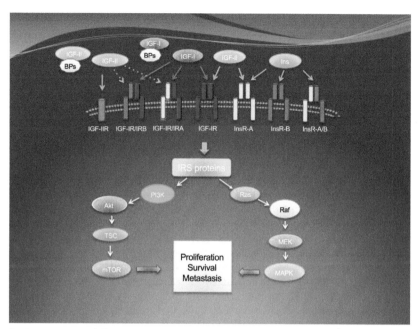

Fig. 1. Components of the IGF axis. The IGF axis is composed of 2 IGF ligands, IGF1 (or IGF-I) and IGF2 (or IGF-II). They bind one of the different IGF binding proteins (BPs). The majority of circulating IGF is bound to IGFBP-3 and a molecule called acid-labile subunit. The different combinations of receptors in the axis bind to IGF1 (IGF-I), IGF2 (IGF-II), and insulin with different affinities, as represented by the large or small size of the ligand.

postnatally,[19,27] postnatal human IGF1 level remains at low concentrations. In addition, human IGF2 is not only highly secreted but also functionally relevant beyond birth.

Although IGF2 is also secreted in the liver, this process is not regulated by GH. The IGF2 gene is imprinted. In most tissues, only the paternal allele is expressed. When imprinting of the maternal allele is lost, IGF2 expression is increased. In the case of Beckwith-Wiedemann syndrome, loss of imprinting results in marked IGF2 overexpression resulting in fetal and neonatal overgrowth. Many tumor types harbor biallelic expression of IGF2 via this mechanism, including Wilms tumor, esophageal carcinoma, Ewing sarcoma, rhabdomyosarcoma, colorectal carcinoma, osteosarcoma, prostate adenocarcinoma, hepatocellular carcinoma, and adrenocortical carcinoma.[11,19,28–36]

The bioavailability of IGF1 and IGF2 is highly influenced by their binding to IGF binding proteins (IGFBPs) and the IGF acid-labile subunit (IGFALS). Several factors can increase IGFBP synthesis, including estrogens,[37] retinoids,[38] and vitamin D.[39] In addition, antiproliferative pathways such as transforming growth factor β[38] and p53[40] also increase IGBP concentration. However, there is also some evidence that shows certain IGFBPs could enhance delivery of these growth factors to the tumor microenvironment.[2,41] Hyperinsulinism indirectly increases hepatic IGF1 secretion and increases its availability by decreasing IGFBP levels.[3,42,43]

Oncogenic transcription factors can also regulate IGFBP expression. EWS-FLI1, an aberrant fusion protein responsible for malignant transformation in Ewing sarcoma family of tumors, binds the IGFBP-3 promoter and decreases its expression.[44] Another example is WT1, a tumor suppressor gene that plays a significant role in the development of Wilms tumor, a pediatric kidney neoplasm. WT1 represses IGF1R expression, thus regulating the activity of the IGF pathway in Wilms tumor.[45]

IGF AXIS IN CANCER

Epidemiologic evidence suggests that obesity and type 2 diabetes, both clinical conditions in which hyperinsulinism is present, are associated with increased cancer risk.[3,46,47] At least for some tumor subtypes, the same holds true if elevated IGF1 level is detected.[48–51] Correlation between IGF1R expression and worse outcome has been suggested in different tumor contexts, including colorectal carcinoma, breast cancer, and melanoma.[52–54]

IGF1R is highly expressed and biologically active in many neoplastic processes. However, gene amplifications were found relatively recently.[55,56] Increased IGF1R copy number was found in small cell lung cancer.[57] In addition, a high level gain of IGF1R at 15q26 was recently described in pediatric high-grade gliomas,[58] a disease in which IGF2 signaling has a growth-promoting role.[59] Recent studies also suggest elevated insulin receptor A (IR-A) expression in cancer cells.[60,61]

IGF1R is often necessary for oncogene-mediated malignant transformation.[62–64] In Ewing sarcoma, IGF1R activity is necessary for transformation of fibroblasts with the EWS/FLI1 fusion transcript, as described in 1997. More recently, silencing of the fusion protein revealed that several microRNAs that negatively regulate expression of proteins in the IGF axis are silenced by EWS/FLI1.[65]

A remarkable aspect of IGF1R biology is its association with resistance to cytotoxic chemotherapy, radiation therapy, and targeted agents.[66] Resistance to cytotoxic agents is documented across tumor types. One of the mechanisms by which this occurs is decreased intracellular concentration of the agent via activation of adenosine triphosphate–dependent efflux pumps such as P-glycoprotein, encoded by the multidrug resistance (MDR) gene. In patients with gastric carcinoma, IGF1R was found to correlate with overexpression of MDR-associated protein 1 and with poor clinical prognosis.[67]

Many preclinical studies have shown sensitization of cancer cell lines to chemotherapy agents by silencing or blocking IGF1R. Although there is some suggestion about AKT activation playing a role in this process, many of the mechanisms involved are still under investigation. In breast cancer cells, IGF1R blockade improved the response to paclitaxel (Taxol) and doxorubicin.[68] Similar results were obtained with non–small cell lung cancer (NSCLC) cells treated with etoposide and carboplatin,[69] atypical teratoid rhabdoid tumor cells treated with doxorubicin and cisplatin,[70] and gastric cancer cells treated with 5-fluorouracil.[71] Other examples include osteosarcoma,[72,73] colorectal carcinoma,[74] mesothelioma,[75] and esophageal carcinoma.[76] A recent study showed increased sensitivity of glioblastoma cell lines to carmustine and cisplatin when the tumor suppressor gene WT1 was silenced.[77] As described earlier, WT1 negatively regulates IGF1R expression. In hepatocellular carcinoma, IGF1 reduces the cell sensitivity to doxorubicin by changing the redox potential via upregulation of glutathione transferase expression.[78] Silencing of the IGF1R gene enhances sensitivity to DNA-damaging agents such as mitoxantrone, etoposide, and nitrogen mustard in prostate cancer cells.[79] An attractive hypothesis to explain this observation considers IGF signaling as a modulator of XRCC5, a DNA double-strand break repair protein involved in nonhomologous end-joining recombination.[80]

Given its link to DNA repair pathway, it is not surprising that IGF1R inhibition can enhance the effect of radiation therapy. IGF1R knockdown results in decreased

ATM expression,[81] whereas defective ATM kinase activity is associated with reduced expression of IGF1R. Both conditions lead to increased radiosensitivity.[82,83] These findings are consistent with clinical data in breast cancer in which a higher rate of tumor recurrence after surgery and radiation was seen in patients whose primary tumors showed high IGF1R expression.[54]

There are examples of cooperation between hormonal therapy and IGF1 axis inhibition. Antiestrogens, such as tamoxifen, are widely used for the management of estrogen receptor–positive breast cancer. However, 40% of patients do not respond to this treatment. Several factors play a role in tamoxifen resistance. IGF1R is known to cross talk with the estrogen receptor pathway and could be responsible for the resistant phenotype. Tamoxifen-resistant breast cancer cell lines have been shown to have an increased expression of IGF2, which is able to trigger growth and survival signaling via IGF1R.[66,84,85] Moreover, IGF1R inhibitors have been able to inhibit growth of tamoxifen-resistant breast cancer cell lines in vitro.[86,87]

IGF1R inhibition can be combined with other molecularly targeted agents. Some cancer types coexpress IGF1R and epidermal growth factor receptor (EGFR).[88] EGFR family members mediate proliferation, differentiation, and survival in malignant cells. About 40% to 80% of NSCLCs have EGFR overexpression,[89] and 30% of breast cancers overexpress human epidermal growth factor receptor 2 (HER-2).[90,91] EGFR inhibitors such as erlotinib and gefitinib have been successfully developed, but resistance to therapy often follows initial response. EGFR/IGFR heterodimers that activate the IGF1R signaling pathway have been found after treating NSCLC cell lines with gefitinib.[92,93] In addition, IGF1R silencing markedly increased apoptosis of gefitinib-treated cell lines.[93] IGF1R has also been found to be a factor in breast cancer resistance to trastuzumab,[94] and there is evidence to suggest that HER-2 phosphorylation is influenced by IGF1R signaling.[95]

TARGETING IGF1R
GH Antagonists

Pegvisomant is a genetically engineered GH receptor antagonist used in the treatment of acromegaly.[96] Although there is preclinical evidence of some antitumor activity, its clinical use as an antineoplastic agent has been limited.[97,98] Somatostatin, the physiologic antagonist of GH, has also been proposed as an anticancer agent in the past.[99]

Ligand Antagonists

IGFPB3 naturally binds the ligands of the IGF axis and decreases their bioavailability in the circulation. Recombinant IGFBP-3 has been proposed as a way to decrease IGF1R signaling, and it showed activity in preclinical models.[100,101]

MEDI-573 is a human neutralizing IGF1/IGF2 monoclonal antibody that inhibits binding of the growth factors to IGF1R and IR-A. It seems to inhibit IGF1R signaling with virtually no effect in insulin activation of IR-A. Preclinical data show inhibition of tumor growth in vivo using xenografts of high-expressing IGF1R/IR-A cells.[102]

Receptor Antagonists

Several neutralizing antibodies against the IGF1R receptor have been extensively studied, and they continue to be evaluated in many clinical trials. A list of the different currently available agents is shown in **Table 2**. There was a significant concern regarding hyperglycemia, because blockade of IGF1R causes a compensatory increase in the levels of GH, which can induce insulin resistance and stimulation of gluconeogenesis.[2] However, hyperglycemia has not been found to be a significant

Table 2
Monoclonal antibodies against IGF1R

	Agent		Ongoing Trials[a]	Toxicities
AMG 479 (Amgen, Thousand Oaks, CA, USA)	Ganitumab	Fully human monoclonal IgG1	EWS, DSRCT, ovarian carcinoma, CRC, NSCLC; pancreatic carcinoma (phase III)	Thrombocytopenia, hyperglycemia, neutralizing antibodies
RG1507 (Roche, Basel, Switzerland)	—	Fully human monoclonal IgG1	Development discontinued	Hyperglycemia, lymphopenia, CVA
IMC-A12 (ImClone, New York, NY, USA)	Cixutumumab	Fully human monoclonal IgG1	ACC, thymic carcinoma, SCLC, soft tissue sarcomas, osteosarcoma, EWS, HCC, breast cancer, head and neck carcinoma, prostate cancer, hepatocellular carcinoma, islet cell cancer, pancreatic cancer	Hyperglycemia, anemia, infusion reaction
MK-0646 (Merck, Whitehouse Station, NJ, USA)	Dalotuzumab	Humanized mouse monoclonal IgG1	NSCLC, SCLC, CRC, pancreatic carcinoma, breast cancer, neuroendocrine tumors	Thrombocytopenia, GI bleeding, pneumonitis, increased transaminase levels
CP-751871 (Pfizer, New York, NY, USA)	Figitumumab	Fully human monoclonal IgG2	CRC, NSCLC, SCLC, breast cancer; phase III (lung cancer) terminated due to lack of benefit	Hyperglycemia, anemia, cholestasis, hyperuricemia
SCH717454 (Schering-Plough, Kenilworth, NJ, USA)	Robatumumab	Fully human monoclonal IgG1	CRC, EWS, osteosarcoma	—
AVE1642 (Sanofi-Aventis, Paris, France)	—	Humanized mouse monoclonal IgG1	Breast cancer, multiple myeloma, hepatocellular carcinoma	Hyperglycemia, hypersensitivity

Abbreviations: ACC, adrenocortical carcinoma; CRC, colorectal carcinoma; CVA, cerebral vascular accident; DSRCT, desmoplastic small round cell tumor; EWS, Ewing sarcoma; GI, gastrointestinal; HCC, hepatocellular carcinoma; SCLC, small cell lung cancer.

[a] Clinicaltrials.gov.

problem in clinical trials using IGF1R blocking antibodies. Available antibodies are either of IgG1 or IgG2 isotype. Isotype differences in terms of side effects, given the different capacity to bind Fc gamma receptors, have not been clearly established yet.[103]

The IGF1 axis has clear biological implications in Ewing sarcoma, and it is not surprising that promising responses have been documented in this group of patients. Durable responses have been achieved in patients with this disease treated with RG1507.[19] In a phase I trial of RG1507 in patients with advanced solid tumors, the drug was well tolerated. Two patients with Ewing sarcoma had confirmed partial responses, and in 13 patients (2 of them with Ewing sarcoma) the disease became stable.[104] In a recent multicenter phase II study of RG1507 in 115 patients with refractory Ewing sarcoma family of tumors, the overall response rate was 10% (1 complete response and 10 partial responses), with a median duration of 29 months. In addition, 8 patients had unconfirmed partial responses.[105] Although the response was overall modest, it is possible that it reflects the need to find an accurate predictive biomarker to determine the patients who are likely to respond to IGF1R blockade. A phase I trial with a different IGF1R blocking antibody, AMG 479, documented a confirmed complete response and a partial response in 2 patients with Ewing sarcoma.[106] Similar results were achieved in a phase I trial of figitumumab in patients with sarcomas.[107]

Another tumor in which blocking IGF1R might be a reasonable strategy is gastrointestinal stromal tumor (GIST).[108–111] Both wild type and KIT-mutant GIST present high expression of IGF1R, and preclinical activity against these tumors has been promising. Clinical trials to further evaluate this hypothesis are in progress.

A randomized phase III trial of figitumumab in combination with paclitaxel and carboplatin versus paclitaxel and carboplatin in patients with NSCLC was permanently suspended at 681 patients because the futility analysis favored the paclitaxel-carboplatin arm,[112] despite promising previous phase II trials.[113] The study showed that figitumumab does not improve overall survival and increases the risk for severe toxicities, even for patients with nonadenocarcinoma histology. However, patients with circulating levels of IGF1 of greater than 1 ng/mL showed improved overall survival, which again stresses the need of appropriate predictive pharmacodynamic biomarkers in targeted therapy trials.

As mentioned earlier, IGF1R plays a role in resistance to chemotherapy and radiation therapy. Taking advantage of IGF1R inhibition while treating patients with cytotoxic agents and/or radiation therapy is being actively explored. In breast cancer models, there is evidence to support combination of IGF1R inhibitors and EGFR inhibitors, given the cross talk that these 2 relevant pathways have.[94,114,115] Moreover, adding downstream signaling inhibition to the receptor blockade to potentiate antitumor effect is a strategy that is being used in several trials in solid tumors. mTOR inhibitors, such as rapamycin, are an interesting choice, because the PI3K/AKT/mTOR pathway is regulated by receptor tyrosine kinases such as IGF1R. In addition, mTOR inhibition induces AKT activation via an IGF-dependent mechanism, supporting the rationale for this combination.[116] Initial results are encouraging, and several trials are under development.[117]

Small Molecule Inhibitors

Tyrosine kinase inhibitors targeting IGF1R have been recently developed. A list of these small molecule inhibitors is depicted in **Table 3**. Most of them target insulin receptors in addition to IGF1R. Even though this could bring opportunity for occurrence of metabolic side effects, it is also a chance to improve therapeutic efficacy, given the cross talk between IGF1R and insulin receptors.[2,3,15] With one notable exception, these drugs are in early phases of development. Linsitinib efficacy in

Table 3
Small molecule inhibitors targeting IGF1R

Agent	Specificity	Ongoing Trials[a]	Toxicities
XL228 (Exelixis, South San Francisco, CA, USA)	IGF1R, SFK, BCR-ABL, FGFR1-3, AURK A, AURK B	Phase I (advanced malignancies/CML)	Hyperglycemia, anorexia, fatigue
OSI906 (Linsitinib) (Astellas, Deerfield, IL, USA)	Reversible ATP-competitive inhibitor IGF1R/IR	NSCLC, ovarian cancer, breast cancer, head and neck carcinoma, HCC, SCLC (phase II), ACC (phase III)	Increased GH and IGF1R concentrations, hyperinsulinemia, hyperglycemia, QTc prolongation, nausea
BIIB022 (Biogen, Cambridge, MA, USA)	—	Phase I, phase Ib (HCC, NSCLC)	Headache, fatigue, nausea, QTc prolongation, hypertension, GI bleed, glucose level fluctuation
AXL 1717 (picropodophyllin) (Axelar, Stockholm, Sweden)	Non-ATP-competitive autophosphorylation inhibitor at Y1136	High IGF1R selectivity (no IR inhibition) Phase I	—
BMS-754807 (Bristol-Myers, New York, NY, USA)	Reversible, ATP-competitive inhibitor IGF1R/IR, MET, RON, TrkA, TrkB, AURK A, AURK B	Phase I/II (solid tumors), breast cancer (phase II)	Hypoglycemia, hyperglycemia, fatigue
INSM18 (nordihydroguaiaretic acid) (Insmed, Monmouth Junction, NJ, USA)	—	IGF1R/HER-2, 5α-reductase, 15-lipoxygenase, PDGFR Phase II: prostate cancer	—

Abbreviations: ACC, adrenocortical carcinoma; ATP, adenosine triphosphate; CML, chronic myelogenous leukemia; GI, gastrointestinal; HCC, hepatocellular carcinoma; PDGFR, platelet-derived growth factor receptor; SCLC, small cell lung cancer; QTc, corrected QT interval.
[a] Clinicaltrials.gov.

adrenocortical carcinoma, a disease with high dependence on IGF signaling, is being evaluated in a phase III trial. These drugs can become an attractive therapeutic tool, given a potentially tolerable toxicity profile, the possibility of oral administration, and the theoretical advantage of multitarget inhibition. However, much has to be learned about these agents and the tumor context in which their efficacy can be maximized.

Metformin

Although metformin is not a new targeted agent, its mechanism of action is closely related to the IGF axis. Initially used as an antidiabetic drug that reduces both glucose and insulin plasma concentrations, the role of this agent in cancer therapy is an exciting area of current research that is beyond the limits of this review and has been described elsewhere.[118] Patients treated with metformin seem to have a lower incidence of cancer than untreated controls in epidemiologic studies.[119–121] This biguanide affects tumor growth by reducing insulin secretion and by inhibiting AMPK-LKB1. Modulation of the IGF axis with a combination of drugs including metformin is promising and is currently under intense investigation.

CHALLENGES AND FUTURE DIRECTIONS

Almost 30 years after the IGF1 precursor[122] was sequenced, major advances are being witnessed in the understanding of IGF1 biology and the development of new and more sophisticated anticancer drugs exploiting this pathway. One of the greatest challenges for the future is the identification of predictive biomarkers to assist in patient selection. IGF1 levels, IGFBP-3 levels, and novel metabolic imaging techniques are just a few examples of the tools being used at the moment.[123,124]

As these agents are being administered to a higher number of patients, it is likely that unforeseen toxicities will become apparent. For example, there is the potential risk of central nervous system toxicity with prolonged exposure to IGF1R blocking agents, because IGF1 is known to provide a neuroprotective effect in the brain.[125]

Determining the most effective ways to combine IGF1R-targeted therapy with either cytotoxic chemotherapy or other targeted agents remains a challenge. As with other newly developed targeted therapies, mechanisms of acquired resistance to IGF1R blockade will be seen, and understanding these mechanisms will be a key for future development of these agents.

REFERENCES

1. Daughaday WH, Hall K, Raben MS, et al. Somatomedin: proposed designation for sulphation factor. Nature 1972;235:107.
2. Pollak M. Insulin and insulin-like growth factor signalling in neoplasia. Nat Rev Cancer 2008;8:915–28.
3. Gallagher EJ, LeRoith D. Minireview: IGF, insulin, and cancer. Endocrinology 2011;152:2546–51.
4. Riedemann J, Macaulay VM. IGF1R signalling and its inhibition. Endocr Relat Cancer 2006;13(Suppl 1):S33–43.
5. Pollak M. Insulin-like growth factor-related signaling and cancer development. Recent Results Cancer Res 2007;174:49–53.
6. De Meyts P. Insulin and its receptor: structure, function and evolution. Bioessays 2004;26:1351–62.
7. Benyoucef S, Surinya KH, Hadaschik D, et al. Characterization of insulin/IGF hybrid receptors: contributions of the insulin receptor L2 and Fn1 domains

and the alternatively spliced exon 11 sequence to ligand binding and receptor activation. Biochem J 2007;403:603–13.

8. Belfiore A. The role of insulin receptor isoforms and hybrid insulin/IGF-I receptors in human cancer. Curr Pharm Des 2007;13:671–86.

9. Laube F. Mannose-6-phosphate/insulin-like growth factor-II receptor in human melanoma cells: effect of ligands and antibodies on the receptor expression. Anticancer Res 2009;29:1383–8.

10. Scott CD, Firth SM. The role of the M6P/IGF-II receptor in cancer: tumor suppression or garbage disposal? Horm Metab Res 2004;36:261–71.

11. Jeyaratnaganthan N, Hojlund K, Kroustrup JP, et al. Circulating levels of insulin-like growth factor-II/mannose-6-phosphate receptor in obesity and type 2 diabetes. Growth Horm IGF Res 2010;20:185–91.

12. Samani AA, Yakar S, LeRoith D, et al. The role of the IGF system in cancer growth and metastasis: overview and recent insights. Endocr Rev 2007;28: 20–47.

13. Denley A, Bonython ER, Booker GW, et al. Structural determinants for high-affinity binding of insulin-like growth factor II to insulin receptor (IR)-A, the exon 11 minus isoform of the IR. Mol Endocrinol 2004;18:2502–12.

14. Favelyukis S, Till JH, Hubbard SR, et al. Structure and autoregulation of the insulin-like growth factor 1 receptor kinase. Nat Struct Biol 2001;8: 1058–63.

15. Buck E, Mulvihill M. Small molecule inhibitors of the IGF-1R/IR axis for the treatment of cancer. Expert Opin Investig Drugs 2011;20:605–21.

16. Shelton JG, Steelman LS, White ER, et al. Synergy between PI3K/Akt and Raf/MEK/ERK pathways in IGF-1R mediated cell cycle progression and prevention of apoptosis in hematopoietic cells. Cell Cycle 2004;3:372–9.

17. Levine AJ, Feng Z, Mak TW, et al. Coordination and communication between the p53 and IGF-1-AKT-TOR signal transduction pathways. Genes Dev 2006;20: 267–75.

18. Pollak MN. Insulin-like growth factors and neoplasia. Novartis Found Symp 2004;262:84–98 [discussion: 98–107, 265–8].

19. Kim SY, Wan X, Helman LJ. Targeting IGF-1R in the treatment of sarcomas: past, present and future. Bull Cancer 2009;96:E52–60.

20. Amiel SA, Sherwin RS, Hintz RL, et al. Effect of diabetes and its control on insulin-like growth factors in the young subject with type I diabetes. Diabetes 1984;33:1175–9.

21. Leung KC, Doyle N, Ballesteros M, et al. Insulin regulation of human hepatic growth hormone receptors: divergent effects on biosynthesis and surface translocation. J Clin Endocrinol Metab 2000;85:4712–20.

22. Busund LT, Ow KT, Russell P, et al. Expression of insulin-like growth factor mitogenic signals in adult soft-tissue sarcomas: significant correlation with malignant potential. Virchows Arch 2004;444:142–8.

23. Loeper S, Ezzat S. Acromegaly: re-thinking the cancer risk. Rev Endocr Metab Disord 2008;9:41–58.

24. Steuerman R, Shevah O, Laron Z. Congenital IGF1 deficiency tends to confer protection against post-natal development of malignancies. Eur J Endocrinol 2011;164:485–9.

25. Guevara-Aguirre J, Balasubramanian P, Guevara-Aguirre M, et al. Growth hormone receptor deficiency is associated with a major reduction in pro-aging signaling, cancer, and diabetes in humans. Sci Transl Med 2011;3: 70ra13.

26. Wu Y, Cui K, Miyoshi K, et al. Reduced circulating insulin-like growth factor I levels delay the onset of chemically and genetically induced mammary tumors. Cancer Res 2003;63:4384–8.
27. LeRoith D, Roberts CT Jr. The insulin-like growth factor system and cancer. Cancer Lett 2003;195:127–37.
28. Cui H, Cruz-Correa M, Giardiello FM, et al. Loss of IGF2 imprinting: a potential marker of colorectal cancer risk. Science 2003;299:1753–5.
29. Zhang L, Zhou W, Velculescu VE, et al. Gene expression profiles in normal and cancer cells. Science 1997;276:1268–72.
30. Giordano TJ, Kuick R, Else T, et al. Molecular classification and prognostication of adrenocortical tumors by transcriptome profiling. Clin Cancer Res 2009;15:668–76.
31. Ravenel JD, Broman KW, Perlman EJ, et al. Loss of imprinting of insulin-like growth factor-II (IGF2) gene in distinguishing specific biologic subtypes of Wilms tumor. J Natl Cancer Inst 2001;93:1698–703.
32. Xu W, Fan H, He X, et al. LOI of IGF2 is associated with esophageal cancer and linked to methylation status of IGF2 DMR. J Exp Clin Cancer Res 2006;25:543–7.
33. Zhan S, Shapiro DN, Helman LJ. Loss of imprinting of IGF2 in Ewing's sarcoma. Oncogene 1995;11:2503–7.
34. Li Y, Meng G, Huang L, et al. Hypomethylation of the P3 promoter is associated with up-regulation of IGF2 expression in human osteosarcoma. Hum Pathol 2009;40:1441–7.
35. Fu VX, Dobosy JR, Desotelle JA, et al. Aging and cancer-related loss of insulin-like growth factor 2 imprinting in the mouse and human prostate. Cancer Res 2008;68:6797–802.
36. Wu J, Qin Y, Li B, et al. Hypomethylated and hypermethylated profiles of H19DMR are associated with the aberrant imprinting of IGF2 and H19 in human hepatocellular carcinoma. Genomics 2008;91:443–50.
37. Huynh H, Yang X, Pollak M. Estradiol and antiestrogens regulate a growth inhibitory insulin-like growth factor binding protein 3 autocrine loop in human breast cancer cells. J Biol Chem 1996;271:1016–21.
38. Gucev ZS, Oh Y, Kelley KM, et al. Insulin-like growth factor binding protein 3 mediates retinoic acid- and transforming growth factor beta2-induced growth inhibition in human breast cancer cells. Cancer Res 1996;56:1545–50.
39. Rozen F, Yang XF, Huynh H, et al. Antiproliferative action of vitamin D-related compounds and insulin-like growth factor-binding protein 5 accumulation. J Natl Cancer Inst 1997;89:652–6.
40. Buckbinder L, Talbott R, Velasco-Miguel S, et al. Induction of the growth inhibitor IGF-binding protein 3 by p53. Nature 1995;377:646–9.
41. Duan C, Ren H, Gao S. Insulin-like growth factors (IGFs), IGF receptors, and IGF-binding proteins: roles in skeletal muscle growth and differentiation. Gen Comp Endocrinol 2010;167:344–51.
42. Frystyk J, Vestbo E, Skjaerbaek C, et al. Free insulin-like growth factors in human obesity. Metabolism 1995;44:37–44.
43. Grinspoon S, Clemmons D, Swearingen B, et al. Serum insulin-like growth factor-binding protein-3 levels in the diagnosis of acromegaly. J Clin Endocrinol Metab 1995;80:927–32.
44. Prieur A, Tirode F, Cohen P, et al. EWS/FLI-1 silencing and gene profiling of Ewing cells reveal downstream oncogenic pathways and a crucial role for repression of insulin-like growth factor binding protein 3. Mol Cell Biol 2004;24:7275–83.

45. Werner H, Shen-Orr Z, Rauscher FJ 3rd, et al. Inhibition of cellular proliferation by the Wilms' tumor suppressor WT1 is associated with suppression of insulin-like growth factor I receptor gene expression. Mol Cell Biol 1995;15:3516–22.

46. Coughlin SS, Calle EE, Teras LR, et al. Diabetes mellitus as a predictor of cancer mortality in a large cohort of US adults. Am J Epidemiol 2004;159:1160–7.

47. Calle EE, Rodriguez C, Walker-Thurmond K, et al. Overweight, obesity, and mortality from cancer in a prospectively studied cohort of U.S. adults. N Engl J Med 2003;348:1625–38.

48. Ahlgren M, Melbye M, Wohlfahrt J, et al. Growth patterns and the risk of breast cancer in women. N Engl J Med 2004;351:1619–26.

49. Chan JM, Stampfer MJ, Giovannucci E, et al. Plasma insulin-like growth factor-I and prostate cancer risk: a prospective study. Science 1998;279:563–6.

50. Diorio C, Pollak M, Byrne C, et al. Insulin-like growth factor-I, IGF-binding protein-3, and mammographic breast density. Cancer Epidemiol Biomarkers Prev 2005;14:1065–73.

51. Gualberto A, Pollak M. Emerging role of insulin-like growth factor receptor inhibitors in oncology: early clinical trial results and future directions. Oncogene 2009;28:3009–21.

52. All-Ericsson C, Girnita L, Seregard S, et al. Insulin-like growth factor-1 receptor in uveal melanoma: a predictor for metastatic disease and a potential therapeutic target. Invest Ophthalmol Vis Sci 2002;43:1–8.

53. Hakam A, Yeatman TJ, Lu L, et al. Expression of insulin-like growth factor-1 receptor in human colorectal cancer. Hum Pathol 1999;30:1128–33.

54. Turner BC, Haffty BG, Narayanan L, et al. Insulin-like growth factor-I receptor overexpression mediates cellular radioresistance and local breast cancer recurrence after lumpectomy and radiation. Cancer Res 1997;57:3079–83.

55. Hellawell GO, Turner GD, Davies DR, et al. Expression of the type 1 insulin-like growth factor receptor is up-regulated in primary prostate cancer and commonly persists in metastatic disease. Cancer Res 2002;62:2942–50.

56. Law JH, Habibi G, Hu K, et al. Phosphorylated insulin-like growth factor-I/insulin receptor is present in all breast cancer subtypes and is related to poor survival. Cancer Res 2008;68:10238–46.

57. Badzio A, Wynes MW, Dziadziuszko R, et al. Increased insulin-like growth factor 1 receptor protein expression and gene copy number in small cell lung cancer. J Thorac Oncol 2010;5:1905–11.

58. Bax DA, Mackay A, Little SE, et al. A distinct spectrum of copy number aberrations in pediatric high-grade gliomas. Clin Cancer Res 2010;16:3368–77.

59. Soroceanu L, Kharbanda S, Chen R, et al. Identification of IGF2 signaling through phosphoinositide-3-kinase regulatory subunit 3 as a growth-promoting axis in glioblastoma. Proc Natl Acad Sci U S A 2007;104:3466–71.

60. Belfiore A, Pandini G, Vella V, et al. Insulin/IGF-I hybrid receptors play a major role in IGF-I signaling in thyroid cancer. Biochimie 1999;81:403–7.

61. Frasca F, Pandini G, Sciacca L, et al. The role of insulin receptors and IGF-I receptors in cancer and other diseases. Arch Physiol Biochem 2008;114:23–37.

62. Sell C, Rubini M, Rubin R, et al. Simian virus 40 large tumor antigen is unable to transform mouse embryonic fibroblasts lacking type 1 insulin-like growth factor receptor. Proc Natl Acad Sci U S A 1993;90:11217–21.

63. Martin MJ, Melnyk N, Pollard M, et al. The insulin-like growth factor I receptor is required for Akt activation and suppression of anoikis in cells transformed by the ETV6-NTRK3 chimeric tyrosine kinase. Mol Cell Biol 2006;26:1754–69.

64. Toretsky JA, Kalebic T, Blakesley V, et al. The insulin-like growth factor-I receptor is required for EWS/FLI-1 transformation of fibroblasts. J Biol Chem 1997;272: 30822–7.

65. McKinsey EL, Parrish JK, Irwin AE, et al. A novel oncogenic mechanism in Ewing sarcoma involving IGF pathway targeting by EWS/Fli1-regulated microRNAs. Oncogene 2011;30(49):4910–20.

66. Casa AJ, Dearth RK, Litzenburger BC, et al. The type I insulin-like growth factor receptor pathway: a key player in cancer therapeutic resistance. Front Biosci 2008;13:3273–87.

67. Ge J, Chen Z, Wu S, et al. Expression levels of insulin-like growth factor-1 and multidrug resistance-associated protein-1 indicate poor prognosis in patients with gastric cancer. Digestion 2009;80:148–58.

68. Beech DJ, Parekh N, Pang Y. Insulin-like growth factor-I receptor antagonism results in increased cytotoxicity of breast cancer cells to doxorubicin and taxol. Oncol Rep 2001;8:325–9.

69. Warshamana-Greene GS, Litz J, Buchdunger E, et al. The insulin-like growth factor-I receptor kinase inhibitor, NVP-ADW742, sensitizes small cell lung cancer cell lines to the effects of chemotherapy. Clin Cancer Res 2005;11: 1563–71.

70. D'Cunja J, Shalaby T, Rivera P, et al. Antisense treatment of IGF-IR induces apoptosis and enhances chemosensitivity in central nervous system atypical teratoid/rhabdoid tumours cells. Eur J Cancer 2007;43:1581–9.

71. Min Y, Adachi Y, Yamamoto H, et al. Insulin-like growth factor I receptor blockade enhances chemotherapy and radiation responses and inhibits tumour growth in human gastric cancer xenografts. Gut 2005;54:591–600.

72. Luk F, Yu Y, Walsh WR, et al. IGF1R-targeted therapy and its enhancement of doxorubicin chemosensitivity in human osteosarcoma cell lines. Cancer Invest 2011;29:521–32.

73. Wang YH, Xiong J, Wang SF, et al. Lentivirus-mediated shRNA targeting insulin-like growth factor-1 receptor (IGF-1R) enhances chemosensitivity of osteosarcoma cells in vitro and in vivo. Mol Cell Biochem 2010;341:225–33.

74. Dallas NA, Xia L, Fan F, et al. Chemoresistant colorectal cancer cells, the cancer stem cell phenotype, and increased sensitivity to insulin-like growth factor-I receptor inhibition. Cancer Res 2009;69:1951–7.

75. Kai K, D'Costa S, Sills RC, et al. Inhibition of the insulin-like growth factor 1 receptor pathway enhances the antitumor effect of cisplatin in human malignant mesothelioma cell lines. Cancer Lett 2009;278:49–55.

76. Liu YC, Leu CM, Wong FH, et al. Autocrine stimulation by insulin-like growth factor I is involved in the growth, tumorigenicity and chemoresistance of human esophageal carcinoma cells. J Biomed Sci 2002;9:665–74.

77. Chen MY, Clark AJ, Chan DC, et al. Wilms' tumor 1 silencing decreases the viability and chemoresistance of glioblastoma cells in vitro: a potential role for IGF-1R de-repression. J Neurooncol 2011;103:87–102.

78. Lee JY, Han CY, Yang JW, et al. Induction of glutathione transferase in insulin-like growth factor type I receptor-overexpressed hepatoma cells. Mol Pharmacol 2007;72:1082–93.

79. Rochester MA, Riedemann J, Hellawell GO, et al. Silencing of the IGF1R gene enhances sensitivity to DNA-damaging agents in both PTEN wild-type and mutant human prostate cancer. Cancer Gene Ther 2005;12:90–100.

80. Cosaceanu D, Budiu RA, Carapancea M, et al. Ionizing radiation activates IGF-1R triggering a cytoprotective signaling by interfering with Ku-DNA binding and

by modulating Ku86 expression via a p38 kinase-dependent mechanism. Oncogene 2007;26:2423–34.

81. Macaulay VM, Salisbury AJ, Bohula EA, et al. Downregulation of the type 1 insulin-like growth factor receptor in mouse melanoma cells is associated with enhanced radiosensitivity and impaired activation of Atm kinase. Oncogene 2001;20:4029–40.

82. Peretz S, Jensen R, Baserga R, et al. ATM-dependent expression of the insulin-like growth factor-I receptor in a pathway regulating radiation response. Proc Natl Acad Sci U S A 2001;98:1676–81.

83. Shahrabani-Gargir L, Pandita TK, Werner H. Ataxia-telangiectasia mutated gene controls insulin-like growth factor I receptor gene expression in a deoxyribonucleic acid damage response pathway via mechanisms involving zinc-finger transcription factors Sp1 and WT1. Endocrinology 2004;145:5679–87.

84. Wakeling AE, Nicholson RI, Gee JM. Prospects for combining hormonal and nonhormonal growth factor inhibition. Clin Cancer Res 2001;7:4350s–5s [discussion: 4411s–2s].

85. Knowlden JM, Hutcheson IR, Barrow D, et al. Insulin-like growth factor-I receptor signaling in tamoxifen-resistant breast cancer: a supporting role to the epidermal growth factor receptor. Endocrinology 2005;146:4609–18.

86. Parisot JP, Hu XF, DeLuise M, et al. Altered expression of the IGF-1 receptor in a tamoxifen-resistant human breast cancer cell line. Br J Cancer 1999;79:693–700.

87. Nicholson RI, Gee JM. Oestrogen and growth factor cross-talk and endocrine insensitivity and acquired resistance in breast cancer. Br J Cancer 2000;82: 501–13.

88. Cunningham MP, Essapen S, Thomas H, et al. Coexpression of the IGF-IR, EGFR and HER-2 is common in colorectal cancer patients. Int J Oncol 2006; 28:329–35.

89. Mendelsohn J. The epidermal growth factor receptor as a target for cancer therapy. Endocr Relat Cancer 2001;8:3–9.

90. Slamon DJ, Clark GM, Wong SG, et al. Human breast cancer: correlation of relapse and survival with amplification of the HER-2/neu oncogene. Science 1987;235:177–82.

91. Press MF, Bernstein L, Thomas PA, et al. HER-2/neu gene amplification characterized by fluorescence in situ hybridization: poor prognosis in node-negative breast carcinomas. J Clin Oncol 1997;15:2894–904.

92. Morgillo F, Woo JK, Kim ES, et al. Heterodimerization of insulin-like growth factor receptor/epidermal growth factor receptor and induction of survivin expression counteract the antitumor action of erlotinib. Cancer Res 2006;66:10100–11.

93. Morgillo F, Kim WY, Kim ES, et al. Implication of the insulin-like growth factor-IR pathway in the resistance of non-small cell lung cancer cells to treatment with gefitinib. Clin Cancer Res 2007;13:2795–803.

94. Lu Y, Zi X, Zhao Y, et al. Insulin-like growth factor-I receptor signaling and resistance to trastuzumab (Herceptin). J Natl Cancer Inst 2001;93:1852–7.

95. Balana ME, Labriola L, Salatino M, et al. Activation of ErbB-2 via a hierarchical interaction between ErbB-2 and type I insulin-like growth factor receptor in mammary tumor cells. Oncogene 2001;20:34–47.

96. Thankamony GN, Dunger DB, Acerini CL. Pegvisomant: current and potential novel therapeutic applications. Expert Opin Biol Ther 2009;9:1553–63.

97. Dagnaes-Hansen F, Duan H, Rasmussen LM, et al. Growth hormone receptor antagonist administration inhibits growth of human colorectal carcinoma in nude mice. Anticancer Res 2004;24:3735–42.

98. McCutcheon IE, Flyvbjerg A, Hill H, et al. Antitumor activity of the growth hormone receptor antagonist pegvisomant against human meningiomas in nude mice. J Neurosurg 2001;94:487–92.

99. Hejna M, Schmidinger M, Raderer M. The clinical role of somatostatin analogues as antineoplastic agents: much ado about nothing? Ann Oncol 2002;13:653–68.

100. Jerome L, Alami N, Belanger S, et al. Recombinant human insulin-like growth factor binding protein 3 inhibits growth of human epidermal growth factor receptor-2-overexpressing breast tumors and potentiates herceptin activity in vivo. Cancer Res 2006;66:7245–52.

101. Alami N, Page V, Yu Q, et al. Recombinant human insulin-like growth factor-binding protein 3 inhibits tumor growth and targets the Akt pathway in lung and colon cancer models. Growth Horm IGF Res 2008;18:487–96.

102. Gao J, Chesebrough JW, Cartlidge SA, et al. Dual IGF-I/II-neutralizing antibody MEDI-573 potently inhibits IGF signaling and tumor growth. Cancer Res 2011; 71:1029–40.

103. Schneider-Merck T, Lammerts van Bueren JJ, Berger S, et al. Human IgG2 antibodies against epidermal growth factor receptor effectively trigger antibody-dependent cellular cytotoxicity but, in contrast to IgG1, only by cells of myeloid lineage. J Immunol 2010;184:512–20.

104. Kurzrock R, Patnaik A, Aisner J, et al. A phase I study of weekly R1507, a human monoclonal antibody insulin-like growth factor-I receptor antagonist, in patients with advanced solid tumors. Clin Cancer Res 2010;16:2458–65.

105. Pappo AS, Patel SR, Crowley J, et al. R1507, a monoclonal antibody to the insulin-like growth factor 1 receptor, in patients with recurrent or refractory Ewing sarcoma family of tumors: results of a phase II Sarcoma Alliance for Research through Collaboration study. J Clin Oncol 2011;29(34):4541–7.

106. Tolcher AW, Sarantopoulos J, Patnaik A, et al. Phase I, pharmacokinetic, and pharmacodynamic study of AMG 479, a fully human monoclonal antibody to insulin-like growth factor receptor 1. J Clin Oncol 2009;27:5800–7.

107. Olmos D, Postel-Vinay S, Molife LR, et al. Safety, pharmacokinetics, and preliminary activity of the anti-IGF-1R antibody figitumumab (CP-751,871) in patients with sarcoma and Ewing's sarcoma: a phase 1 expansion cohort study. Lancet Oncol 2010;11:129–35.

108. Pantaleo MA, Astolfi A, Nannini M, et al. The emerging role of insulin-like growth factor 1 receptor (IGF1r) in gastrointestinal stromal tumors (GISTs). J Transl Med 2010;8:117.

109. Braconi C, Bracci R, Cellerino R. Molecular targets in gastrointestinal stromal tumors (GIST) therapy. Curr Cancer Drug Targets 2008;8:359–66.

110. Janeway KA, Zhu MJ, Barretina J, et al. Strong expression of IGF1R in pediatric gastrointestinal stromal tumors without IGF1R genomic amplification. Int J Cancer 2010;127:2718–22.

111. Tarn C, Rink L, Merkel E, et al. Insulin-like growth factor 1 receptor is a potential therapeutic target for gastrointestinal stromal tumors. Proc Natl Acad Sci U S A 2008;105:8387–92.

112. Jassem J, Langer CJ, Karp DD, et al. Randomized, open label, phase III trial of figitumumab in combination with paclitaxel and carboplatin versus paclitaxel and carboplatin in patients with non-small cell lung cancer (NSCLC). J Clin Oncol 2010;28(Suppl; abstr 7500). Available at: http://meeting.ascopubs.org/cgi/content/abstract/28/15_suppl/7500. Accessed January 31, 2012.

113. Karp DD, Paz-Ares LG, Novello S, et al. Phase II study of the anti-insulin-like growth factor type 1 receptor antibody CP-751,871 in combination with

paclitaxel and carboplatin in previously untreated, locally advanced, or metastatic non-small-cell lung cancer. J Clin Oncol 2009;27:2516–22.

114. Buck E, Eyzaguirre A, Rosenfeld-Franklin M, et al. Feedback mechanisms promote cooperativity for small molecule inhibitors of epidermal and insulin-like growth factor receptors. Cancer Res 2008;68:8322–32.

115. Guix M, Faber AC, Wang SE, et al. Acquired resistance to EGFR tyrosine kinase inhibitors in cancer cells is mediated by loss of IGF-binding proteins. J Clin Invest 2008;118:2609–19.

116. Wan X, Harkavy B, Shen N, et al. Rapamycin induces feedback activation of Akt signaling through an IGF-1R-dependent mechanism. Oncogene 2007;26: 1932–40.

117. Naing A, Kurzrock R, Burger A, et al. Phase I trial of cixutumumab combined with temsirolimus in patients with advanced cancer. Clin Cancer Res 2011;17: 6052–60.

118. Pollak M. Metformin and other biguanides in oncology: advancing the research agenda. Cancer Prev Res (Phila) 2010;3:1060–5.

119. Monami M, Colombi C, Balzi D, et al. Metformin and cancer occurrence in insulin-treated type 2 diabetic patients. Diabetes Care 2011;34:129–31.

120. Chen TM, Lin CC, Huang PT, et al. Metformin associated with lower mortality in diabetic patients with early stage hepatocellular carcinoma after radiofrequency ablation. J Gastroenterol Hepatol 2011;26:858–65.

121. Bo S, Ciccone G, Rosato R, et al. Cancer mortality reduction and metformin. A retrospective cohort study in type 2 diabetic patients. Diabetes Obes Metab 2012;14(1):23–9.

122. Jansen M, van Schaik FM, Ricker AT, et al. Sequence of cDNA encoding human insulin-like growth factor I precursor. Nature 1983;306:609–11.

123. Heskamp S, van Laarhoven HW, Molkenboer-Kuenen JD, et al. ImmunoSPECT and immunoPET of IGF-1R expression with the radiolabeled antibody R1507 in a triple-negative breast cancer model. J Nucl Med 2010;51:1565–72.

124. Gualberto A, Pollak M. Clinical development of inhibitors of the insulin-like growth factor receptor in oncology. Curr Drug Targets 2009;10:923–36.

125. Freude S, Schilbach K, Schubert M. The role of IGF-1 receptor and insulin receptor signaling for the pathogenesis of Alzheimer's disease: from model organisms to human disease. Curr Alzheimer Res 2009;6:213–23.

Targeting Angiogenesis in Gynecologic Cancers

Behrouz Zand, MD[a], Robert L. Coleman, MD[a,b],
Anil K. Sood, MD[a,b,c],*

KEYWORDS

- Angiogenesis • Gynecologic cancer • Antiangiogenic drugs • Bevacizumab

KEY POINTS

- Recent insights at the molecular and cellular levels are paving the way for a more directed approach to target mechanisms driving tumorigenesis, such as angiogenesis.
- Antiangiogenic drugs have shown promise for treatment of gynecologic cancers in phase II and phase III trials.
- Clinical responses to antiangiogenesis drugs have been transitory, followed by progressive disease likely due to acquired resistance to such drugs.

Gynecologic malignancies, including cancers of the uterus, ovaries, cervix, fallopian tubes, vagina, and vulva, carry an estimated incidence of 83,750 cases per year and estimated mortality rate of more than 27,000 women per year.[1] Endometrial cancer is the most common gynecologic malignancy. Ovarian cancer, however, remains the most common cause of mortality from a gynecologic cancer. The reason for this is attributed to the advanced stage of ovarian cancer at the time of diagnosis, frequent

Behrouz Zand is supported by NCI-DHHS-NIH T32 Training Grant (T32 CA101642). Portions of this work were supported by the Gynecologic Cancer Foundation, the National Institutes of Health (CA 109298, P50 CA083639, P50 CA098258, CA128797, RC2GM092599, and U54 CA151668), the Ovarian Cancer Research Fund, Inc. (Program Project Development Grant), the DOD (OC073399, W81XWH-10-1-0158, and BC085265), Baylor College of Medicine and the MD Anderson Cancer Center Multidisciplinary Research Program, the Zarrow Foundation, the Marcus Foundation, the Blanton-Davis Ovarian Cancer Research Program, the Laura and John Arnold Foundation, the RGK Foundation, and the Betty Ann Asche Murray Distinguished Professorship.
[a] Department of Gynecologic Oncology and Reproductive Medicine, The University of Texas MD Anderson Cancer Center, 1155 Herman Pressler, Unit 1362, Houston, TX 77030, USA
[b] Center for RNA Interference and Non-Coding RNAs, The University of Texas MD Anderson Cancer Center, Houston, TX 77030, USA
[c] Department of Cancer Biology, The University of Texas MD Anderson Cancer Center, Houston, TX 77030, USA
* Corresponding author. Department of Cancer Biology, The University of Texas MD Anderson Cancer Center, 1155 Herman Pressler, Unit 1362, Houston, TX 77030.
E-mail address: asood@mdanderson.org

recurrences, and the emergence of drug resistance. Advances in surgery, chemotherapy, and patient care have improved outcomes for gynecologic malignancies, but overall survival (OS) rates seem to have plateaued.[2] Therefore, new therapies and therapeutic approaches are needed to improve the outlook for women with gynecologic cancers. Recent insights at the molecular and cellular levels are paving the way for a more directed approach to target mechanisms driving tumorigenesis, such as angiogenesis. This article reviews the roles of new and emerging antiangiogenesis drugs, summarizes the data obtained from clinical trials of antiangiogenic agents, and discusses trials under way to address the role of such strategies in gynecologic cancers.

ANGIOGENESIS

Development of new blood supply is essential for the development and maintenance of any tissue or organ.[3,4] For cancer to grow beyond 1 mm³ in size, it is necessary for the tumor to develop a sufficient blood supply.[4] Over the past several years, it has become apparent that neovascularization of tumors is a highly complex and regulated process. Classically, there are 2 distinct types of angiogenesis that have been described. The first is sprouting, which involves branching of new blood vessels from pre-existing blood vessels. The second type is splitting or nonsprouting angiogenesis, which involves the splitting of a lumen of an existing vessel. Unlike physiologic angiogenesis, tumor angiogenesis involves endothelial cells that fail to become quiescent.[5] These cells proliferate and grow uncontrollably and have a different phenotype from physiologic vasculature. Morphologically, the tumor vasculature is characterized by irregularly shaped vessels, which are dilated, tortuous, and disorganized.[6,7]

Recently, other mechanisms of tumor vascularization have been discovered. These include the recruitment of endothelial progenitor cells (EPCs), vessel co-option, vasculogenic mimicry, and lymphangiogenesis. EPCs are circulating cells in the blood that can form new blood vessels. The mobilization and recruitment of EPCs is promoted by several growth factors, chemokines, and cytokines produced during tumor growth.[8] Vessel co-option is a process whereby tumor cells can grow along existing blood vessels without evoking an angiogenic response in such vascular places, such as the brain or lungs.[9] Vasculogenic mimicry is the process of tumor cell plasticity, mainly in aggressive tumors, in which tumor cells dedifferentiate to an endothelial phenotype and make tube-like structures.[9] This mechanism provides an alternate route for tumor vascularization that may be independent of traditional angiogenesis processes. The majority of antiangiogenesis treatments, however, are currently tailored toward the sprouting biology of angiogenesis.

The establishment of angiogenesis relies on several proangiogenic factors, such as vascular endothelial growth factor (VEGF), basic fibroblast growth factor, platelet-derived growth factor (PDGF), ephrins, and their receptors. Tumor cells can produce proangiogenic factors for vessel formation. The vessel density and circulating tumor levels of proangiogenic factors VEGF and PDGF are poor prognostic indicators for many solid tumors, including ovarian, endometrial, and cervical carcinomas.[10–12] Due to their critical role in angiogenesis, proangiogenic factors are attractive therapeutic targets and highly studied in the area of cancer therapeutics.

BEVACIZUMAB

VEGF is a major proangiogenic factor and of the best characterized. It consists of family proteins of which VEGFA (synonymously called VEGF) is the dominant angiogenic factor.[13] It was originally known as vascular permeability factor/VEGF and its mechanism in angiogenesis was unclear.[14] Significant progress in angiogenesis research has elucidated that there are 3 VEGF receptors, with VEGFR-2 most significant for angiogenesis in most solid tumors.[13] On VEGF binding to its receptor on endothelial cells, a cascade of signaling events is activated that results in transcriptional activation of genes responsible for endothelial cell growth. Moreover, activated endothelial cells produce matrix metalloproteinases, which break down the extracellular matrix to allow migration of endothelial cells for new blood vessel formation.[15,16]

Among the various strategies for targeting VEGF, perhaps the most advanced is the monoclonal antibody bevacizumab. Bevacizumab is a humanized monoclonal antibody directed against human VEGF. It binds to VEGF to block its interaction with VEGF receptors (VEGFR-1 and VEGFR-2), with resultant inhibition of angiogenesis and endothelial cell proliferation.[17] It was the first drug the US Food and Drug Administration (FDA) approved for targeting tumor angiogenesis. Currently, bevacizumab is approved for a variety of solid tumors (eg, colorectal, renal cell, and nonsquamous non–small cell lung cancers and glioblastoma).[18]

Based on encouraging preclinical results, bevacizumab has been investigated clinically in ovarian cancer patients, both in frontline and recurrent disease settings. Response rates among women with recurrent disease ranged from 16% to 24% in initial phase II trials, with median survival of 10.7 to 17 months when bevacizumab was administered either as a single agent or in combination with cyclophosphamide.[19–21] In a phase II study of recurrent ovarian and primary peritoneal cancer, patients received single-agent bevacizumab every 3 weeks until disease progression or significant toxicity. Of the 62 evaluable patients, 21% had a clinical response, including 2 complete responses. Median progression-free survival (PFS) and OS rates were 4.7 and 17 months, respectively. This regimen was well tolerated, and no association was made between prior platinum sensitivity and hazard to progression or death.[19] In a phase II bevacizumab monotherapy study by Cannistra and colleagues,[20] 44 patients with platinum-resistant epithelial ovarian cancer and peritoneal serous cancer received single-agent bevacizumab every 3 weeks for 5 cycles. Overall response rate was 16%, and median PFS was 4.4 months. This study was terminated early due to a higher than expected incidence of bowel perforation of 11%. More of the toxicities of bevacizumab are discussed later. From these studies, it is apparent that bevacizumab has single-agent activity against ovarian cancer, and subsequent studies addressed its efficacy in combination with cytotoxic agents.

In a phase II study by Penson and colleagues,[22] 62 patients with primary epithelial ovarian, fallopian tube, uterine papillary serous, or primary peritoneal cancer were evaluated using carboplatin and paclitaxel in combination with bevacizumab. All 3 agents were given every 21 days for 6 to 8 cycles followed by bevacizumab every 3 weeks for 1 year. All patients had a CT scan after surgery and before chemotherapy and 45% of the study population had suboptimal cytoreduction (>1 cm residual disease). Radiographic responses were documented in 21 (75%) of 28 women with measurable disease, with CA-125 responses in 76% of patients. The median PFS was 29.8 months. These efficacy results were favorable compared with historical controls.[23] Another phase II study of patients with primary advanced-stage ovarian, peritoneal, or fallopian tube cancer used a treatment protocol of carboplatin/paclitaxel plus bevacizumab for 6 cycles and resulted in an overall 80% response rate. The toxicities were overall well tolerated and no gastrointestinal perforations occurred. Two patients had grade 3 hypertension.[24] A recent phase II, single-institution, open-label trial of intravenous (IV) bevacizumab in combination with intraperitoneal chemotherapy for patients with untreated primary advanced-stage ovarian cancer, however,

suggested that bowel toxicity may be exacerbated with this route of administration.[25]
Table 1 summarizes selected phase II trials with bevacizumab in gynecologic cancers.

There are several phase III clinical trials under way or recently completed in ovarian cancer. The Gynecologic Oncology Group (GOG) 218 and International Collaboration on Ovarian Neoplasms (ICON) 7 are 2 randomized phase III studies that include combination chemotherapy with maintenance therapy. In GOG 218, 1873 women with previously untreated advanced epithelial ovarian, primary peritoneal, or fallopian tube carcinoma showed that women who received bevacizumab in combination with paclitaxel and carboplatin, and continued on bevacizumab maintenance therapy for a total duration of 15 months, had a median PFS of 14.1 months compared with 10.3 months in women who received chemotherapy alone (hazard ratio [HR] 0.72, $P<.0001$).[26] ICON7 included 1528 women with previously untreated epithelial ovarian, primary peritoneal, or fallopian tube carcinoma. Women who received bevacizumab in combination with paclitaxel and carboplatin and continued use of bevacizumab maintenance for a total duration of up to 12 months had a median PFS of 18.3 months compared with 16 months in women who received chemotherapy alone (HR 0.79, $P = .001$).[27]

Several studies were also launched in the setting of relapsed ovarian cancer. The GOG 213 (NCT00565851) and OCEANS (NCT00434642) studies are evaluating chemotherapy and bevacizumab combinations (paclitaxel/carboplatin and gemcitabine/carboplatin, respectively) in patients with recurrent platinum-sensitive disease. The OCEANS study recently reported safety and efficacy data in 484 patients stratified

Table 1
Phase II trials of bevacizumab in gynecologic cancers

Study	Therapy	No. of Patients	Selection Criteria	SD (%)	PR (%)	CR (%)	Median PFS (Mo)/ Median OS (Mo)
Monk et al,[30] 2009	Bev	46	Recur CxCa	NA	10.9	0	3.40/7.29
Burger et al,[19] 2007	Bev	62	Recur OvaCa	51.6	17.7	3.2	4.7/16.9
Cannistra et al,[20] 2007	Bev	44	Ovaca	61.4	15.9	0	4.4/10.7
Aghajanian et al,[29] 2011	Bev	52	Recur EndoCa	NA	1.9	11.5	4.2/10.6
Micha et al,[24] 2007	CPB/PTX + bev	20	OvaCa	5	50	30	NA/NA
Penson et al,[22] 2010	CPB/PTX + bev	62	OvaCa	21	55	21	29.8/NA
Garcia et al,[21] 2008	Cyclo + bev	70	Recur OvaCa	63	24	0	7.2/16.9
Konner et al,[25] 2011	IV/IP PTX + IP CDDP + bev	41	OvaCa	NA	NA	NA	28.6/NA

Abbreviations: bev, bevacizumab; CDDP, cisplatin; CPB, carboplatin; CR, complete response; CxCa, cervical cancer; Cyclo, cyclophosphamide; EndoCa, endometrial cancer; IV, intravenous; IP, intraperitoneal; NA, not available; OvaCa, epithelial ovarian cancer; PR, partial response; PTX, paclitaxel; Recur, recurrent disease; SD, stable disease.

by length of platinum-free interval and performance of secondary surgery.[28] Unique in this design was the ability to maintain bevacizumab therapy to progression after 6 to 10 cycles of concomitant therapy with gemcitabine and carboplatin. No gastrointestinal perforations were observed on either arm of this placebo-controlled trial. Grade 3 hypertension and proteinuria were more frequently observed in the bevacizumab arm.The median PFS of the experimental arm was 12.4 months, however, and compared favorably with 8.4 months in the control arm (HR 0.484; 95% CI, 0.39–0.61; $P<.0001$). OS was immature at this report. The AURELIA trial is evaluating the addition of bevacizumab to paclitaxel, topotecan, and liposomal doxorubicin in patients with platinum-resistant ovarian cancer. **Table 2** shows the completed, ongoing, and future phase III trials of bevacizumab in gynecologic cancers.

Phase II studies have also reported some response with use of bevacizumab alone in the setting of persistent or recurrent endometrial and cervical cancer. In patients with recurrent endometrial cancer, bevacizumab treatment resulted in a response rate of 13.5% (1 complete response and 7 partial responses) with a median PFS of 3.4 months and OS of 7.29 months.[29] In patients with persistent or recurrent squamous cell carcinoma of the cervix, 23.9% had progression-free interval disease for

Table 2			
Phase III trials of bevacizumab in gynecologic cancers			
Trial	**Site of Disease**	**Drug Regimens**	**Date**
GOG 218	OvaCa	CPB + PTX vs CBP + PTX + bev vs CBP + PTX + bev, then maintenance bev	Sep 2005 to Oct 2008
ICON7	OvaCa	CBP + PTX with and without bev, then maintenance bev	Opened Apr 2006
GOG 252	OvaCa	IV vs IP platinum + PTX with IV bev, then maintenance bev	Opened Aug 2009
GOG 262	OvaCa	Dose dense PTX with bev	Opened Feb 2010
GOG 213	Platinum-sensitive recur OvaCa	CBP + PTX with and without bev, then maintenance bev	Opened Dec 2007
OCEANS	Platinum-sensitive recur OvaCa	CBP + GCB with and without bev	2007–2011
AURELIA	Platinum-resistant OvaCa	PTX + TPT + LD with and without bev	Opened Oct 2009
GCIG	Stage II–IV or recur MucOvaCa	CBP + PTX with and without bev, then maintenance bev vs OX + CAP with and without bev, then maintenance bev	Opened Jan 2010
GOG 240	Stage IVB, recur CxCa	CDDP + PTX with and without bev vs TPT/PTX with and without bev	Opened Apr 2009

Abbreviations: bev, bevacizumab; CAP, capecitabine; CBP, carboplatin; CDDP, cisplatin; CxCa, cervical cancer; EndoCa, endometrial cancer; GCB, gemcitabine; IV, intravenous; IP, intraperitoneal; LD, liposomal doxorubicin; MucOvaCa, mucinous ovarian cancer; OvaCa, epithelial ovarian cancer; OX, oxiplatin; PTX, paclitaxel; recur, recurrent disease; TPT, topotecan.

6 months and 10.9% had a partial response. The median PFS was 3.40 months and OS of 7.29 months. This compared favorably with historical GOG phase II trials in this setting.[30] **Table 1** provides a summary of selected phase II trials with bevacizumab in gynecologic cancers.

Although anti-VEGF treatments show some promise, there are concerns related to toxicity. The toxicities associated with bevacizumab have been documented from various trials and include hypertension, proteinuria, hemorrhage, neutropenia, venous thromboembolism, pulmonary embolus, congestive heart failure, myocardial infarction, and cerebrovascular ischemia. Hypertension is one the most common side effects of bevacizumab. The pathogenesis of bevacizumab-induced hypertension is not thoroughly understood. It is thought that VEGF antagonism can cause a decrease in nitric-oxide production by inhibition of nitric oxide synthase. Suppression of nitric oxide leads to vasoconstriction and decreased sodium ion renal excretion leading to high blood pressure.[31] The occurrence of hypertension is dose dependent. For example, the overall incidence of hypertension in patients receiving low-dose (3, 5, or 7.5 mg/kg/dose) versus higher-dose (10 or 15 mg/kg/dose) single-agent bevacizumab is 2.7% to 32% and 17.6% to 36%, respectively.[32] This bevacizumab toxicity may be useful as a clinical response parameter in patients. Among breast non–small cell lung cancer patients or colorectal cancer patients treated with bevacizumab, those with grades 2–4 hypertension had longer median survival compared with those without such elevation in blood pressure.[33–35] Perren and colleagues[27] and Scartozzi and colleagues[35] showed that in metastatic colorectal patients treated with bevacizumab, the median PFS was 14.5 months for patients showing bevacizumab-related hypertension, whereas it was 3.1 months in those without hypertension ($P = .04$). Although hypertension may be a good clinical measure of treatment response, bevacizumab-induced hypertension must be treated to avoid cardiovascular injury. Furthermore, permanent discontinuation of bevacizumab is recommended in patients who have hypertensive crisis.[36]

Proteinuria in response to bevacizumab can occur as a result of interference with VEGF-dependent glomerular endothelial injury.[37] It can also occur due to thrombotic microangiopathy. The proteinuria is typically asymptomatic and detected incidentally. Monitoring by use of regular urine dipstick should be considered. Those with dipstick reading of 2 g or more should undergo 24-hour urine total protein collection. Bevacizumab should be stopped if a patient is excreting at least 2 g of protein in a 24-hour period. Treatment may resume if the patient recovers within 3 weeks and has no sign of nephrotic syndrome.[36]

There is evidence of increased risk of arterial thromboembolic events associated with bevacizumab therapy. In a pooled data analysis of 1745 patient with metastatic colorectal cancer, non–small cell lung cancer, or breast cancer from 5 randomized trials, the addition of bevacizumab to chemotherapy was associated with increased risk of arterial thromboembolic events (overall incidence was 3.8% with bevacizumab vs 1.7% with chemotherapy). There was no difference with regard to venous thromboembolic events between the 2 groups.[38]

One of the most worrisome complications of bevacizumab in the setting of gynecologic cancers is intestinal perforation. Two phase II trials of bevacizumab in the treatment of ovarian cancer were stopped early due to a high rate of intestinal perforation (11%–15%).[20,39] Other studies have shown smaller incidence of intestinal perforation of approximately 4% to 5% in ovarian cancer.[40,41] Perforations are thought more prevalent in those with acute diverticulitis, intra-abdominal abscess, gastrointestinal obstruction, tumor at perforation site, abdominal carcinomatosis, and previous abdominal or pelvic radiotherapy.[42,43] Therefore, careful patient selection to reduce risk should be considered by limiting or excluding bevacizumab treatment in patients with clinical symptoms of bowel obstruction, rectosigmoid involvement on examination physical examination, and bowel involvement on CT.[44] There is an increased risk of wound healing complications in patients receiving bevacizumab. It is recommended that there is a 30-day window between discontinuation of bevacizumab and major surgery to lower the risk of surgical wound or bowel anastomosis complications.[36]

VEGF TRAP (AFLIBERCEPT)

VEGF Trap (aflibercept) is a protein that contains the VEGF binding regions of VEGFR-1 and VEGFR-2 fused to the Fc portion of human IgG1. It acts as a high-affinity soluble VEGFR decoy receptor and, therefore, inhibits the activity of VEGF.[45] Aflibercept is composed of entirely human protein sequences, and has a higher affinity to VEGF than bevacizumab. Furthermore, it can bind to placenta growth factor. The interactions between placenta growth factor and neuropilin-1 and neuropilin-2 provide additional regulation of tumor-associated vasculature.[46] Two randomized phase 2 studies were done in patients with recurrent ovarian cancer.[47,48] Results of these studies showed that in heavily pretreated patients, single-agent aflibercept could induce tumor response, delay progression, prevent reaccumulation of ascites, and prolong the time for the need for a paracentesis.

Coleman and colleagues[49] recently reported a combined phase I/II trial of docetaxel plus aflibercept in patients with recurrent ovarian, primary peritoneal, or fallopian tube cancer. In the phase II portion, patients were given aflibercept (6 mg/kg) and docetaxel (75 mg/m^2) every 3 weeks. Of the 46 patients enrolled in the phase II trial, 33 had platinum-resistant disease and 13 were platinum sensitive. Of the 46 patients enrolled in the phase II trial, 11 (24%) had a complete response, 14 had a partial response (30%), and 11 (24%) had stable disease. Median PFS was 6.4 months and median OS was 26.6 months. Similar to bevacizumab, aflibercept treatment was associated with fatigue, hypertension, and proteinuria.

SMALL MOLECULE TYROSINE KINASE INHIBITORS

Tyrosine kinases are widely considered of therapeutic interest because of their role in growth factor signaling. Small molecule tyrosine kinase inhibitors (SMTKIs) inhibit VEFGRs directly rather than binding the VEGF ligand as seen with bevacizumab.

Sorafenib

Sorafenib is an inhibitor of VEGFR-1, VEGFR-2, VEGFR-3, PDGF receptor (PDGFR)-β, and Raf-1 tyrosine kinase activity.[50] It is currently FDA approved for treatment of unresectable hepatocellular carcinoma and advanced renal cell carcinoma.[51,52] Matei and colleagues[53] evaluated sorafenib alone (400 mg orally twice daily) in patients with recurrent ovarian cancer or primary peritoneal cancer; 24% of the patients had stable disease for 6 months and 3.4% of patients had a partial response. This modest response was further hindered by substantial toxicity. These included significant grade 3 or 4 toxicities, such as rash, hand-foot syndrome, and metabolic, gastrointestinal, cardiovascular, and pulmonary toxicities. These investigators did not recommended continuation of monotherapy with sorafenib for recurrent ovarian and primary peritoneal cancer. Sorafenib has been evaluated in a phase II trial in combination with gemcitabine in recurrent ovarian cancer and found to have a rate of stable disease at 60% with a 4.7% partial response rate. The median time to progression was 5.4 months, and the median OS was 13.0 months.[54] To determine the efficacy and toxicity of the sorafenib and topotecan combination in platinum-resistant ovarian cancer, a combined analysis of phase I/II showed a partial responses rate of 16.7%; however, only one patient (7%) had a partial response in the phase II portion. The overall stable disease rate was 46.7%. The median PFS was 3.7 months (95% CI, 3.0–5.5) and median OS was 14.0 months.[55] Currently, a phase II trial of sorafenib in combination with carboplatin/paclitaxel for first-line treatment of ovarian cancer is under way.[56]

Nimeiri and colleagues[57] evaluated patients with advanced uterine carcinoma and carcinosarcoma in a phase II trial with sorafenib (400 mg orally twice daily). The results were modest, showing a partial response rate of 5%, and 42.5% achieved stable disease. The 6-month PFS rate was 29%, and the median OS was 11.4 months.

Sunitinib

Sunitinib, also a multikinase inhibitor, blocks VEGFR-1, VEGFR-2, VEGFR-3, PDGFR-β, and RET.[58] It is currently FDA approved for advanced renal cell carcinoma and gastrointestinal stromal tumors.[58] A phase II trial of patients with recurrent epithelial ovarian and primary peritoneal cancer using monotherapy sunitinib resulted in a partial response rate of 3.3%; 53% of patients had stable disease. Overall median PFS was 4.1 months. Common adverse events included fatigue, gastrointestinal symptoms, hand-foot syndrome, and hypertension.[59]

A multicenter phase II study was performed to evaluate the activity of sunitinib in women with locally advanced or metastatic cervical cancer. Sunitinib (50 mg/d) was administered in 6-week cycles (4 weeks on treatment followed by 2 weeks off treatment). Approximately 84% of patients had stable disease, and the median time to progression was 3.5 months. Fatigue, diarrhea, nausea, taste alteration, hypertension, mucositis, and heartburn were the most common nonhematological adverse events. Hematological toxicity was mostly grade 1 or 2 although grade 3 lymphopenia was reported in 7 patients and grade 4 in one. The biggest concern in this study was a high fistula rate of 26.3%, which included rectovaginal, enterocutaneous, and bladder-peritoneal. The investigators did not recommend continuation of sunitinib monotherapy in this clinical setting for a phase III trial.[60] In phase II studies of patients with recurrent uterine leiomyosarcoma, sunitinib monotherapy resulted in a partial response rate of 8.7%. The PFS rate at 6 months was 17.4%. The median PFS was 1.5 months and the trial failed to meet the objective response.[61]

Overall, the side-effect profile of sorafenib and sunitinib seems similar to that of bevacizumab. One additional side effect seen with these SMTKIs is hand-foot syndrome. A combination of antiangiogenic agents has been shown to improve efficacy; however, it comes at an added cost of increased toxicity. In a study of combined sorafenib and bevacizumab, there was a 43% response rate in ovarian cancer patients. The combination therapy increased toxicity, however, necessitating the need for dose reduction of sorafenib.[62]

Cediranib

Cediranib is a tyrosine kinase inhibitor (TKI) of VEGFR-1, VEGFR-2, VEGFR-3, PDGFR-α, and c-kit. In a phase II study of cediranib monotherapy for recurrent ovarian cancer, peritoneal cancer, and fallopian tube cancer, there was a partial response rate of 17%, 13% had stable disease, and there were no complete responses. Median PFS was 5.2 months, and 17% were free of progression at 6 months. Eleven patients (23%) were removed from the study because of toxicities before 2 cycles. Grade 3 toxicities (>20% of patients) included hypertension (46%), fatigue (24%), and diarrhea (13%). Grade 2 hypothyroidism occurred in 43% of patients. Grade 4 toxicities included CNS hemorrhage (n = 1), hypertriglyceridemia/hypercholesterolemia (n = 1), and dehydration/elevated creatinine (n = 1). No bowel perforations or fistulas occurred.[63] Currently, the ICON6 study, in a phase III trial, is investigating the role of combination daily cediranib with carboplatin/paclitaxel or carboplatin/gemcitabine for 6 cycles followed by at least 18 months or until progression of daily cediranib for recurrent platinum-sensitive ovarian cancer.[64]

Pazopanib

Pazopanib is an inhibitor of VEGFR-1, VEGFR-2, VEGFR-3, PDGFR-α, PDGFR-β, and c-kit. Pazopanib is FDA approved for the treatment of patients with advanced renal cell carcinoma. In a phase II trial of recurrent ovarian, fallopian tube, and primary peritoneal cancer, the CA-125 response rate was 31%. No patients with measurable disease had a partial or complete response. The PFS at 6 months was 17%. The most common side effects were diarrhea, fatigue, and nausea. The most common adverse events leading to discontinuation of study drug were grade 3 ALT (8%) and AST (8%) elevation. Only one grade 4 toxicity (peripheral edema) was reported.[65] Currently, pazopanib is being investigated as maintenance therapy in a double-blind, placebo-controlled, phase III clinical study in women who have achieved a partial or complete response to primary platinum-based adjuvant chemotherapy in ovarian cancer (NCT00866697).

In advanced and recurrent cervical cancer, a phase II trial evaluated a combination of daily oral pazopanib and oral lapatinib (dual anti–epidermal growth factor receptor [EGFR] and anti-HER2/neu TKI) versus daily oral pazopanib or daily oral lapatinib monotherapy. Randomization of 228 patients resulted in 78 patients (34%) assigned to the lapatinib arm, 74 patients (33%) to the pazopanib arm, and 76 patients (33%) to the combination arm. Combination therapy arm was discontinued, however, due to higher rate of toxicity and discontinuation of drugs. Also, the futility boundary was crossed for combination therapy versus lapatinib monotherapy. PFS improved with pazopanib compared with lapatinib (median PFS, 17.1 weeks vs 18.1 weeks; HR 0.66; 90% CI, 0.48 to 0.91; $P<.013$). OS was 11.6 weeks longer in the pazopanib arm compared with the lapatinib arm (median OS, 50.7 weeks vs 39.1 weeks; HR 0.67; 90% CI, 0.46 to 0.99; $P = .045$).[66]

BIBF 1120

BIBF 1120 is a potent inhibitor of VEGFR as well as PDGF and fibroblast growth factor receptor. In a randomized phase II placebo-controlled trial, patients who had just completed chemotherapy for relapsed ovarian cancer, with evidence of response, but at high risk of further early recurrence were treated with BIBF 1120. The study drug was taken continuously (28-day cycles) for 9 cycles (36 weeks) or until disease progression or patient withdrawal. The 36-week PFS 26-week rates were 16.3% and 5.0% in the BIBF 1120 and placebo groups, respectively (HR 0.65; 95% CI, 0.42 to 1.02; $P = .06$). Toxicity was also well tolerated.[67] This has prompted a phase III trial (NCT01015118) where BIBF 1120 will be combined with carboplatin/paclitaxel as front-line chemotherapy in ovarian cancer. **Table 3** summarizes studies involving these SMTKIs.

EPIDERMAL GROWTH FACTOR RECEPTOR ANTIBODIES AND TYROSINE KINASE INHIBITORS

Given the heterogeneity, the redundancy of aberrant pathways, and the contribution of microenvironment to the survival, growth, and metastasis of solid tumors, it is attractive to target multiple pathways that can contribute to angiogenesis.[68] Experimental

Table 3
Clinical trials of SMTKIs

Study	Therapy	No. of Patients	Selection Criteria	SD (%)	PR (%)	CR (%)	Median PFS (mo)/ Median OS (mo)
Matei et al,[53] 2011	Sora	71	Recur OvaCa	33.9	3.4	0	2.1/16.33
Nimeiri et al,[57] 2010	Sora	56	Recur UC or UCS	42.5[a] 25[b]	5[a] 0[b]	0[a] 0[b]	3.2/11.4[a] 1.8/5.0[b]
Welch et al,[54] 2010	Sora + GCB	33	Recur OvaCa	23.3	4.7	0	5.4/13.0
Ramasubbaiah et al,[55] 2011	Sora + TPT	30	Recur OvaCa	46.7	16.7	0	3.7/14.0
Mackay et al,[60] 2010	Suni	19	LACC or MCC	84	0	0	3.5/NA
Biagi et al,[59] 2011	Suni	30	Recur OvaCa	36.7	3.3	0	4.1/NA
Matulonis et al,[63] 2009	Cedi	46	Recur OvaCa	13	17	0	5.2/NA
Friedlander et al,[65] 2010	Pazo	17	Recur OvaCa	18	18	0	NA/NA
Monk et al,[66] 2010	Pazo vs Lap	Pazo = 74 Lap = 78	LACC and Recur cervix	43 44	8 4	1 1	18.1/50.7 17.1/39.1

Abbreviations: Cedi, cediranib; CR, complete response; GCB, gemcitabine; LACC, locally advanced cervical cancer; Lap, lapatinib; MCC, metastatic cervical cancer; NA, not available; OvaCa, epithelial ovarian cancer; Pazo, pazopanib; PR, partial response; Recur, recurrent disease; SD, stable disease; Sora, sorafenib; Suni, sunitinib; TPT, topotecan; UC, uterine carcinoma; UCS, uterine carcinosarcoma.
[a] Uterine carcinoma.
[b] Uterine carcinosarcoma.

evidence has shown that these pathways are functionally linked and has demonstrated a role for VEGF in the acquired resistance to anti-EGFR drugs when these receptors are pharmacologically blocked.[64,69] Combined inhibition of EGFR and VEGF signaling interferes with a molecular feedback loop responsible for acquired resistance to anti-ErbB agents and promotes apoptosis while ablating tumor-induced angiogenesis.[68,70]

Like VEGF, EGFR is a tyrosine kinase receptor in the cell membrane. EGFR is in a family of 4 members: EGFR (Her1), ErbB2 (Her2), ErbB3 (Her3), and ErbB4 (Her4).[71] The ligand, epidermal growth factor (EGF) and transforming growth factor α, binds to EGFR, which then dimerizes the receptor and turns on the signaling cascade pathways to cause cellular proliferation, motility, invasion, apoptosis, and angiogenesis. EGFR family members can also be activated by other signaling proteins independent of exogenous EGF ligands. These include other receptor tyrosine kinases, such as insulinlike growth factor 1 receptor.[72] EGFR is overexpressed in 60% of ovarian cancers, 60% to 80% of endometrial cancers, 73% of cervical carcinomas, and 68% of vulvar malignancies. It has been shown associated with advanced cancer stage and poorer prognosis.[61,73–77] Tumor-associated endothelial cells can express EGFR, and EGFR expression can induce VEGF expression in cancer cells.[78] In vivo studies of EGFR have shown increased sensitivity of tumors to chemotherapy and radiation therapy.[79,80] EGFR and ErbB2 generally induce cytostatic effects in vitro and rarely cause apoptosis.[81,82] In vivo studies, however, show anti-EGFR treatment leads to tumor regression,[5] likely due to EFGR affecting host-tumor reactions leading to cell death. For the strategy to block EGFR activity, 2 types of inhibitors are currently used: (1) monoclonal antibodies and (2) EGFR TKIs.

Monoclonal Antibodies

Cetuximab is a monoclonal antibody against EGFR and has shown improved survival in patients with head/neck and colorectal carcinoma.[83,84] In a phase II trial of relapsed platinum-sensitive ovarian cancer patients who underwent combination therapy of cetuximab and carboplatin, 26 (92.9%) had EGFR-positive tumors, and the response rate in this group included 9 who demonstrated an objective response (3 complete responses and 6 partial responses) and 8 with stable disease. The response rate did not meet criteria for opening a second stage of accrual.[85] In a phase II trial of front-line treatment for advanced ovarian cancer, cetuximab was combined with carboplatin and paclitaxel. The median PFS was 14.4 months, and PFS at 18 months was 38.8%. This combination did not demonstrate prolongation of PFS when compared with historical data.[86] Finally, cetuximab monotherapy was evaluated in a phase II trial of recurrent/persistent ovarian cancer where minimal activity was found with this strategy. One of 25 patients achieved partial remission and 9 patients had stable disease. The median PFS was 2.1 months.[87]

In cervical cancer, cetuximab therapy has had minimal to no effect in recent phase II clinical trials. In a phase II trial of advanced squamous cell or adenocarcinoma of the cervix, cetuximab was combined with cisplatin and topotecan chemotherapy. There were no complete responses, and the partial response and stable disease rate was 32%. This study was stopped due to excess toxicity from the treatments.[88] In another phase II study in advanced cervical cancer, cetuximab was combined with cisplatin. There was a 29.6% partial response rate and 4.8% complete response rate. Based on these results, phase III development was not recommended because there was no additional benefit with cetuximab therapy.[89] Using cetuximab as monotherapy was largely ineffective in advanced cervical cancer. In a phase II trial of squamous and nonsquamous cell recurrent cervical cancer, there were no partial or complete responses with cetuximab monotherapy.[90]

Two other EGFR monoclonal antibodies studied in gynecologic cancers are matuzumab and trastuzumab. Matuzumab monotherapy was evaluated in a phase II trial of recurrent platinum refractory ovarian cancer or primary peritoneal cancer. In this study, there were no partial or complete responses. The stable disease rate was 16.2%, and median PFS was 1.9 months.[91] In 2008, matuzumab was discontinued due to poor efficacy in clinical trials.[18] Trastuzumab is an anti-Her2 antibody and has been studied in phase II trials in ovarian and endometrial cancers. Her2 gene amplification has been found to directly correlate with poor clinical outcomes in many malignancies, including breast cancer.[92] Data regarding Her2 overexpression and its association with prognosis in ovarian cancer are controversial. Early studies suggested that Her2 overexpression in ovarian cancer was a frequent event; however, subsequent studies using techniques for validation suggest that Her2 overexpression and amplification frequency in ovarian cancer are much rarer.[93] Furthermore, overexpression of Her2 has been associated with a worse prognosis in some studies but not others.[94,95] In a phase II trial of persistent or refractory ovarian cancer, 1 patient had a complete response and 2 patients had a partial response. Furthermore, immunohistochemistry revealed only 11.4% had Her2-positive cancers.[96] In a prospective cohort study of mucinous ovarian cancers, Her2 amplification was present in 18.2% of patients, although it was not of prognostic significance.[95] In advanced endometrial cancer, HER-2 overexpression via immunohistochemistry and HER-2 gene amplification via fluorescence in situ hybridization were detected in 44% (104 of 234) and 12% (21 of 182) of specimens, respectively.[97] The results of trastuzumab in endometrial cancer have been disappointing. In a phase II trial of advanced or recurrent Her2-positive endometrial cancer, trastuzumab treatment resulted in no objective responses and the trial was stopped early due to poor accrual.[98]

EGFR Tyrosine Kinase Inhibitors

EGFR TKIs act intracellularly by competing with ATP binding in the catalytic region of the kinase domain, thereby inhibiting enzymatic activity and its downstream effects.[72] Although these TKIs can target EGFR, many can also target mutant receptors, like EGFRvIII, that lack the critical extracellular regulatory region targeted by some of the antibodies.[72]

Gefitinib (Iressa or ZD1839) has been evaluated in several phase II trials in gynecologic cancers. Posadas and colleagues[99] evaluated 24 patients with platinum refractory ovarian cancer. No objective responses occurred. Approximately 37% of patients had stable disease for greater than 2 months. A phase II trial of persistent or recurrent ovarian cancer with gefitinib showed a partial response of 3.7%. In a phase II trial of recurrent or metastatic cervical cancer, gefitinib monotherapy was evaluated. The majority (86.7%) of patient biopsies expressed high levels of EGFR (2+ or 3+ staining intensity). No patients had an objective response from treatment, and 20% of patients had stable disease. The most common drug-related side effects were diarrhea, acne, vomiting, and nausea.[100]

Another EGFR TKI is erlotinib and has shown minimal activity in gynecologic cancers. In a phase II trial of recurrent or progressive ovarian cancer positive for EGFR, no complete responses and 6% partial response rate occurred with erlotinib therapy.[36] In a phase II trial of recurrent or refractory ovarian cancer, erlotinib and bevacizumab combination therapy was evaluated. The complete response rate and partial response rate with this combination was 7.7% each. Due to the lack of improvement compared with bevacizumab therapy alone and 2 incidents of fatal gastric perforations, the study was stopped.[39] In a phase II trial of recurrent cervical cancer patients treated with erlotinib, there were no objective responses, with 4 (16%) achieving stable disease; only 1 patient had a PFS greater than or equal to 6 months (4%). Erlotinib was well tolerated with the most common drug-related adverse events gastrointestinal toxicities, fatigue, and rash.[101] A summary of clinical trials in gynecologic cancers with EGFR inhibition is in **Table 4**.

In summary, clinical trials using anti-EGFR therapy have shown limited activity in gynecologic cancers. Given the high expression of EGFR in gynecologic malignancies, future studies using it in combination with cytotoxic therapy may be beneficial. Furthermore, determining reliable biomarkers to assess patient responsiveness can help monitor EGFR dependent malignancies.

ALTERNATIVE TARGETS AND STRATEGIES

Although the studies (discussed previously) have revealed an arsenal of molecular drugs that can target angiogenesis, tumor progression eventually occurs and no difference in OS has been accomplished with current clinical trials in antiangiogenesis drugs. Therefore, different strategies and targets for angiogenesis are needed. One strategy that may hold promise to fight tumor progression includes agents that target components of the tumor microenvironment. For example, pericytes are cells surrounding endothelial cells and are required for microvascular stability and function.

Table 4
Phase II clinical trials of EGFR inhibitors in gynecologic cancers

Study	Therapy	No. of Patients	Selection Criteria	SD (%)	PR (%)	CR (%)	Median PFS/Median OS	Comments
Schilder et al,[80] 2009	Cetux	25	Recur OvaCa	36	4	0	1.8/13	—
Santin et al,[90] 2011	Cetux	35	Recur CxCa	31.4	0	0	1.97/6.7	—
Secord et al,[85] 2008	Cetux + CBP	26	Recur platinum-sensitive OvaCa	11.5	23	11.5	9.4/NA	32% Acniform rash, 18% grade 3–4 hypersensitivity reaction
Konner et al,[86] 2008	Cetux + PTX + CBP	40	OvaCa	NA	NA	NA	14.4/NA	Did not demonstrate prolongation of PFS when compared with historical data
Kurtz et al,[88] 2009	CSP + TPT + cetux	19	Advance CxCa	32	32	0	5.7/7.2	Study stopped due to excess toxicity (myelosuppression)
Farley et al,[89] 2011	CSP + cetux	27	Advanced or recur CxCa	NA	29.6	3.7	3.91/8.77	No additional benefit compared with cisplatin alone
Seiden et al,[91] 2007	Matzu	37	Recur platinum refractory OvaCa	16.2	0	0	1.9/10.3	—
Fleming et al,[98] 2010	Matzu	33	Advanced or recur EndoCa	36.3	0	0	1.81–1.84/6.8–7.85	—
Posadas et al,[99] 2007	Gefi	24	Platinum-refractory OvaCa	37	0	0	NA/NA	—
Schilder et al,[87] 2009	Gefi	27	Recur OvaCa	36	0	0	1.87/13	—
Goncalves et al,[100] 2008	Gefi	28	Recur or met CxCa	20	0	0	1.22/3.51	—
Gordon et al,[113] 2005	Erlo	34	Recur OvaCa	44	6	0	4.58/8.00	—
Nimeiri al,[39] 2008	Erlo + bev	13	Recur OvaCa	54	7.7	7.7	4.1/11.0	—
Schilder et al,[101] 2009	Erlo	28	Recur CxCa	16	0	0	1.87/4.96	—

Abbreviations: bev, bevacizumab; CBP, carboplatin; cetux, cetuximab; CSP, cisplatin; CxCa, cervical cancer; Erlo, Erlotinib; Gefi, gefitinib; Matzu, matuzumab; NA, not available; OvaCa, epithelial ovarian cancer; PTX, paclitaxel; Recur, recurrent disease.

Based on the known role of PDGF-BB/PDGFR-β in pericyte regulation, highly specific inhibitors against PDGF-B were tested in ovarian cancer models with the agent AX102. A combination of bevacizumab with AX102 was more effective than bevacizumab alone and resulted in 76% and 88% inhibition of tumor growth.[102] Therefore, dual targeting of endothelial cells and pericytes holds potential as an antivascular therapeutic approach in ovarian carcinoma.

Other targets identified in the tumor vasculature include the enhancer of zeste homolog 2 (EZH2) and focal adhesion kinase (FAK). EZH2 has been identified as a key regulator of tumor angiogenesis. EZH2 silencing in the tumor-associated endothelial cells using small interfering RNA resulted in significant growth inhibition in an orthotopic ovarian cancer model. EZH2 silencing in tumor endothelial cells also resulted in decreased angiogenesis.[103] FAK plays a critical role in ovarian cancer cell survival and in various steps in the metastatic cascade. Treatment with FAK small interfering RNA–dioleoylphosphatidylcholine plus docetaxel resulted in decreased microvessel density, decreased expression of VEGF and matrix metalloproteinase 9, and increased apoptosis of tumor-associated endothelial cells and tumor cells.[104] As research into the field of angiogenesis continues to rapidly advance, more molecular targets will be identified and new antiangiogenesis targets will be available to combat tumor growth.

AMG 386 is an investigational, angiopoietin antagonist peptide-Fc fusion protein that selectively binds Ang1 and Ang2, prevents their interaction with Tie2, and inhibits tumor endothelial cell proliferation and tumor growth.[105] Results from a randomized, double-blind, placebo-controlled phase II study to evaluate the safety and tolerability of AMG 386 (3 or 10 mg/kg IV weekly) in combination with paclitaxel (80 mg/m^2 IV weekly [3 weeks on/1 week off]) in patients with advanced recurrent epithelial ovarian, primary peritoneal, or fallopian tube cancer were recently presented at the American Society of Clinical Oncology 2010 annual meeting. The addition of AMG 386 to paclitaxel demonstrated dose-responsive improvements in PFS together with a manageable safety profile distinct from that of VEGF inhibition.[106] Cabozantinib (XL-184) is an oral, potent inhibitor of MET and VEGFR-2. MET overexpression has been observed in variety of solid tumors, including advanced ovarian cancer.[107] MET drives more invasive and aggressive behavior of tumor cells, resulting in metastasis.[107,108] MET is further up-regulated by the hypoxic conditions created by VEGF pathway inhibitors, which leads to promotion of metastasis.[107,108] Results from a phase II trial of cabozantinib (100 mg/d orally for 12 weeks) with advanced progressive epithelial ovarian cancer showed a high clinical response (overall 24%).[109] Due to these promising results, AMG 386 and cabozantinib are entering phase III trials.

SUMMARY

Antiangiogenic drugs have shown promise for treatment of gynecologic cancers in phase II and phase III trials. Several targets in angiogenesis pathways have been identified and drugs targeting these areas have been and are under evaluation. Currently, bevacizumab, especially in ovarian cancer, seems to hold the most promising results. Whether other agents, such as aflibercept or SMTKIs, will have similar or better success requires additional work.

Unfortunately, the clinical responses to antiangiogenesis drugs have been transitory, followed by progressive disease. This is likely due to inherent or acquired resistance to such drugs.[110] Therefore, an important area of ongoing research involves identification of reliable predictive markers and understanding the mechanisms of resistance to antiangiogenesis agents.[108,111,112] The authors expect that a deeper understanding of such biology will result in better therapeutic approaches that can improve the outcome of patients suffering from gynecologic or other malignancies.

REFERENCES

1. Jemal A, Siegel R, Xu J, et al. Cancer statistics, 2010. CA Cancer J Clin 2010; 60(5):277–300.
2. Bast RC Jr, Hennessy B, Mills GB. The biology of ovarian cancer: new opportunities for translation. Nat Rev Cancer 2009;9(6):415–28.
3. Achen MG, Stacker SA. The vascular endothelial growth factor family; proteins which guide the development of the vasculature. Int J Exp Pathol 1998;79(5): 255–65.
4. Folkman J. What is the evidence that tumors are angiogenesis dependent? J Natl Cancer Inst 1990;82(1):4–6.
5. Hanahan D, Folkman J. Patterns and emerging mechanisms of the angiogenic switch during tumorigenesis. Cell 1996;86(3):353–64.
6. Baluk P, Hashizume H, McDonald DM. Cellular abnormalities of blood vessels as targets in cancer. Curr Opin Genet Dev 2005;15(1):102–11.
7. Nagy JA, Chang SH, Shih SC, et al. Heterogeneity of the tumor vasculature. Semin Thromb Hemost 2010;36(3):321–31.
8. Ahn GO, Brown J. Role of endothelial progenitors and other bone marrow-derived cells in the development of the tumor vasculature. Angiogenesis 2009;12(2):159–64.
9. Döme B, Hendrix MJ, Paku S, et al. Alternative vascularization mechanisms in cancer: pathology and therapeutic implications. Am J Pathol 2007;170(1): 1–15.
10. Kaku T, Kamura T, Kinukawa N, et al. Angiogenesis in endometrial carcinoma. Cancer 1997;80(4):741–7.
11. Bremer GL, Tiebosch AT, van der Putten HW, et al. Tumor angiogenesis: an independent prognostic parameter in cervical cancer. Am J Obstet Gynecol 1996; 174(1 Pt 1):126–31.
12. Alvarez AA, Krigman HR, Whitaker RS, et al. The prognostic significance of angiogenesis in epithelial ovarian carcinoma. Clin Cancer Res 1999;5(3): 587–91.
13. Ellis LM, Hicklin DJ. VEGF-targeted therapy: mechanisms of anti-tumour activity. Nat Rev Cancer 2008;8(8):579–91.
14. Dvorak HF, Brown LF, Detmar M, et al. Vascular permeability factor/vascular endothelial growth factor, microvascular hyperpermeability, and angiogenesis. Am J Pathol 1995;146(5):1029–39.
15. Mignatti P, Rifkin DB. Plasminogen activators and matrix metalloproteinases in angiogenesis. Enzyme Protein 1996;49(1–3):117–37.
16. Cierniewski CS, Malinowski M, Bednarek R, et al. Adhesive and proteolytic phenotype of migrating endothelial cells induced by thymosin beta-4. Ann N Y Acad Sci 2007;1112:123–39.
17. Samant RS, Shevde LA. Recent advances in anti-angiogenic therapy of cancer. Oncotarget 2011;2(3):122–34.
18. Available at: http://www.takeda.com/press/article_29042.html. Accessed February 18, 2008.
19. Burger RA, Sill MW, Monk BJ, et al. Phase II trial of bevacizumab in persistent or recurrent epithelial ovarian cancer or primary peritoneal cancer: a Gynecologic Oncology Group Study. J Clin Oncol 2007;25(33):5165–71.

20. Cannistra SA, Matulonis UA, Penson RT, et al. Phase II study of bevacizumab in patients with platinum-resistant ovarian cancer or peritoneal serous cancer. J Clin Oncol 2007;25(33):5180–6.

21. Garcia AA, Hirte H, Fleming G, et al. Phase II clinical trial of bevacizumab and low-dose metronomic oral cyclophosphamide in recurrent ovarian cancer: a trial of the California, Chicago, and Princess Margaret Hospital phase II consortia. J Clin Oncol 2008;26(1):76–82.

22. Penson RT, Dizon DS, Cannistra SA, et al. Phase II study of carboplatin, paclitaxel, and bevacizumab with maintenance bevacizumab as first-line chemotherapy for advanced mullerian tumors. J Clin Oncol 2010;28(1):154–9.

23. McGuire WP, Hoskins WJ, Brady MF, et al. Cyclophosphamide and cisplatin compared with paclitaxel and cisplatin in patients with stage III and stage IV ovarian cancer. N Engl J Med 1996;334(1):1–6.

24. Micha JP, Goldstein BH, Rettenmaier MA, et al. A phase II study of outpatient first-line paclitaxel, carboplatin, and bevacizumab for advanced-stage epithelial ovarian, peritoneal, and fallopian tube cancer. Int J Gynecol Cancer 2007;17(4): 771–6.

25. Konner JA, Grabon DM, Gerst SR, et al. Phase II study of intraperitoneal paclitaxel plus cisplatin and intravenous paclitaxel plus bevacizumab as adjuvant treatment of optimal stage II/III epithelial ovarian cancer. J Clin Oncol 2011; 29(35):4662–8.

26. Burger RA, Brady MF, Bookman MA, et al. Phase III trial of bevacizumab in the primary treatment of advanced epithelial ovarian cancer (EOC), primary peritoneal (PPC) or Fallopian tube cancer (FTC): a gynecologic oncology group study. J Clin Oncol 2010;28(Suppl 20):946s.

27. Perren T, Swart AM, Pfisterer J, et al. ICON7: a phase III Gynaecologic Cancer InterGroup (GCIG) trial of adding bevacizumab to standard chemotherapy in women with newly diagnosed epithelial ovarian (EOC), primary peritoneal (PPC) or Fallopian tube cancer (FTC). Paper presented at: Oral presentation at ESMO. Milan (Italy), October 8-12, 2010.

28. Aghajanian C, Finkler NJ, Rutherford T. OCEANS: a randomized, double-blinded, placebo-controlled phase III trial of chemotherapy with or without bevacizumab (BEV) in patients with platinum-sensitive recurrent epithelial ovarian (EOC), primary peritoneal (PPC), or fallopian tube cancer (FTC). Paper presented at: 2011 ASCO Annual Meeting Proceedings. Chicago (IL), June 3-7, 2011.

29. Aghajanian C, Sill MW, Darcy KM, et al. Phase II trial of bevacizumab in recurrent or persistent endometrial cancer: a Gynecologic Oncology Group study. J Clin Oncol 2011;29(16):2259–65.

30. Monk BJ, Sill MW, Burger RA, et al. Phase II trial of bevacizumab in the treatment of persistent or recurrent squamous cell carcinoma of the cervix: a gynecologic oncology group study. J Clin Oncol 2009;27(7):1069–74.

31. van Heeckeren WJ, Ortiz J, Cooney MM, et al. Hypertension, proteinuria, and antagonism of vascular endothelial growth factor signaling: clinical toxicity, therapeutic target, or novel biomarker? J Clin Oncol 2007;25(21):2993–5.

32. Zhu X, Wu S, Dahut WL, et al. Risks of proteinuria and hypertension with bevacizumab, an antibody against vascular endothelial growth factor: systematic review and meta-analysis. Am J Kidney Dis 2007;49(2):186–93.

33. Schneider BP, Wang M, Radovich M, et al. Association of vascular endothelial growth factor and vascular endothelial growth factor receptor-2 genetic polymorphisms with outcome in a trial of paclitaxel compared with paclitaxel plus

bevacizumab in advanced breast cancer: ECOG 2100. J Clin Oncol 2008; 26(28):4672–8.

34. Dahlberg SE, Sandler AB, Brahmer JR, et al. Clinical course of advanced non-small-cell lung cancer patients experiencing hypertension during treatment with bevacizumab in combination with carboplatin and paclitaxel on ECOG 4599. J Clin Oncol 2010;28(6):949–54.

35. Scartozzi M, Galizia E, Chiorrini S, et al. Arterial hypertension correlates with clinical outcome in colorectal cancer patients treated with first-line bevacizumab. Ann Oncol 2009;20(2):227–30.

36. Gordon MS, Cunningham D. Managing patients treated with bevacizumab combination therapy. Oncology 2005;69(Suppl 3):25–33.

37. Ostendorf T, Kunter U, Eitner F, et al. VEGF(165) mediates glomerular endothelial repair. J Clin Invest 1999;104(7):913–23.

38. Scappaticci FA, Skillings JR, Holden SN, et al. Arterial thromboembolic events in patients with metastatic carcinoma treated with chemotherapy and bevacizumab. J Natl Cancer Inst 2007;99(16):1232–9.

39. Nimeiri HS, Oza AM, Morgan RJ, et al. Efficacy and safety of bevacizumab plus erlotinib for patients with recurrent ovarian, primary peritoneal, and fallopian tube cancer: a trial of the Chicago, PMH, and California Phase II Consortia. Gynecol Oncol 2008;110(1):49–55.

40. Diaz JP, Tew WP, Zivanovic O, et al. Incidence and management of bevacizumab-associated gastrointestinal perforations in patients with recurrent ovarian carcinoma. Gynecol Oncol 2010;116(3):335–9.

41. Han ES, Monk BJ. What is the risk of bowel perforation associated with bevacizumab therapy in ovarian cancer? Gynecol Oncol 2007;105(1):3–6.

42. Stone RL, Sood AK, Coleman RL. Collateral damage: toxic effects of targeted antiangiogenic therapies in ovarian cancer. Lancet Oncol 2010;11(5):465–75.

43. Rutkowski P, Ruka W. Emergency surgery in the era of molecular treatment of solid tumours. Lancet Oncol 2009;10(2):157–63.

44. Simpkins F, Belinson JL, Rose PG. Avoiding bevacizumab related gastrointestinal toxicity for recurrent ovarian cancer by careful patient screening. Gynecol Oncol 2007;107(1):118–23.

45. Holash J, Davis S, Papadopoulos N, et al. VEGF-Trap: a VEGF blocker with potent antitumor effects. Proc Natl Acad Sci U S A 2002;99(17):11393–8.

46. Kim ES, Serur A, Huang J, et al. Potent VEGF blockade causes regression of coopted vessels in a model of neuroblastoma. Proc Natl Acad Sci U S A 2002;99(17):11399–404.

47. Tew WP, Colombo N, Ray-Coquard I, et al. VEGF-Trap for patients (pts) with recurrent platinum-resistant epithelial ovarian cancer (EOC): preliminary results of a randomized, multicenter phase II study. J Clin Oncol 2007;25(18S) [abstract: 5508].

48. Gotlieb WH, Amant F, Advani S, et al. Intravenous aflibercept for treatment of recurrent symptomatic malignant ascites in patients with advanced ovarian cancer: a phase 2, randomised, double-blind, placebo-controlled study. Lancet Oncol 2012;13(2):154–62.

49. Coleman RL, Duska LR, Ramirez PT, et al. Phase 1-2 study of docetaxel plus aflibercept in patients with recurrent ovarian, primary peritoneal, or fallopian tube cancer. Lancet Oncol 2011;12(12):1109–17.

50. Wilhelm S, Carter C, Lynch M, et al. Discovery and development of sorafenib: a multikinase inhibitor for treating cancer. Nat Rev Drug Discov 2006;5(10): 835–44.

51. Kane RC, Farrell AT, Saber H, et al. Sorafenib for the treatment of advanced renal cell carcinoma. Clin Cancer Res 2006;12(24):7271–8.

52. Kane RC, Farrell AT, Madabushi R, et al. Sorafenib for the treatment of unresectable hepatocellular carcinoma. Oncologist 2009;14(1):95–100.

53. Matei D, Sill MW, Lankes HA, et al. Activity of sorafenib in recurrent ovarian cancer and primary peritoneal carcinomatosis: a gynecologic oncology group trial. J Clin Oncol 2011;29(1):69–75.

54. Welch SA, Hirte HW, Elit L, et al. Sorafenib in combination with gemcitabine in recurrent epithelial ovarian cancer: a study of the Princess Margaret Hospital Phase II Consortium. Int J Gynecol Cancer 2010;20(5):787–93.

55. Ramasubbaiah R, Perkins SM, Schilder J, et al. Sorafenib in combination with weekly topotecan in recurrent ovarian cancer, a phase I/II study of the Hoosier Oncology Group. Gynecol Oncol 2011;123(3):499–504.

56. Hainsworth JD, Numnum TM, Rao GG. A randomized phase II study of paclitaxel/carboplatin with or without sorafenib in the first-line treatment of patients with stage III/IV epithelial ovarian cancer. Presented at ASCO. Chicago (IL), June 4-6, 2010.

57. Nimeiri HS, Oza AM, Morgan RJ, et al. A phase II study of sorafenib in advanced uterine carcinoma/carcinosarcoma: a trial of the Chicago, PMH, and California Phase II Consortia. Gynecol Oncol 2010;117(1):37–40.

58. Izzedine H, Buhaescu I, Rixe O, et al. Sunitinib malate. Cancer Chemother Pharmacol 2007;60(3):357–64.

59. Biagi JJ, Oza AM, Chalchal HI, et al. A phase II study of sunitinib in patients with recurrent epithelial ovarian and primary peritoneal carcinoma: an NCIC Clinical Trials Group Study. Ann Oncol 2011;22(2):335–40.

60. Mackay HJ, Tinker A, Winquist E, et al. A phase II study of sunitinib in patients with locally advanced or metastatic cervical carcinoma: NCIC CTG Trial IND.184. Gynecol Oncol 2010;116(2):163–7.

61. Hensley ML, Sill MW, Scribner DR Jr, et al. Sunitinib malate in the treatment of recurrent or persistent uterine leiomyosarcoma: a Gynecologic Oncology Group phase II study. Gynecol Oncol 2009;115(3):460–5.

62. Azad NS, Posadas EM, Kwitkowski VE, et al. Combination targeted therapy with sorafenib and bevacizumab results in enhanced toxicity and antitumor activity. J Clin Oncol 2008;26(22):3709–14.

63. Matulonis UA, Berlin S, Ivy P, et al. Cediranib, an oral inhibitor of vascular endothelial growth factor receptor kinases, is an active drug in recurrent epithelial ovarian, fallopian tube, and peritoneal cancer. J Clin Oncol 2009;27(33):5601–6.

64. Raja FA, Griffin CL, Qian W, et al. Initial toxicity assessment of ICON6: a randomised trial of cediranib plus chemotherapy in platinum-sensitive relapsed ovarian cancer. Br J Cancer 2011;105(7):884–9.

65. Friedlander M, Hancock KC, Rischin D, et al. A Phase II, open-label study evaluating pazopanib in patients with recurrent ovarian cancer. Gynecol Oncol 2010;119(1):32–7.

66. Monk BJ, Mas Lopez L, Zarba JJ, et al. Phase II, open-label study of pazopanib or lapatinib monotherapy compared with pazopanib plus lapatinib combination therapy in patients with advanced and recurrent cervical cancer. J Clin Oncol 2010;28(22):3562–9.

67. Ledermann JA, Hackshaw A, Kaye S, et al. Randomized phase II placebo-controlled trial of maintenance therapy using the oral triple angiokinase inhibitor BIBF 1120 after chemotherapy for relapsed ovarian cancer. J Clin Oncol 2011; 29(28):3798–804.

68. Tortora G, Ciardiello F, Gasparini G. Combined targeting of EGFR-dependent and VEGF-dependent pathways: rationale, preclinical studies and clinical applications. Nat Clin Pract Oncol 2008;5(9):521–30.

69. Ellis LM. Epidermal growth factor receptor in tumor angiogenesis. Hematol Oncol Clin North Am 2004;18(5):1007–21, viii.

70. Viloria-Petit A, Crombet T, Jothy S, et al. Acquired resistance to the antitumor effect of epidermal growth factor receptor-blocking antibodies in vivo: a role for altered tumor angiogenesis. Cancer Res 2001;61(13):5090–101.

71. Yarden Y. The EGFR family and its ligands in human cancer. Signalling mechanisms and therapeutic opportunities. Eur J Cancer 2001;37(Suppl 4):S3–8.

72. Siwak DR, Carey M, Hennessy BT, et al. Targeting the epidermal growth factor receptor in epithelial ovarian cancer: current knowledge and future challenges. J Oncol 2010;2010:568938.

73. Zagouri F, Bozas G, Kafantari E, et al. Endometrial cancer: what is new in adjuvant and molecularly targeted therapy? Obstet Gynecol Int 2010;2010: 749579.

74. Growdon WB, Boisvert SL, Akhavanfard S, et al. Decreased survival in EGFR gene amplified vulvar carcinoma. Gynecol Oncol 2008;111(2):289–97.

75. Kersemaekers AM, Fleuren GJ, Kenter GG, et al. Oncogene alterations in carcinomas of the uterine cervix: overexpression of the epidermal growth factor receptor is associated with poor prognosis. Clin Cancer Res 1999; 5(3):577–86.

76. Kim JW, Kim YT, Kim DK, et al. Expression of epidermal growth factor receptor in carcinoma of the cervix. Gynecol Oncol 1996;60(2):283–7.

77. Oonk MH, de Bock GH, van der Veen DJ, et al. EGFR expression is associated with groin node metastases in vulvar cancer, but does not improve their prediction. Gynecol Oncol 2007;104(1):109–13.

78. Kim SJ, Uehara H, Karashima T, et al. Blockade of epidermal growth factor receptor signaling in tumor cells and tumor-associated endothelial cells for therapy of androgen-independent human prostate cancer growing in the bone of nude mice. Clin Cancer Res 2003;9(3):1200–10.

79. Liang K, Ang KK, Milas L, et al. The epidermal growth factor receptor mediates radioresistance. Int J Radiat Oncol Biol Phys 2003;57(1):246–54.

80. Schilder RJ, Pathak HB, Lokshin AE, et al. Phase II trial of single agent cetuximab in patients with persistent or recurrent epithelial ovarian or primary peritoneal carcinoma with the potential for dose escalation to rash. Gynecol Oncol 2009;113(1):21–7.

81. Mendelsohn J, Baselga J. Epidermal growth factor receptor targeting in cancer. Semin Oncol 2006;33(4):369–85.

82. Baselga J, Arteaga CL. Critical update and emerging trends in epidermal growth factor receptor targeting in cancer. J Clin Oncol 2005;23(11):2445–59.

83. Bernier J. Cetuximab in the treatment of head and neck cancer. Expert Rev Anticancer Ther 2006;6(11):1539–52.

84. Mittmann N, Au HJ, Tu D, et al. Prospective cost-effectiveness analysis of cetuximab in metastatic colorectal cancer: evaluation of National Cancer Institute of Canada Clinical Trials Group CO.17 trial. J Natl Cancer Inst 2009;101(17): 1182–92.

85. Secord AA, Blessing JA, Armstrong DK, et al. Phase II trial of cetuximab and carboplatin in relapsed platinum-sensitive ovarian cancer and evaluation of epidermal growth factor receptor expression: a Gynecologic Oncology Group study. Gynecol Oncol 2008;108(3):493–9.

86. Konner J, Schilder RJ, DeRosa FA, et al. A phase II study of cetuximab/pacli-taxel/carboplatin for the initial treatment of advanced-stage ovarian, primary peritoneal, or fallopian tube cancer. Gynecol Oncol 2008;110(2):140–5.

87. Schilder RJ, Sill MW, Chen X, et al. Phase II study of gefitinib in patients with relapsed or persistent ovarian or primary peritoneal carcinoma and evaluation of epidermal growth factor receptor mutations and immunohistochemical expression: a Gynecologic Oncology Group Study. Clin Cancer Res 2005; 11(15):5539–48.

88. Kurtz JE, Hardy-Bessard AC, Deslandres M, et al. Cetuximab, topotecan and cisplatin for the treatment of advanced cervical cancer: a phase II GINECO trial. Gynecol Oncol 2009;113(1):16–20.

89. Farley J, Sill MW, Birrer M, et al. Phase II study of cisplatin plus cetuximab in advanced, recurrent, and previously treated cancers of the cervix and evalua-tion of epidermal growth factor receptor immunohistochemical expression: a Gynecologic Oncology Group study. Gynecol Oncol 2011;121(2):303–8.

90. Santin AD, Sill MW, McMeekin DS, et al. Phase II trial of cetuximab in the treat-ment of persistent or recurrent squamous or non-squamous cell carcinoma of the cervix: a Gynecologic Oncology Group study. Gynecol Oncol 2011;122(3): 495–500.

91. Seiden MV, Burris HA, Matulonis U, et al. A phase II trial of EMD72000 (matuzu-mab), a humanized anti-EGFR monoclonal antibody, in patients with platinum-resistant ovarian and primary peritoneal malignancies. Gynecol Oncol 2007; 104(3):727–31.

92. Hayes DF, Thor AD, Dressler LG, et al. HER2 and response to paclitaxel in node-positive breast cancer. N Engl J Med 2007;357(15):1496–506.

93. Farley J, Fuchiuji S, Darcy KM, et al. Associations between ERBB2 amplification and progression-free survival and overall survival in advanced stage, suboptimally-resected epithelial ovarian cancers: a Gynecologic Oncology Group Study. Gynecol Oncol 2009;113(3):341–7.

94. Sheng Q, Liu J. The therapeutic potential of targeting the EGFR family in epithe-lial ovarian cancer. Br J Cancer 2011;104(8):1241–5.

95. McAlpine J, Wiegand K, Vang R, et al. HER2 overexpression and amplification is present in a subset of ovarian mucinous carcinomas and can be targeted with trastuzumab therapy. BMC Cancer 2009;9(1):433.

96. Bookman MA, Darcy KM, Clarke-Pearson D, et al. Evaluation of monoclonal humanized anti-HER2 antibody, trastuzumab, in patients with recurrent or refractory ovarian or primary peritoneal carcinoma with overexpression of HER2: a phase II trial of the Gynecologic Oncology Group. J Clin Oncol 2003; 21(2):283–90.

97. Grushko TA, Filiaci VL, Mundt AJ, et al. An exploratory analysis of HER-2 ampli-fication and overexpression in advanced endometrial carcinoma: a Gynecologic Oncology Group study. Gynecol Oncol 2008;108(1):3–9.

98. Fleming GF, Sill MW, Darcy KM, et al. Phase II trial of trastuzumab in women with advanced or recurrent, HER2-positive endometrial carcinoma: a Gynecologic Oncology Group study. Gynecol Oncol 2010;116(1):15–20.

99. Posadas EM, Liel MS, Kwitkowski V, et al. A phase II and pharmacodynamic study of gefitinib in patients with refractory or recurrent epithelial ovarian cancer. Cancer 2007;109(7):1323–30.

100. Goncalves A, Fabbro M, Lhomme C, et al. A phase II trial to evaluate gefitinib as second- or third-line treatment in patients with recurring locoregionally advanced or metastatic cervical cancer. Gynecol Oncol 2008;108(1):42–6.

101. Schilder RJ, Sill MW, Lee YC, et al. A phase II trial of erlotinib in recurrent squamous cell carcinoma of the cervix: a Gynecologic Oncology Group Study. Int J Gynecol Cancer 2009;19(5):929–33.
102. Lu C, Shahzad MM, Moreno-Smith M, et al. Targeting pericytes with a PDGF-B aptamer in human ovarian carcinoma models. Cancer Biol Ther 2010;9(3): 176–82.
103. Lu C, Han HD, Mangala LS, et al. Regulation of tumor angiogenesis by EZH2. Cancer Cell 2010;18(2):185–97.
104. Halder J, Kamat AA, Landen CN Jr, et al. Focal adhesion kinase targeting using in vivo short interfering RNA delivery in neutral liposomes for ovarian carcinoma therapy. Clin Cancer Res 2006;12(16):4916–24.
105. Herbst RS, Hong D, Chap L, et al. Safety, pharmacokinetics, and antitumor activity of AMG 386, a selective angiopoietin inhibitor, in adult patients with advanced solid tumors. J Clin Oncol 2009;27(21):3557–65.
106. Karlan BY, Oza AM, Richardson GE, et al. Randomized, double-blind, placebo-controlled phase II study of AMG 386 combined with weekly paclitaxel in patients with recurrent ovarian cancer. J Clin Oncol 2012;30(4):362–71.
107. Eder JP, Vande Woude GF, Boerner SA, et al. Novel therapeutic inhibitors of the c-Met signaling pathway in cancer. Clin Cancer Res 2009;15(7):2207–14.
108. Bergers G, Hanahan D. Modes of resistance to anti-angiogenic therapy. Nat Rev Cancer 2008;8(8):592–603.
109. Buckanovich R, Berger R, Sella A, et al. Activity of cabozantinib (XL184) in advanced ovarian cancer patients (pts): results from a phase II randomized discontinuation trial (RDT). Paper presented at: ASCO. Chicago (IL), June 3-7, 2011.
110. Hanahan D, Weinberg RA. Hallmarks of cancer: the next generation. Cell 2011; 144(5):646–74.
111. Azam F, Mehta S, Harris AL. Mechanisms of resistance to antiangiogenesis therapy. Eur J Cancer 2010;46(8):1323–32.
112. Ebos JM, Lee CR, Kerbel RS. Tumor and host-mediated pathways of resistance and disease progression in response to antiangiogenic therapy. Clin Cancer Res 2009;15(16):5020–5.
113. Gordon AN, Finkler N, Edwards RP, et al. Efficacy and safety of erlotinib HCl, an epidermal growth factor receptor (HER1/EGFR) tyrosine kinase inhibitor, in patients with advanced ovarian carcinoma: results from a phase II multicenter study. Int J Gynecol Cancer 2005;15(5):785–92.

Targeting the Hedgehog Pathway
Role in Cancer and Clinical Implications of Its Inhibition

Deirdre J. Cohen, MD

KEYWORDS

- Hedgehog • Therapeutics • Cancer • Drugs • Pathway

KEY POINTS

- The Hh pathway is a vital signaling pathway in embryogenesis and more recently has been implicated in the pathogenesis of a vast variety of malignancies.
- The key components of the pathway include the Hh ligands Sonic, Indian, and Desert, which bind the receptor PTCH, thereby relieving its inhibition of the receptor SMO, leading to downstream signaling via the GLI transcription factors.
- There are multiple models for aberrant Hh pathway activation, including both ligand dependent and independent, as well as a role in tumor stem cell maintenance.
- Hh pathway inhibition is an active area of research, with strong preclinical rationale and proof of concept in malignancies, such as basal cell carcinoma, which have constitutive activation of the Hh pathway.
- Novel pathway inhibitors have been or are currently being developed to antagonize the Hh pathway and provide a molecularly targeted approach to cancer treatment.

The Hedgehog (Hh) pathway is a signaling cascade that is evolutionally highly conserved and plays an important role in embryonic pattern formation and stem cell response to tissue damage.[1,2] The Hh gene was originally identified in 1980 by Christiane Nusslein-Volhard and Eric F. Wieschaus, developmental biologists studying the segmentation pattern of *Drosophila melanogaster* (fruit fly) embryos.[3] Their genetic analysis found that loss of the gene encoding the secreted protein that is a key regulator of the pathway in fruit flies gives rise to a mutant embryonic phenotype with spiky projections similar to the appearance of a hedgehog. Three Hh homolog genes have since been identified in vertebrates and are termed Sonic hedgehog (Shh) after the popular video game character, and Indian hedgehog (Ihh) and Desert hedgehog (Dhh), both after existing species of hedgehogs. The Hh family of proteins serve a variety of functions in vertebrate embryogenesis, including body patterning, cell migration, growth, differentiation, and survival. This signaling is context dependent, varying based on the receiving cell type, can be short range and long range, and is concentration dependent, typical of a morphogen.[2,4] The fundamental regulatory

Financial disclosure: The author has nothing to disclose.
Division of GI Oncology, NYU Cancer Institute, 160 East 34th Street, New York, NY 10016, USA
E-mail address: Deirdre.Cohen@nyumc.org

Hematol Oncol Clin N Am 26 (2012) 565–588
doi:10.1016/j.hoc.2012.01.005
0889-8588/12/$ – see front matter © 2012 Elsevier Inc. All rights reserved.

role Hh plays in development is underscored by the consequences of pathway misregulation or inhibition, which have been shown to cause severe birth defects, including holoprosencephaly, cyclopia, and microcephaly.[5–7] In adults, the pathway is much less active and widespread. It is mainly involved in tissue maintenance and repair, including the skin, bone, and intestine.[8–10]

Given the pivotal role the Hh pathway plays in embryonic development in terms of proliferation and differentiation, it is not surprising that it has also been implicated in tumorigenesis and tumor growth acceleration in a vast variety of malignancies. The initial connection between aberrant Hh pathway signaling and cancer was made in a rare condition called Gorlin syndrome, in which patients develop numerous basal cell carcinomas (BCCs) during their lifetimes and are predisposed to other types of malignancies, including medulloblastoma and rhabdomyosarcoma. These patients were noted to have mutations in components of the Hh pathway, leading to its constitutive activation.[11] Other types of cancers, including for example breast, prostate, pancreas, colon, lung, and chronic myelogenous leukemia (CML), have subsequently been shown to have inappropriate Hh pathway activation. Given that misregulation of the Hh pathway has been implicated in such a wide array of disparate malignancies, targeting its signaling has been an active area of research over the past 2 decades. In this article, I summarize the mechanism of Hh pathway signal transduction, discuss the models of pathway activation, review the clinical data using Hh inhibitors, and discuss challenges to the development of pathway inhibitors.

PATHWAY SIGNAL TRANSDUCTION

Signaling within the Hh pathway begins with the secretion of 1 of the 3 Hh proteins: Sonic, Indian, or Desert. The Hh protein undergoes extensive processing, with many modifications and is an unusual secreted protein in that it harbors 2 covalently linked lipid adducts.[12] The precursor protein undergoes initial autoprocessing to release its N-terminal fragment. This peptide is subsequently modified by covalent binding of a cholesterol molecule on its C terminus, conferring a high affinity for the plasma membrane and precluding its further release and spread.[13] The N-terminus then undergoes palmitoylation mediated by an acyl transferase encoded by HHAT.[14] Thus, the ultimate secreted morphogen is termed Hh-Np ("p" standing for processed).[13] The subsequent secretion of the processed protein involves several molecules for its movement, extracellular transport, and release—the best characterized being the large multipass transmembrane protein Dispatched (DISP). It appears that DISP is essential for Hh signaling, as animals with mutations in DISP have accumulation of Hh in producing cells and therefore downstream signaling of the pathway is lost.[15,16]

Once secreted from the producing cell, Hh binds on the receiving cell to the Patched protein (PTCH), a 12-transmembrane protein, and initiates the signaling cascade. The simplest model is that Hh binds PTCH, alleviating PTCH inhibition of the 7-transmembrane G-protein-coupled receptor–like protein Smoothened (SMO), thereby enabling signal transduction to the nucleus (**Fig. 1**). Conversely, in the absence of ligand binding, PTCH catalytically inhibits the activity of SMO; however, the exact mechanism of the interaction is unclear. It is known from tissue-cultured cells that PTCH inhibits SMO at substoichiometric concentrations.[17] One proposed mechanism for PTCH inhibition of SMO may involve the transport by PTCH of a small molecule regulator of SMO movement or activity. Candidates for this small molecule include PI4P, lipoproteins, and provitamin D3.[18–21] Another possible mechanism is that PTCH represses SMO by affecting its localization to the cell surface. Specifically, it is thought that PTCH prevents SMO translocation into the primary cilium, a microtubule-based antennalike structure that emanates from the surface of virtually all cells in the mammalian body. The primary cilium is a sensory organelle that receives both mechanical and chemical signals from other cells and the environment, and transmits these signals to the nucleus to elicit a cellular response.[22] It has been shown to play a pivotal role in the Hh transduction pathway. For example, mutations in intraflagellar transport, which normally functions in retrograde and anterograde movement of molecules within the primary cilium, results in mice with Hh loss-of-function phenotypes.[23,24] When exposed to Hh ligand, PTCH, which is normally present in the cilia, becomes internalized, thereby allowing SMO to move from internal vesicles all the way up along the shaft of the cilium.

Once Hh binds to PTCH and thereby alleviates repression of SMO, a signaling cascade is initiated through activation of the GLI family of zinc transcription factors, thereby translating the extracellular stimulus into defined transcriptional programs in a context-dependent and cell-type specific manner. Unlike *Drosophila*, which have a single GLI protein that is encoded by the cubitus interruptus gene, vertebrates have 3 GLI transcriptions factors (GLI 1–3). GLI2 and 3 are bifunctional transcription factors, functioning as either activators or repressors depending on their modification, processing, and nuclear trafficking.[1] Because GLI1 lacks the N-terminal repressor domain, it functions exclusively as an activator.[25] It is also most highly dependent on active Hh signaling and therefore is the most often used surrogate for pathway

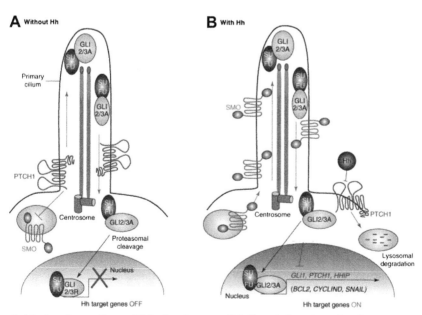

Fig. 1. Hh signaling pathway. (*A*) In the absence of Hh ligands (inactivated pathway), PTCH1 is localized on the primary cilium and suppresses SMO, preventing downstream activation of GLI transcription factors and thereby signal transduction. (*B*) In the presence of Hh ligand binding to PTCH1, PTCH1 becomes internalized and degraded allowing for SMO to move into the primary cilium and activate GLI, leading to upregulation of target genes including GLI1, PTCH1, and HHIP. (*Reprinted from* Scales SJ, de Sauvage FJ. Mechanisms of Hedgehog pathway activation in cancer and implications for therapy. Trends Pharmacol Sci 2009;30(6):303–12; with permission.)

activation. GLI family members are phosphorylated by protein kinase A (PKA) and glycogen synthase 3 (GSK3) in the absence of Hh signaling, but are relieved from PKA/GSK3-mediated phosphorylation in the presence of Hh signaling.[26,27] In the absence of Hh activation, GLI2 is degraded, owing to phosphorylation-mediated ubiquitylation, and GLI3 is processed into a repressor.[28] Once the Hh pathway is activated, GLI family members are stabilized, translocated into the nucleus, and bind the consensus binding site (5'-TGGGTGGTC-3') in the target gene promoter.[29–31] Hh signaling seems to be dependent on the relative balance of GLI activator and repressor forms.[32] The activity of GLI transcription factors is regulated at several different levels, including nuclear-cytoplasmic shuttling, ubiquitination, protein degradation, and the transcriptional activity of GLI molecules.[33] One well-characterized negative regulator of Hh signaling is the Suppressor of Fused (SUFU) protein, which acts as a tumor suppressor gene. It associates with and inhibits GLI molecule function and is required for GLI3 processing.[34–36] The Hh target genes are numerous and involved in a wide variety of cellular functions, including control of cell proliferation, survival, epithelial-to-mesenchymal transition (EMT), maintenance of stemness, and cell fate determination.[28] In addition, GLI, PTCH, and Hh-interacting protein are not only components of the pathway, but are also target genes themselves and involved in several regulatory feedback loops.

LINKING THE Hh PATHWAY AND HUMAN CANCER

Similar to its role in *Drosophila*, the Hh pathway in humans was initially implicated in embryogenesis and development as an essential signaling pathway. Unlike in the embryo or neonate, Hh activation was found to be much more limited in the adult and restricted to areas of tissue damage and repair. More recently, however, aberrant Hh pathway signaling has been implicated in cancer formation and growth. The link was first made in 1996 when mutations in PTCH were discovered to be associated with a rare hereditary form of BCC, called basal cell nevus syndrome or Gorlin syndrome.[37,38] Gorlin syndrome is an autosomal dominant genetic disease in which patients develop numerous BCCs during their lifetime and are at an increased risk of other tumors, including medulloblastoma, a tumor of the cerebellar progenitor cells, and rhabdomyosarcoma, a muscle tumor. These patients have a germline mutation in 1 allele of the PTCH gene, and basal-cell tumors from these patients lack the remaining normal PTCH gene. Without functional PTCH, SMO is freed from repression and the Hh pathway becomes constitutively active. The association between the Hh pathway and tumorigenesis was further supported by the identification of aberrant activation in sporadic BCCs. Most BCC tumors have either inactivating mutations in PTCH1 (>85%) or, less commonly, activating mutations in SMO.[39–42] Since the initial connection between the Hh pathway and carcinogenesis in BCCs, aberrant signaling and/or reactivation of the cascade have been noted in a wide and disparate number of cancers, including both solid tumor and hematologic malignancies.

MODELS OF PATHWAY ACTIVATION IN CANCER

There are 3 basic models that have been proposed for Hh pathway activity in cancer (**Fig. 2**).[5] The first elucidated was the Hh ligand-independent cancers, such as BCCs, and were termed type I cancers. These tumors have pathway-activating mutations that lead to constitutive activation of the Hh pathway. Type II cancers are ligand-dependent and autocrine (or juxtacrine), so that Hh is both produced and responded

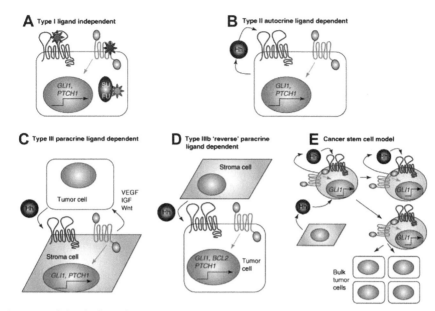

Fig. 2. Models of Hh pathway activation in cancer. (*A*) Type I ligand-independent cancers harbor inactivating (*green star*) mutations in the negative PTCH1 or SUFU, or activating mutations (*red star*) in SMO, leading to pathway activation in a cell-autonomous manner even in the absence of ligand and expression of target genes such as GLI1 and PTCH1. (*B*) Type II ligand-dependent autocrine cancers secrete Hh and respond to it, leading to cell-autonomous pathway activation. (*C*) Type III ligand-dependent paracrine cancers secrete Hh, which binds to PTCH1 on stromal cells, leading to pathway activation in that cell type and feedback of other growth or survival signals (such as IGF, VEGF, and Wnt) to the tumor. (*D*) Type IIIb "reverse paracrine" tumors receive Hh secreted from stromal cells, such as the bone marrow or lymph nodes, which leads to pathway activation in the tumor, upregulating survival genes such as BCL2 in addition to GLI1 and PTCH1. (*E*) The cancer stem cell model postulates that Hh signaling occurs only in self-renewing putative cancer stem cells (*yellow*), which either produce their own Hh ligand or receive it from stromal cells, including the vasculature. A subset of the cancer stem cells will then differentiate into Hh pathway–negative tumor cells that comprise the bulk of the tumor. Key: PTCH1, red; SMO, green; SUFU, brown; Hh, purple; nucleus, light blue; receiving cell, white rectangle; stromal cells, gray diamonds; cancer stem cells, yellow circles. (*Reprinted from* Scales SJ, de Sauvage FJ. Mechanisms of Hedgehog pathway activation in cancer and implications for therapy. Trends Pharmacol Sci 2009;30(6):303–12; with permission.)

to by the same (or neighboring) tumor cells, whereas Type III cancers are also ligand dependent, but use paracrine signaling. In this model, Hh is produced by the tumor epithelium and received by the surrounding stroma (analogous to epithelial-to-mesenchymal transition in early development), which then feeds back growth and/or survival signals to the tumor. A variation to this model has recently been described, termed "reverse paracrine" signaling or Type IIIb, where Hh is secreted from stromal cells to the receiving cells in a tumor.

In addition to the aforementioned 3 models, there is an alternative model that implicates aberrant Hh pathway activation in cancer stem cells (CSCs).[17,43–45] CSCs comprise a small subset of cells in a tumor that are characterized by being able to self-renew and initiate tumor spread. They are typically resistant to chemotherapy, possibly contributing to relapse.[46] Similar to its role in normal stem cell activity, the Hh pathway has been shown to be active in several types of CSCs, including breast, glioma, pancreatic, multiple myeloma, and CML.[47–52] The exact mechanism of Hh deregulation within CSCs is still unclear and may rely on autocrine, paracrine, and/ or ligand-independent signaling. What is clear, however, is that Hh inhibition appears to deplete this tumorigenic population in animal models and therefore holds great potential promise in the clinic.

DISCOVERY OF THE FIRST Hh INHIBITOR: CYCLOPAMINE

The discovery of the first Hh pathway inhibitor is an interesting story and dates back to the 1950s when an increased incidence of congenital malformations, including cyclopia, was noted in newborn lambs. These teratogenic effects were linked to pregnant ewes consuming a corn lily plant (*Veratrum californicum*).[53] Analysis of the plant led to isolation and identification of the principal teratogen, termed cyclopamine, a steroidal alkaloid. Following the discovery of the Hh pathway first in *Drosophila* and later in humans and the understanding that mutations within this signaling cascade can lead to deformities, such as holoprosencephaly, which can include cyclopic features, Cooper and colleagues[54] demonstrated that cyclopamine acts through inhibition of the Hh pathway. The elucidation of cyclopamine as an Hh pathway inhibitor took decades and has since served as a powerful tool to help understand the role the Hh pathway plays in diseases, including cancer.

Cyclopamine inhibits the Hh pathway by binding to, and inactivating SMO.[55] It has been used extensively in preclinical studies; however, because of its low affinity, poor oral bioavailability, and suboptimal pharmacokinetics, it has not moved forward in the clinic. Furthermore, in addition to inactivating SMO, cyclopamine may also have "off-target" effects, as cells without the SMO receptor have been shown to undergo apoptosis and often very high concentrations of cyclopamine are required to inhibit cell proliferation.[56] Given the multiple impediments to the clinical use of cyclopamine, as well as the potential importance of the Hh pathway in a vast array of pathologies, additional inhibitors with improved pharmacologic properties have since been identified via high-throughput screening of small-molecule libraries. Although the screens were designed to probe the entire Hh signaling cascade, most of the identified inhibitors have been reported to target SMO itself. SMO seems to be the most druggable component of the pathway, whereas other components are more structurally complex and inaccessible.

Hh PATHWAY INHIBITORS

Among the various Hh pathway inhibitors (HPIs), vismodegib (GDC-0449; Curis/Genentech) is the farthest along in development. Vismodegib is a synthetic small-molecule inhibitor of the Hh pathway that binds to and inhibits SMO. It was designed to be more potent and have more favorable pharmaceutical properties than the steroidal alkaloid cyclopamine.[5,56,57] Phase I clinical testing is completed and vismodegib is now being evaluated in multiple phase II studies, some of which have recently been reported, including colon, ovarian, and BCCs (see later in this article). Other synthetic SMO inhibitors include BMS-833923 (XL139; Exelexis/Bristol-Myers Squibb), LDE225 and LEQ506 (Novartis), PF-04449913 (Pfizer), and LY2940680 (Eli Lily), which have either completed or are nearing completion of phase I testing. IPI-926 (Infinity) is the only semisynthetic SMO inhibitor currently in clinical testing. It was derived from cyclopamine and demonstrates improved potency and physiochemical properties, including acid stability and aqueous solubility.[58] Phase I single-agent findings have been reported and currently combination phase I and phase II testing is ongoing for chondrosarcoma, and pancreatic and head and neck cancers (**Table 1**).

Although there are definite differences among the various SMO inhibitors in terms of structure, they otherwise have similar profiles. They are all oral selective small molecule inhibitors with high potency (half maximal effective concentration <20 nM), long half-lives (24–168 hours), and a very manageable side-effect profile.[59–62] The most common toxicities include fatigue, dysgeusia, myalgias, alopecia, and nausea, which may be a class effect. They also have all shown to have exposure-dependent target inhibition as measured by GLI expression.

Apart from SMO inhibitors, there are other Hh pathway components that are being targeted for inhibition. One of the more challenging targets has been the Hh pathway ligand Shh, an extracellular protein that is upstream of SMO and undergoes extensive lipid modification, making it a challenge to access. The macrocylic small molecule robotnikinin is the first reported inhibitor of Shh.[63] It was discovered through a small-molecule microarray-based screen of a bacterially expressed biologically active Shh N-terminal fragment (ShhN) and then subsequently optimized for better binding and dissociation time. It binds to ShhN at concentrations between 1.56 and 25.00 µM with a Kd value of 3.1 µM. It was shown to block transcription of Hh pathway targets in primary keratinocytes treated with Shh compared with that seen in mock-treated controls. It did not prevent transcription triggered by small-molecule agonists of SMO, suggesting that the compound acts earlier in the pathway than SMO. Although still in preclinical development, robotnikinin and other small-molecule inhibitors of Shh may ultimately play an important role in the treatment of ligand-dependent tumors. There are multiple other inhibitors that act downstream of SMO on various different facets of the Hh pathway. Inhibition of GLI-mediated transcription is an attractive target, as it is theoretically efficacious irrespective of the mode of Hh pathway activation. Two low-molecular-weight compounds, GANT58 and GANT61, have been identified, which act at the nucleus to block GLI function.[64] Although they are from different chemical classes, they both are potent and selective inhibitors of GLI with a half maximal inhibitory concentration of ~5 µM. Furthermore, they both block cell growth in an in vivo xenograft prostate cancer model. More recently, 4 additional Hh pathway inhibitors, which act downstream of SMO, have been characterized. Termed HPI-1 through HPI-4, each has a unique mechanism of action, involved in GLI processing, GLI activation, and primary cilia formation, suggesting that multiple steps in GLI regulation are pharmacologically targetable.[65]

Additionally, 2 well-known and widely used agents approved by the Food and Drug Administration (FDA) for separate indications have been shown to inhibit the Hh pathway. Both itraconazole, a commonly used antifungal, and arsenic trioxide, an important treatment for acute promyelocytic leukemia, have demonstrated preclinical evidence for Hh pathway inhibition. Arsenic trioxide's mechanism of action is thought to be through inhibition of GLI transcriptional effectors, blocking Hh-induced ciliary accumulation of GLI2 and thereby reducing steady-state levels,[66] whereas itraconazole has been shown to act at the level of SMO by a mechanism that is distinct from that of cyclopamine and other known SMO antagonists, and prevents the ciliary accumulation of SMO normally caused by Hh stimulation.[67] There is currently a clinical trial under way with itraconazole in patients with BCCs, building on this new understanding of an established drug (see **Table 1**).

Table 1
Hedgehog pathway inhibitors currently in clinical trials for cancer

Drug	Tumor Target	Other Agent(s)	Phase	Design	ClinicalTrials.gov Identifier
GDC-0449	Pancreas	—	II (single arm)	Preoperative GDC-0449	NCT01096732
	Pancreas	Gemcitabine, nab-paclitaxel	II (single arm)	Metastatic disease treated with GDC-0449 + chemotherapy	NCT01088815
	Pancreas	Gemcitabine	Unspecified	Pilot study to investigate pancreatic stem cells before & after treatment with GDC-0449 + gemcitabine	NCT01195415
	Pancreas	Erlotinib, gemcitabine	I	Metastatic disease treated with GDC-0449 + erlotinib ± gemcitabine	NCT00878163
	Pancreas	Gemcitabine	II (randomized, placebo controlled)	Metastatic disease treated with gemcitabine ± GDC-0449	NCT01064622
	Small cell lung cancer	Cisplatin (cis), etoposide (E)	II (randomized)	Three arms: cis+E, cis+E+ GDC-0449, cis+E + cixutumumab	NCT00887159
	Gastroesophageal	5-Fluoruracil, oxaliplatin	II (randomized, placebo controlled)	Advanced gastroesophageal cancer treated with FOLFOX ± GDC-0449	NCT00982592
	Prostate	Leuprolide acetate or goserelin	Ib/II (randomized)	Preoperative GDC-0449 + androgen ablation compared with androgen ablation alone followed by radical prostatectomy for locally advanced prostate adenocarcinoma	NCT01163084
	Medulloblastoma	—	I	Recurrent or refractory medulloblastoma in pediatric patients	NCT00822458
	Medulloblastoma	—	II (single arm)	Recurrent or refractory medulloblastoma in pediatric patients, stratified by IHC for Hh pathway	NCT01239316
	Medulloblastoma	—	II (single arm)	Recurrent or refractory disease treated with GDC-0449	NCT00939484
	Sarcoma	RO4929097	Ib/II	Advanced or metastatic sarcomas treated with combination GDC-0449 + gamma secretase inhibitor	NCT01154452

Drug	Cancer	Combination	Phase	Description	NCT
	Chondrosarcoma	—	II	Metastatic or unresectable chondrosarcoma treated with GDC-0449	NCT01267955
	Multiple myeloma	—	Ib	High-risk myeloma in first remission following autologous stem cell transplantation	NCT01330173
	Basal Cell Carcinoma (BCC)	—	II	2-cohort trial evaluating the efficacy & safety of GDC-0449 in operable BCC	NCT01201915
	BCC	—	II (single arm)	Locally advanced or metastatic BCC	NCT01367665
IPI-926	Pancreas	Gemcitabine	Ib/II	Metastatic disease patients randomized in phase II to gemcitabine ± IPI-926	NCT01130142
	Pancreas	5-Fluorouracil, irinotecan, oxaliplatin (FOLFIRINOX)	I	Advanced disease treated with FOLFIRINOX + IPI-926	NCT01383538
	Head and neck	Cetuximab	I	Advanced disease treated with combined cetuximab + IPI-926	NCT01255800
	Chondrosarcoma	—	II (randomized, placebo controlled)	Unresectable disease treated with IPI-926 or placebo	NCT01310816
	Myelofibrosis	—	II	Single-arm study with primary end point of response rate	NCT01371617
LDE225	BCC	—	II	Randomized double-blind study of efficacy and safety of 2 dose levels of LDE225 in unresectable disease	NCT01327053
	BCC	—	II (randomized, placebo controlled)	Adult patients with nevoid BCC syndrome	NCT01350115
	Pancreas	Gemcitabine	I/II	Neoadjuvant combination therapy in borderline resectable pancreatic cancer	NCT01431794

(continued on next page)

Table 1
(continued)

Drug	Tumor Target	Other Agent(s)	Phase	Design	ClinicalTrials.gov Identifier
BMS-833923	CML	Dasatinib	I	Dose-finding study in CML patients with resistance or suboptimal response to a prior TKI	NCT01218477
	Gastroesophageal	Cisplatin, capecitabine	Ib	1st line treatment of advanced disease	NCT00909402
	Small cell lung cancer (SCLC)	Carboplatin, etoposide	Ib	Extensive stage SCLC treated with BMS-833923 + carboplatin + etoposide followed by maintenance BMS-833923	NCT00927875
PF-04449913	CML/hematologic malignancies	Dasatinib or bosutinib	I	PF-04449913 in select hematologic malignancies or in combination with dasatinib or bosutinib in CML	NCT00953758
	Solid tumors	—	I	Advanced solid tumors treated with single agent	NCT01286467
LY2940680	Solid tumors	—	I	Advanced solid tumors treated with single agent	NCT01226485
Itraconazole	BCC	—	Pilot	To determine if 3 weeks of oral or topical itraconazole reduces BCC biomarkers	NCT01108094
	SCLC	Pemetrexed	Randomized phase II	Previously treated SCLC treated with pemetrexed ± itraconazole	NCT00769600

LIGAND-INDEPENDENT TUMORS AND Hh INHIBITION
Basal Cell Carcinoma

Since the initial recognition in 1996 of the link between Gorlin syndrome and aberrant activation of the Hh pathway, much has been learned about Hh mutation–driven tumors and their treatment. Following the identification of germline-inactivating mutations in the PTCH gene in patients with Gorlin syndrome, sporadic BCCs were subsequently also found to have mutations in the Hh pathway. Further research has established that upregulation of Hh signaling is the pivotal abnormality in all BCCs.[11] Specifically, nearly 90% have identifiable mutations in at least one allele of PTCH (loss of function mutation) and an additional 10% have activating mutations in SMO (gain-of-function mutation), with rare mutations also found in SUFU.[42,68] These mutations lead to constitutive activation of the Hh pathway with increased cell proliferation and tumor formation. Various preclinical models have confirmed the role of aberrant Hh pathway activation in BCCs. For example, overexpression of SHH, GLI, or SMO in the skin of otherwise normal mice produces lesions that are BCC-like in histologic appearance and phenotypic markers.[68–70] Furthermore, mice that are heterozygous for PTCH are more susceptible to UV-induced BCC.[71] These same models have also helped to confirm the efficacy of HPIs in blocking tumor cell growth. For example, SMO antagonists have been shown to suppress proliferation and induce apoptosis of basaloid nests in BCC model systems, while having no effect on normal skin cells.[72] Given the strong preclinical evidence demonstrating the Hh pathway as the key oncogenic pathway driving the formation and maintenance of BCCs, attempts at pathway inhibition downstream of the causative mutation were soon made in the clinic.

One of the first tested HPIs in the clinic for the treatment of BCCs was a topical SMO antagonist called CUR61414. Based on promising results with use of the topical compound in mice, a phase I randomized, double-blind placebo-controlled study was undertaken in superficial or nodular BCCs from 2005 to 2006.[73] The primary end point was the safety and tolerability of a multidose regimen of CUR61414 at various concentrations applied topically for up to 28 days. A secondary objective included clinical activity as measured by the percentage of tumors with complete clearance. A total of 42 patients were enrolled and there were no serious adverse events (SAEs) reported. Most adverse events (AEs) were skin-related and of mild severity. In terms of response, none of the patients had a complete tumor clearance, defined as both clinical and histopathologic. Unlike in the mouse, the treatment failed to reduce GLI or PTCH expression in 8 patients tested, suggesting a differential potency in human versus mouse SMO and/or inadequate drug concentrations in BCCs owing to low penetration or rapid clearance. Although this initial study was not successful in validating Hh inhibition as a useful method for treating BCC, subsequent studies have been more promising.

The first support of proof of concept was reported by Von Hoff and colleagues[59,74] in a phase I trial investigating the safety and tolerability of vismodegib in patients with a variety of solid tumors that were refractory to standard therapy. The study had an open-label, multicenter, 2-stage design in which vismodegib was dose escalated until dose-limiting toxicity, disease progression, or lack of benefit, as determined by the investigator. In the initial stage, vismodegib was escalated from 150 mg daily to 270 mg daily and then to 540 mg daily. There were no dose-limiting side effects observed, and the dosage of 150 mg daily was chosen as the recommended phase 2 dosage because higher dosages did not result in an increased plasma concentration of the drug. There were 3 patients with BCC enrolled in the first stage, 2 of whom were noted to have a clinical benefit. As a result, the second stage included a cohort of patients with advanced BCC in addition to a cohort of patients with solid tumors, a group that was enriched with patients with BCC. In total, there were 33 patients with BCC enrolled in the study. Of the 18 patients with metastatic BCC tumors, the overall response rate (RR) was 50% (95% confidence interval [CI]: 29–71), and of the 15 patients with locally advanced BCC, the RR was 60% (95% CI: 33–83). The treatment was very well tolerated, without any dose-limiting or grade 5 AEs. A single grade 4 AE (asymptomatic hyponatremia) occurred. The most common grade 2 and 3 AEs included fatigue, myalgias, weight loss, dysgeusia, and hyponatremia. Pharmacodynamic studies demonstrated down modulation of the Hh pathway as measured by a decrease in GLI1 expression in nonaffected skin biopsies taken pretreatment and on treatment. Furthermore, GLI1 mRNA was overexpressed in BCC tumors when compared with control normal skin or lung tumor ($P<.001$ for all comparisons). When tumor tissue was analyzed for mutations in the PTCH1 gene, 9 of 10 specimens were found to harbor the mutation, further supporting PTCH's role as a tumor suppressor, with its loss of activity driving oncogenesis.

This study was the first to confirm the participation of the Hh pathway in BCC and suggests that its inhibition would be a valuable treatment for inoperable BCC. As a result, a phase II, international, single-arm, multicenter, 2-cohort, open-label study was conducted in 104 patients with advanced BCC, including 71 with locally advanced (laBCC) disease and 33 with metastatic disease (mBCC).[75] Patients received 150 mg vismodegib daily until disease progression or intolerable toxicity. The primary end point was overall response rate, as assessed by an independent review facility, with secondary end points including investigator-assessed overall response rate (ORR), progression-free survival (PFS), overall survival (OS), and duration of response in all evaluable patients. The ORR, as assessed by an independent review facility, showed vismodegib substantially shrank tumors or healed visible lesions, with an observed RR of 43% in the laBCC cohort and 30% in the mBCC cohort. Study investigators assessed the ORR to be 55%, with 60% in the laBCC cohort, and 46% in mBCC cohort. The clinical benefit rate (defined as patients who experienced response, as well as those who experienced prolonged stable disease for more than 24 weeks) showed vismodegib shrank tumors or healed visible lesions, or prevented them from growing any further in 75% of patients with laBCC and 76% of patients with mBCC, as assessed by independent review. The median duration of PFS by independent review for both patients with mBCC and patients with laBCC was 9.5 months. Treatment was generally well tolerated and the most common AEs included muscle spasms, hair loss, altered taste sensation, weight loss, fatigue, nausea, decreased appetite, and diarrhea; however, there were 4 SAEs thought to be related to treatment, including cholestasis, dehydration with syncope, pneumonia with heart failure, and pulmonary embolism. Based on these data, vismodegib has recently been FDA approved for the treatment of adults with metastatic basal cell carcinoma or with locally advanced basal cell carcinoma that has recurred following surgery or who are not candidates for surgery, and who are not candidates for radiation.

In addition to vismodegib, several other SMO antagonists have also demonstrated antitumor activity in BCC. For example, in a phase I study of LDE225 in advanced solid tumors, 1 patient with BCC experienced a complete response (CR) with histologic clearance, 4 patients with BCC had a partial response (PR), and 2 patients with BCC had disease stabilization.[61] IPI-926 also is active in BCC, showing 6 (27%) clinical or radiologic PRs in the 22 patients with Hh-inhibitor naive BCC.[62] In addition to clinical activity, these HPIs have demonstrated convincing pharmacodynamic data, with an exposure-dependent reduction of GLI1 mRNA, verifying that they are hitting their target within the pathway.

Given the mild, but certainly bothersome, side effects that have been reported with the various oral SMO antagonists in the treatment of BCC, topical routes continue to be investigated as a possibly less toxic and equally efficacious modality. Although the initial study of topical CUR61414 did not demonstrate any efficacy in humans,[76] a subsequent study with a different HPI merits promise. Topical LDE225 was developed as a distinct and selective antagonist of SMO with single-digit nanomolar potency. In an exploratory study, 8 patients with nevoid basal cell carcinoma syndrome were enrolled in a double-blind, randomized, vehicle-controlled intraindividual study.[77] Among the 8 patients, there were a total of 27 BCC tumors treated twice daily with 0.75% LDE225 cream or vehicle for 4 weeks. No skin irritation was noted or any clinically significant abnormalities. Of 13 BCCs treated with LDE225, 12 showed a clinical response (3 CR, 9 PR), whereas only 1 of the 14 lesions treated with vehicle demonstrated a clinical response. In addition, a greater than twofold downregulation of Hh target genes was demonstrated in 6 of 8 patients, confirming that the topical SMO inhibitor hits its target.

Medulloblastoma

Medulloblastoma, a rare and aggressive childhood tumor of cerebellar origin, is another malignancy that has demonstrated dependence on the Hh pathway for its pathogenesis. As with BCC, the first indication that the Hh pathway was involved in medulloblastoma came from the fact that patients with Gorlin syndrome have an increased risk of developing this unusual brain tumor, occurring in approximately 5% of these patients. The Hh pathway's role in medulloblastoma is not surprising, given the importance of its signaling in the normal cerebellar maturation process. During development, granule cell precursors must expand, migrate, and differentiate from the external granule-cell layer to form the internal granule-cell layer, a process that is spatially and temporally regulated by activation of the Hh pathway. Disruption of this process, with constitutive activation of the Hh pathway, can result in the development of medulloblastoma.[78] In mouse models heterozygous for the PTCH1 mutation, medulloblastoma occurs in about one-third of mice by 25 weeks of age.[79] In humans, it has been shown that the Hh pathway is activated, often owing to mutations in PTCH1, SMO, or SUFU, in about 30% of medulloblastomas.[80,81] There is also preclinical evidence that inhibition of the Hh pathway leads to regression of medulloblastoma tumors in PTCH mutant mice.[78] The first proof of concept for Hh pathway inhibition in medulloblastoma was reported by Rudin and colleagues.[82] They reported a case of a 26-year-old man with refractory medulloblastoma who was treated with daily vismodegib and had a dramatic PR, with rapid regression of tumor burden and reduction of symptoms. The treatment was well tolerated; however, the patient progressed within 3 months of therapy initiation. Molecular analysis of the patient's tumor pretreatment showed increased expression of Hh target genes and an underlying somatic mutation in PTCH1, suggesting reliance on the Hh pathway. A subsequent analysis of the tumor tissue following progression was undertaken to evaluate the mechanism of treatment resistance. An amino acid substitution at a conserved aspartic acid residue of SMO was identified that had no effect on Hh signaling but disrupted the ability of GDC-0449 to bind SMO and suppress the pathway.[83] This was the first report of a mechanism of resistance to HPIs and will be important in informing future drug development aimed at targeting the Hh pathway. There are currently several ongoing trials investigating HPIs in medulloblastoma in both adults and children. Given the high morbidity associated with treatment of medulloblastoma, as well as the poor outcomes, treatment with HPIs may offer a new therapeutic avenue;

however, caution is necessary because the Hh pathway plays such a crucial role in normal development, and, as a result, the effects of HPIs on children will need to be carefully monitored.

LIGAND-DEPENDENT TUMORS AND Hh INHIBITION
Preclinical

The Hh pathway has been implicated in multiple different solid tumors based on its overexpression rather than an intrinsic mutation. The first identified Hh-overexpressing tumor was small cell lung cancer (SCLC), a tumor that was studied given the essential role Hh is known to play in branching morphogenesis in the developing lung.[84] It was shown that about 25% of human SCLC samples had relatively high expression of both SHH and GLI1 and that the growth of SCLC cell lines could be inhibited in vitro using cyclopamine or a monoclonal anti-Hh antibiody.[85] In an in vivo SCLC xenograft mouse model, cyclopamine also inhibited tumor growth, suggesting that certain tumors depend on tumor cell–derived overproduction of Hh ligand for their growth, functioning in an autocrine fashion. Since then, ligand-dependent growth has been reported in most tumor types, including pancreatic, colon, gastroesophageal, breast, prostate, melanoma, lung, and ovarian cancer. In fact, it is estimated that up to 25% of human tumors may depend on Hh pathway activity for growth.[86]

Although the overexpression of Hh ligands in a variety of tumor types is clear, the extent, timing, and mechanism of action of the Hh pathway is still under active investigation. For example, in different tumor types, Hh signaling is expressed at different points in carcinogenesis. In gastric and prostate cancer, Hh signaling may be important for tumor metastasis, as inhibition of the pathway reduces cell invasiveness and motility.[87–89] The Hh pathway may promote metastases through epithelial-mesenchymal transition (EMT), an important developmental process. By upregulating the transcription factor SNAIL and downregulating E-cadherin, the Hh pathway exerts its effect on EMT and thereby metastasis.[88,89] In pancreatic and esophageal cancers, pathway activation is found in both early and metastatic cancer, suggesting the pathway's importance in tumor development.[90–92] Other lines of evidence suggest that the Hh pathway is mainly involved in CSC proliferation.[50–52,90,93] For example, it has been reported that putative pancreatic CSCs have higher SHH mRNA levels than the normal pancreas, and pretreatment with an SMO antagonist can preferentially deplete the aldehyde dehydrogenase–positive subpopulation of pancreatic tumor cells and inhibit subsequent tumor growth.[47,90] Hh signaling may also have a key role in maintenance of CML CSCs.[49,93] Treatment of CML CSCs with HPIs was reported to inhibit growth both in vitro and in vivo, prolonging time to relapse. Furthermore, many studies have demonstrated that Hh pathway activation is associated with chemotherapy and/or radiotherapy resistance, a quality inherent to a CSCs.[94–96]

Initial preclinical evidence suggested that an autocrine feedback loop was responsible for Hh-induced tumor growth. This was because tumor cells were shown to express Hh ligands in addition to downstream signaling components and their growth could be inhibited both in vitro and in vivo with HPIs.[85,88,92,97–99] In most cases, cyclopamine was the HPI used in these studies, and because doses 2 orders of magnitude greater than the amount required to inhibit Hh signaling in GLI-luciferase reporter assays were used, it is unclear if potential off-target effects of cyclopamine were responsible for the antitumor effect. Furthermore, in a subsequent study it was shown that there is no correlation between GLI1 and PTCH downregulation in tumor cells, even at the high concentrations that caused growth inhibition, again calling into question whether cyclopamine causes growth inhibition via the Hh pathway in an autocrine fahsion.[56] As a result, a paracrine mechanism of action for the Hh pathway in carcinogenesis was put forth. Yauch and colleagues[56] showed in xenograft models that although many human tumors do produce Hh ligands, the target genes upregulated by these ligands are expressed in stromal cells of mouse origin and can be downregulated with HPI treatment. This paracrine model was confirmed in a number of experiments using genetically engineered mouse models in which Hh expression was found in the tumor and Hh signaling (detected by PTCH1-LacZ reporter staining) was seen only in the surrounding myofirboblasts.[100] In addition, genetic ablation of SMO from pancreatic epithelium in a mouse model had no effect on cancer formation; whereas, genetic deletion of SMO in stromal fibroblasts led to slower growth of Hh-expressing colorectal xenografts.[56,101] In human samples from pancreatic, prostate, and colon cancers, Hh has been shown to be expressed in the tumor epithelium, and GLI, conversely, is expressed in the surrounding stroma.[100,102,103] Although there is good evidence for the paracrine model, the mechanism of stromal feedback to the tumor is unclear. Growth factors secreted by the tumor stroma in response to Hh signaling, including insulin-like growth factor 1(IGF-1), angiogenic factors, and Wnt, may directly feedback on the tumor leading to tumor cell proliferation and survival.[56,104] Another possible mechanism is via alteration of the stroma. In a mouse model of pancreatic cancer, the inhibition of Hh signaling enhanced the delivery and response to chemotherapy by depleting tumor–associated stromal tissue.[96]

In addition to autocrine and paracrine models of Hh activation in ligand-dependent tumors, a more recently characterized model of "reverse paracrine" signaling has been demonstrated in hematologic malignancies. In cancers, including multiple myeloma, lymphoma, and leukemia, Hh ligands secreted from the bone marrow stroma seem to be essential to the survival of the malignant B cells in vitro via upregulation of the antiapoptotic factor Bcl2.[49,105] In this model, Hh is thought to provide the appropriate microenvironment for tumor growth; however, this concept has been disputed, as there is some evidence in chronic lymphocytic leukemia (CLL) that SMO and stromal cell–derived Hh ligands play only a minor role in ex vivo cell survival and in fact there may be an intrinsic SMO-independent role of GLI for CLL cell survival.[106]

Clinical

Although there are several ongoing clinical trials testing the concept of Hh pathway inhibition in ligand-dependent malignancies, there are currently only 2 studies that have completed accrual and have reported their results: one in metastatic colorectal cancer and the other in advanced ovarian cancer. The first study is a randomized, placebo-controlled phase II study of vismodegib, an SMO antagonist, combined with chemotherapy in the first-line treatment of patients with metastatic colorectal cancer.[107] The primary end point was PFS and secondary end points included safety of the combination, RR, and OS. There were also embedded correlative laboratory studies including measurement of Hh ligand levels by immunohistochemistry and quantitative reverse transcriptase polymerase chain reaction and correlation with PFS. Patients were stratified based on the chemotherapy regimen chosen (5-fluorouracil, leucovorin, oxaliplatin [mFOLFOX]/bevacizumab or 5-fluorouracil, leucovorin, irinotecan [FOLFIRI]/bevacizumab) and received 150 mg daily of vismodegib/placebo in combination with chemotherapy every 2 weeks. A total of 199 patients were enrolled: 123 in the mFOLFOX/bevacizumab strata and 72 in the FOLFIRI/bevacizumab strata. The study did not meet its primary end point and PFS was not improved with the addition of vismodegib to standard chemotherapy for metastatic colorectal cancer (8.2 vs 9.9 months [mFOLFOX ± vismodegib] and 10.5 vs 10.1 months [FOLFIRI ± vismodegib]). Anorexia, weight loss, dysgeusia, and muscle cramps occurred at a greater frequency in patients treated with vismodegib. Compared with placebo, treatment intensity was lower for all regimen components in the patients treated with vismodegib. Pharmacokinetic analysis for each regimen component, including vismodegib, did not reveal any significant drug-drug interactions. In terms of the biomarker analysis, Hh ligand expression did not predict response to vismodegib, as there was no correlation seen between pathway expression and PFS. The negative results of this trial are in stark contradiction to the preclinical data demonstrating colorectal cancer's seeming dependence on the Hh pathway.[56] There are a variety of possible explanations for why Hh pathway inhibition failed in this setting. For example, patients were not selected based on their tumor's expression of the Hh pathway. Although post hoc analysis was done and did not show a correlation with Hh expression and efficacy of vismodegib, the numbers were relatively small to make any firm conclusions. Second, the timing of pathway inhibition in the metastatic setting may not be optimal for colorectal cancer and perhaps if initiated earlier in the disease course an effect would be seen. At a certain point, cancer cells may have already developed the ability to thrive in a microenvironment-independent manner and therefore would be insensitive to molecular targeted drugs acting by depriving cancer cells of paracrine-acting stimuli. If in fact the pivotal effect of the Hh pathway is on CSCs, then perhaps using standard chemotherapy first to debulk the tumor followed by HPIs may be a better strategy. Finally, the combination with bevacizumab may have obscured the effect of the HPI in colorectal cancer. Recent evidence has shown that in tumor types, such as colorectal cancer, in which the Hh's predominant tumor-promoting effect is through the induction of stromal vascular endothelial growth factor (VEGF)-A, combination with anti-VEGF therapy would not be expected to provide further benefit.[108]

The second completed trial is a phase II randomized, placebo-controlled study of vismodegib as maintenance therapy in patients with ovarian cancer in second or third complete remission.[109] In this study, patients were randomized to treatment with either vismodegib or placebo within 3 to 14 weeks following the most recent chemotherapy. The primary end point was investigator-assessed PFS and secondary end points were safety and measurement of Hh expression in archival tissue. A total of 104 women were enrolled, 81% of whom were in second remission. The hazard ratio for PFS was 0.79 (95% CI, 0.46–1.35); median PFS was 5.8 months for placebo versus 7.5 months for vismodegib. No new safety signals were observed, and the most common AEs included muscle cramps, dysgeusia, and alopecia; however, more patients in the vismodegib arm discontinued treatment compared with the placebo arm, either because of an AE or patient decision. Hh expression was not detected in most of the submitted archival tissue. Once again, Hh pathway inhibition failed in the clinic for treatment of ligand-dependent tumors. In this study, proof of concept was focused on the putative CSC population, as the patients were all in complete remission. Although a negative study, it again must be emphasized that there was no enrichment of the population with Hh high-expressing tumors. Furthermore, the earlier discontinuation of vismodegib secondary to toxicity or patient preference may suggest a lower tolerance to AEs in this setting, an argument for more tolerable HPIs, thereby making them more effective. Finally, perhaps inhibition at SMO is not the most effective way to inhibit the pathway in ligand-dependent tumors and instead focusing on the GLI transcription factors where all the transduction machinery converges or conversely inhibiting the Hh ligands at the very start of the pathway may be more successful.

ONGOING CLINICAL TRIALS

There are numerous ongoing clinical trials in both ligand-independent and ligand-dependent tumors with a variety of HPIs, all of which inhibit at SMO (see **Table 1**). The mutation-driven malignancies under investigation include BCC and medulloblastoma, both adult and pediatric. The ligand-dependent tumors being studied span a vast array of malignancies from pancreatic cancer to chondrosarcoma. These studies are targeting the Hh pathway from different angles. Most are using HPIs in the advanced disease setting, combined with a chemotherapy backbone, hoping to take advantage of the Hh's role in disease progression. Others are more focused on CSCs, trying to target a population that is by definition resistant to chemotherapy and radiation. For example, there are 2 studies combining an HPI with a notch inhibitor, another important pathway in stem cell maintenance. Another study is exploring how HPI in pancreatic cancer affects the number of CSCs and if this number is affected by treatment with chemotherapy in addition to an HPI. There is also a study being conducted in SCLC in which patients are treated with an HPI in combination with chemotherapy to "debulk" the tumor, followed by maintenance with an HPI, targeting the putative CSCs. Finally, there are a number of studies in hematologic malignancies focusing on the proposed "reverse paracrine" model of Hh pathway activity. For example, there is a study in myelofibrosis investigating whether HPI is efficacious in improving RR by specifically targeting the microenvironment. There is also a study examining the efficacy of an HPI in patients with multiple myeloma following autologous stem cell transplantation.

CHALLENGES TARGETING THE Hh PATHWAY

The Hh pathway represents a new opportunity for targeted therapy of multiple malignancies. Proof of concept has been achieved for tumors with mutations, such as BCC. In such tumors where there is a clear constitutive activation of the Hh pathway and it not only initiates but also sustains the tumor's growth, pathway inhibition is clearly an effective treatment; however, similar to many other molecularly targeted treatments, acquired drug resistance can be a problem. The first reported case of resistance occurred in a patient with refractory medulloblastoma who had an initial dramatic response to an SMO inhibitor with tumor regression and symptom resolution; however, within 3 months the patient had evidence of tumor regrowth at multiple sites. Analysis of one of the progressing lesions demonstrated an SMO mutation, resulting in a single amino acid change, and thereby leading to a deficiency in drug-target binding.[83] This case highlights one potential problem in the development of HPIs and demonstrates the importance of understanding mechanisms of drug resistance to design second-generation or complementary inhibitors. There are currently ongoing efforts to identify second-generation SMO inhibitors that display activity in vismodegib-resistant tumors, as well as inhibitors that act downstream of SMO.[110]

In addition to drug resistance resulting from mutations within the Hh pathway, it is also important to consider compensatory upregulation of other signaling pathways as possible mechanisms of resistance. There is evidence for cross talk between the Hh pathway and several other key pathways involved in carcinogenesis, including Wnt, p53, and a variety of growth factors. For example, Hh and Wnt can form a positive or negative feedback loop depending on the tissue context, an important consideration when testing HPIs. Furthermore, regulation of GLI1 expression by transforming growth factor β, Ras, JUN, and p53 has been reported.[101,111–113] When mechanisms of SMO resistance have been studied in vitro, in addition to mutations in SMO or upregulation of GLI, there is also evidence for upregulation of the IGF-1R-PI3K signaling cascade.[114] Given the Hh pathway's many interactions with a multitude of other growth pathways, a combination approach may be a more effective treatment strategy by potentially preventing resistance.

Finally, it is important to carefully monitor the toxicities of HPIs given the critical role the pathway normally plays in development. Careful attention must be paid to the potential teratogenic effects of HPIs and warning given to patients regarding pregnancy prevention. In addition, the use of inhibitors of the Hh pathway in childhood malignancies, such as medulloblastoma, must proceed with extreme caution given that it is unclear what AEs may result in a prepubescent population.

SUMMARY

Since the initial discovery of the Hh pathway by developmental biologists, there has been rapid advancement in our understanding of its role and mechanism of action in normal development and malignancy. Aberrant Hh pathway activation is clearly important in the pathogenesis of many cancers and has become the target for inhibition by several new therapeutic agents. Novel pathway inhibitors have been or are currently being developed to antagonize the Hh pathway and provide a molecularly targeted approach to cancer treatment. The challenge remains how best to identify tumors for this treatment and in what situation to use these inhibitors so they are most effective.

REFERENCES

1. Ingham PW, Nakano Y, Seger C. Mechanisms and functions of Hedgehog signalling across the metazoa. Nat Rev Genet 2011;12(6):393–406.
2. Ingham PW, McMahon AP. Hedgehog signaling in animal development: paradigms and principles. Genes Dev 2001;15(23):3059–87.
3. Nusslein-Volhard C, Wieschaus E. Mutations affecting segment number and polarity in *Drosophila*. Nature 1980;287(5785):795–801.
4. Hooper JE, Scott MP. Communicating with Hedgehogs. Nat Rev Mol Cell Biol 2005;6(4):306–17.
5. Rubin LL, de Sauvage FJ. Targeting the Hedgehog pathway in cancer. Nat Rev Drug Discov 2006;5(12):1026–33.
6. Belloni E, Muenke M, Roessler E, et al. Identification of Sonic hedgehog as a candidate gene responsible for holoprosencephaly. Nat Genet 1996;14(3): 353–6.
7. Roessler E, Belloni E, Gaudenz K, et al. Mutations in the human Sonic Hedgehog gene cause holoprosencephaly. Nat Genet 1996;14(3):357–60.
8. Adolphe C, Narang M, Ellis T, et al. An in vivo comparative study of sonic, desert and Indian hedgehog reveals that hedgehog pathway activity regulates epidermal stem cell homeostasis. Development 2004;131(20):5009–19.
9. van den Brink GR. Hedgehog signaling in development and homeostasis of the gastrointestinal tract. Physiol Rev 2007;87(4):1343–75.
10. Rockel JS, Alman BA. Don't hedge your bets: hedgehog signaling as a central mediator of endochondral bone development and cartilage diseases. J Orthop Res 2011;29(6):810–5.
11. Epstein EH. Basal cell carcinomas: attack of the hedgehog. Nat Rev Cancer 2008;8(10):743–54.

12. Mann RK, Beachy PA. Novel lipid modifications of secreted protein signals. Annu Rev Biochem 2004;73:891–923.

13. Gallet A. Hedgehog morphogen: from secretion to reception. Trends Cell Biol 2011;21(4):238–46.

14. Buglino JA, Resh MD. Identification of conserved regions and residues within Hedgehog acyltransferase critical for palmitoylation of Sonic Hedgehog. PLoS One 2010;5(6):e11195.

15. Kawakami T, Kawcak T, Li YJ, et al. Mouse dispatched mutants fail to distribute hedgehog proteins and are defective in hedgehog signaling. Development 2002;129(24):5753–65.

16. Ma Y, Erkner A, Gong R, et al. Hedgehog-mediated patterning of the mammalian embryo requires transporter-like function of dispatched. Cell 2002;111(1):63–75.

17. Taipale J, Cooper MK, Maiti T, et al. Patched acts catalytically to suppress the activity of Smoothened. Nature 2002;418(6900):892–7.

18. Yavari A, Nagaraj R, Owusu-Ansah E, et al. Role of lipid metabolism in smoothened derepression in hedgehog signaling. Dev Cell 2010;19(1):54–65.

19. Khaliullina H, Panakova D, Eugster C, et al. Patched regulates Smoothened trafficking using lipoprotein-derived lipids. Development 2009;136(24):4111–21.

20. Callejo A, Culi J, Guerrero I. Patched, the receptor of Hedgehog, is a lipoprotein receptor. Proc Natl Acad Sci U S A 2008;105(3):912–7.

21. Bijlsma MF, Spek CA, Zivkovic D, et al. Repression of smoothened by patched-dependent (pro-) vitamin D3 secretion. PLoS Biol 2006;4(8):e232.

22. Michaud EJ, Yoder BK. The primary cilium in cell signaling and cancer. Cancer Res 2006;66(13):6463–7.

23. Huangfu D, Liu A, Rakeman AS, et al. Hedgehog signalling in the mouse requires intraflagellar transport proteins. Nature 2003;426(6962):83–7.

24. Cortellino S, Wang C, Wang B, et al. Defective ciliogenesis, embryonic lethality and severe impairment of the Sonic Hedgehog pathway caused by inactivation of the mouse complex A intraflagellar transport gene Ift122/Wdr10, partially overlapping with the DNA repair gene Med1/Mbd4. Dev Biol 2009;325(1):225–37.

25. Bai CB, Stephen D, Joyner AL. All mouse ventral spinal cord patterning by hedgehog is Gli dependent and involves an activator function of Gli3. Dev Cell 2004;6(1):103–15.

26. Bhatia N, Thiyagarajan S, Elcheva I, et al. Gli2 is targeted for ubiquitination and degradation by beta-TrCP ubiquitin ligase. J Biol Chem 2006;281(28):19320–6.

27. Wang B, Li Y. Evidence for the direct involvement of {beta}TrCP in Gli3 protein processing. Proc Natl Acad Sci U S A 2006;103(1):33–8.

28. Katoh Y, Katoh M. Hedgehog target genes: mechanisms of carcinogenesis induced by aberrant hedgehog signaling activation. Curr Mol Med 2009;9(7): 873–86.

29. Kinzler KW, Vogelstein B. The GLI gene encodes a nuclear protein which binds specific sequences in the human genome. Mol Cell Biol 1990;10(2):634–42.

30. Sasaki H, Hui C, Nakafuku M, et al. A binding site for Gli proteins is essential for HNF-3beta floor plate enhancer activity in transgenics and can respond to Shh in vitro. Development 1997;124(7):1313–22.

31. Kinzler KW, Ruppert JM, Bigner SH, et al. The GLI gene is a member of the Kruppel family of zinc finger proteins. Nature 1988;332(6162):371–4.

32. Ruiz i Altaba A, Mas C, Stecca B. The Gli code: an information nexus regulating cell fate, stemness and cancer. Trends Cell Biol 2007;17(9):438–47.

33. Yang L, Xie G, Fan Q, et al. Activation of the hedgehog-signaling pathway in human cancer and the clinical implications. Oncogene 2010;29(4):469–81.

34. Barnfield PC, Zhang X, Thanabalasingham V, et al. Negative regulation of Gli1 and Gli2 activator function by Suppressor of fused through multiple mechanisms. Differentiation 2005;73(8):397–405.
35. Kise Y, Morinaka A, Teglund S, et al. Sufu recruits GSK3beta for efficient processing of Gli3. Biochem Biophys Res Commun 2009;387(3):569–74.
36. Cheng SY, Bishop JM. Suppressor of Fused represses Gli-mediated transcription by recruiting the SAP18-mSin3 corepressor complex. Proc Natl Acad Sci U S A 2002;99(8):5442–7.
37. Hahn H, Wicking C, Zaphiropoulous PG, et al. Mutations of the human homolog of Drosophila patched in the nevoid basal cell carcinoma syndrome. Cell 1996; 85(6):841–51.
38. Johnson RL, Rothman AL, Xie J, et al. Human homolog of patched, a candidate gene for the basal cell nevus syndrome. Science 1996;272(5268):1668–71.
39. Gailani MR, Stahle-Backdahl M, Leffell DJ, et al. The role of the human homologue of Drosophila patched in sporadic basal cell carcinomas. Nat Genet 1996;14(1):78–81.
40. Reifenberger J, Wolter M, Weber RG, et al. Missense mutations in SMOH in sporadic basal cell carcinomas of the skin and primitive neuroectodermal tumors of the central nervous system. Cancer Res 1998;58(9):1798–803.
41. Xie J, Johnson RL, Zhang X, et al. Mutations of the PATCHED gene in several types of sporadic extracutaneous tumors. Cancer Res 1997;57(12):2369–72.
42. Reifenberger J, Wolter M, Knobbe CB, et al. Somatic mutations in the PTCH, SMOH, SUFUH and TP53 genes in sporadic basal cell carcinomas. Br J Dermatol 2005;152(1):43–51.
43. Zhang Y, Kalderon D. Hedgehog acts as a somatic stem cell factor in the Drosophila ovary. Nature 2001;410(6828):599–604.
44. Takebe N, Harris PJ, Warren RQ, et al. Targeting cancer stem cells by inhibiting Wnt, Notch, and Hedgehog pathways. Nat Rev Clin Oncol 2011;8(2):97–106.
45. Merchant AA, Matsui W. Targeting Hedgehog—a cancer stem cell pathway. Clin Cancer Res 2010;16(12):3130–40.
46. Visvader JE, Lindeman GJ. Cancer stem cells in solid tumours: accumulating evidence and unresolved questions. Nat Rev Cancer 2008;8(10):755–68.
47. Li C, Heidt DG, Dalerba P, et al. Identification of pancreatic cancer stem cells. Cancer Res 2007;67(3):1030–7.
48. Theunissen JW, de Sauvage FJ. Paracrine Hedgehog signaling in cancer. Cancer Res 2009;69(15):6007–10.
49. Dierks C, Beigi R, Guo GR, et al. Expansion of Bcr-Abl-positive leukemic stem cells is dependent on Hedgehog pathway activation. Cancer Cell 2008;14(3): 238–49.
50. Clement V, Sanchez P, de Tribolet N, et al. HEDGEHOG-GLI1 signaling regulates human glioma growth, cancer stem cell self-renewal, and tumorigenicity. Curr Biol 2007;17(2):165–72.
51. Peacock CD, Wang Q, Gesell GS, et al. Hedgehog signaling maintains a tumor stem cell compartment in multiple myeloma. Proc Natl Acad Sci U S A 2007; 104(10):4048–53.
52. Liu S, Dontu G, Mantle ID, et al. Hedgehog signaling and Bmi-1 regulate self-renewal of normal and malignant human mammary stem cells. Cancer Res 2006;66(12):6063–71.
53. Binns W, James LF, Shupe JL, et al. A congenital cyclopian-type malformation in lambs induced by maternal ingestion of a range plant, Veratrum californicum. Am J Vet Res 1963;24:1164–75.

54. Cooper MK, Porter JA, Young KE, et al. Teratogen-mediated inhibition of target tissue response to Shh signaling. Science 1998;280(5369):1603–7.
55. Chen JK, Taipale J, Cooper MK, et al. Inhibition of Hedgehog signaling by direct binding of cyclopamine to Smoothened. Genes Dev 2002;16(21): 2743–8.
56. Yauch RL, Gould SE, Scales SJ, et al. A paracrine requirement for hedgehog signalling in cancer. Nature 2008;455(7211):406–10.
57. Williams JA. Hedgehog signaling pathway as a target for therapeutic intervention in basal cell carcinoma. Drug News Perspect 2003;16(10):657–62.
58. Tremblay MR, Nevalainen M, Nair SJ, et al. Semisynthetic cyclopamine analogues as potent and orally bioavailable hedgehog pathway antagonists. J Med Chem 2008;51(21):6646–9.
59. Von Hoff DD, LoRusso PM, Rudin CM, et al. Inhibition of the hedgehog pathway in advanced basal-cell carcinoma. N Engl J Med 2009;361(12):1164–72.
60. Siu LL, Papadopoulos K, Alberts SR, et al. A first-in-human, phase I study of an oral hedgehog (HH) pathway antagonist, BMS-833923 (XL139), in subjects with advanced or metastatic solid tumors [abstract]. J Clin Oncol 2010;28(15 Suppl): abstr 2501.
61. Tawbi HA, Ahnert JR, Dummer R, et al. Phase I study of LDE225 in advanced solid tumors: updated analysis of safety, preliminary efficacy, and pharmacokinetic-pharmacodynamic correlation. J Clin Oncol 2011;29(15 Suppl):abstr 3062.
62. Rudin CM, Jimeno A, Miller WH, et al. A phase I study of IPI-926, a novel hedgehog pathway inhibitor, in patients (pts) with advanced or metastatic solid tumors. J Clin Oncol 2011;29(15 Suppl):abstr 3014.
63. Stanton BZ, Peng LF, Maloof N, et al. A small molecule that binds Hedgehog and blocks its signaling in human cells. Nat Chem Biol 2009;5(3):154–6.
64. Lauth M, Bergstrom A, Shimokawa T, et al. Inhibition of GLI-mediated transcription and tumor cell growth by small-molecule antagonists. Proc Natl Acad Sci U S A 2007;104(20):8455–60.
65. Hyman JM, Firestone AJ, Heine VM, et al. Small-molecule inhibitors reveal multiple strategies for Hedgehog pathway blockade. Proc Natl Acad Sci U S A 2009;106(33):14132–7.
66. Kim J, Lee JJ, Gardner D, et al. Arsenic antagonizes the Hedgehog pathway by preventing ciliary accumulation and reducing stability of the Gli2 transcriptional effector. Proc Natl Acad Sci U S A 2010;107(30):13432–7.
67. Kim J, Tang JY, Gong R, et al. Itraconazole, a commonly used antifungal that inhibits Hedgehog pathway activity and cancer growth. Cancer Cell 2010;17(4): 388–99.
68. Xie J, Murone M, Luoh SM, et al. Activating Smoothened mutations in sporadic basal-cell carcinoma. Nature 1998;391(6662):90–2.
69. Oro AE, Higgins KM, Hu Z, et al. Basal cell carcinomas in mice overexpressing sonic hedgehog. Science 1997;276(5313):817–21.
70. Nilsson M, Unden AB, Krause D, et al. Induction of basal cell carcinomas and trichoepitheliomas in mice overexpressing GLI-1. Proc Natl Acad Sci U S A 2000;97(7):3438–43.
71. Aszterbaum M, Epstein J, Oro A, et al. Ultraviolet and ionizing radiation enhance the growth of BCCs and trichoblastomas in patched heterozygous knockout mice. Nat Med 1999;5(11):1285–91.
72. Williams JA, Guicherit OM, Zaharian BI, et al. Identification of a small molecule inhibitor of the hedgehog signaling pathway: effects on basal cell carcinoma-like lesions. Proc Natl Acad Sci U S A 2003;100(8):4616–21.

73. Tang T, Tang JY, Li D, et al. Targeting superficial or nodular basal cell carcinoma with topically formulated small molecule inhibitor of smoothened. Clin Cancer Res 2011;17(10):3378–87.

74. LoRusso PM, Rudin CM, Reddy JC, et al. Phase I trial of hedgehog pathway inhibitor vismodegib (GDC-0449) in patients with refractory, locally advanced or metastatic solid tumors. Clin Cancer Res 2011;17(8):2502–11.

75. Sekulic A, Migden M, Oro A, et al. Abstracts of the 7th European Association of Dermato-Oncology (EADO) Congress. J20-23, 2011. Nantes, France. Melanoma Res 2011;21(Suppl):e1–63.

76. Tang JY, Mackay-Wiggan JM, Aszterbaum M, et al. An investigator-initiated, phase II randomized, double-blind, placebo-controlled trial of GDC-0449 for prevention of BCCs in basal cell nevus syndrome (BCNS) patients. Orlando (FL): American Association for Cancer Research; 2011.

77. Skvara H, Kalthoff F, Meingassner JG, et al. Topical treatment of basal cell carcinomas in nevoid basal cell carcinoma syndrome with a smoothened inhibitor. J Invest Dermatol 2011;131(8):1735–44.

78. Romer JT, Kimura H, Magdaleno S, et al. Suppression of the Shh pathway using a small molecule inhibitor eliminates medulloblastoma in Ptc1(+/-)p53(-/-) mice. Cancer Cell 2004;6(3):229–40.

79. Goodrich LV, Milenkovic L, Higgins KM, et al. Altered neural cell fates and medulloblastoma in mouse patched mutants. Science 1997;277(5329):1109–13.

80. Lee Y, Miller HL, Jensen P, et al. A molecular fingerprint for medulloblastoma. Cancer Res 2003;63(17):5428–37.

81. Thompson MC, Fuller C, Hogg TL, et al. Genomics identifies medulloblastoma subgroups that are enriched for specific genetic alterations. J Clin Oncol 2006;24(12):1924–31.

82. Rudin CM, Hann CL, Laterra J, et al. Treatment of medulloblastoma with hedgehog pathway inhibitor GDC-0449. N Engl J Med 2009;361(12):1173–8.

83. Yauch RL, Dijkgraaf GJ, Alicke B, et al. Smoothened mutation confers resistance to a Hedgehog pathway inhibitor in medulloblastoma. Science 2009;326(5952):572–4.

84. Pepicelli CV, Lewis PM, McMahon AP. Sonic hedgehog regulates branching morphogenesis in the mammalian lung. Curr Biol 1998;8(19):1083–6.

85. Watkins DN, Berman DM, Burkholder SG, et al. Hedgehog signalling within airway epithelial progenitors and in small-cell lung cancer. Nature 2003;422(6929):313–7.

86. Lum L, Beachy PA. The Hedgehog response network: sensors, switches, and routers. Science 2004;304(5678):1755–9.

87. Yoo YA, Kang MH, Kim JS, et al. Sonic hedgehog signaling promotes motility and invasiveness of gastric cancer cells through TGF-beta-mediated activation of the ALK5-Smad 3 pathway. Carcinogenesis 2008;29(3):480–90.

88. Karhadkar SS, Bova GS, Abdallah N, et al. Hedgehog signalling in prostate regeneration, neoplasia and metastasis. Nature 2004;431(7009):707–12.

89. Feldmann G, Dhara S, Fendrich V, et al. Blockade of hedgehog signaling inhibits pancreatic cancer invasion and metastases: a new paradigm for combination therapy in solid cancers. Cancer Res 2007;67(5):2187–96.

90. Feldmann G, Fendrich V, McGovern K, et al. An orally bioavailable small-molecule inhibitor of Hedgehog signaling inhibits tumor initiation and metastasis in pancreatic cancer. Mol Cancer Ther 2008;7(9):2725–35.

91. Ma X, Sheng T, Zhang Y, et al. Hedgehog signaling is activated in subsets of esophageal cancers. Int J Cancer 2006;118(1):139–48.

92. Thayer SP, di Magliano MP, Heiser PW, et al. Hedgehog is an early and late mediator of pancreatic cancer tumorigenesis. Nature 2003;425(6960):851–6.

93. Zhao C, Chen A, Jamieson CH, et al. Hedgehog signalling is essential for maintenance of cancer stem cells in myeloid leukaemia. Nature 2009;458(7239): 776–9.

94. Sims-Mourtada J, Izzo JG, Apisarnthanarax S, et al. Hedgehog: an attribute to tumor regrowth after chemoradiotherapy and a target to improve radiation response. Clin Cancer Res 2006;12(21):6565–72.

95. Yoshikawa R, Nakano Y, Tao L, et al. Hedgehog signal activation in oesophageal cancer patients undergoing neoadjuvant chemoradiotherapy. Br J Cancer 2008; 98(10):1670–4.

96. Olive KP, Jacobetz MA, Davidson CJ, et al. Inhibition of Hedgehog signaling enhances delivery of chemotherapy in a mouse model of pancreatic cancer. Science 2009;324(5933):1457–61.

97. Berman DM, Karhadkar SS, Maitra A, et al. Widespread requirement for Hedgehog ligand stimulation in growth of digestive tract tumours. Nature 2003;425(6960):846–51.

98. Qualtrough D, Buda A, Gaffield W, et al. Hedgehog signalling in colorectal tumour cells: induction of apoptosis with cyclopamine treatment. Int J Cancer 2004;110(6):831–7.

99. Stecca B, Mas C, Clement V, et al. Melanomas require HEDGEHOG-GLI signaling regulated by interactions between GLI1 and the RAS-MEK/AKT pathways. Proc Natl Acad Sci U S A 2007;104(14):5895–900.

100. Tian H, Callahan CA, DuPree KJ, et al. Hedgehog signaling is restricted to the stromal compartment during pancreatic carcinogenesis. Proc Natl Acad Sci U S A 2009;106(11):4254–9.

101. Nolan-Stevaux O, Lau J, Truitt ML, et al. GLI1 is regulated through Smoothened-independent mechanisms in neoplastic pancreatic ducts and mediates PDAC cell survival and transformation. Genes Dev 2009;23(1):24–36.

102. Fan L, Pepicelli CV, Dibble CC, et al. Hedgehog signaling promotes prostate xenograft tumor growth. Endocrinology 2004;145(8):3961–70.

103. Bailey JM, Swanson BJ, Hamada T, et al. Sonic hedgehog promotes desmoplasia in pancreatic cancer. Clin Cancer Res 2008;14(19):5995–6004.

104. Yamazaki M, Nakamura K, Mizukami Y, et al. Sonic hedgehog derived from human pancreatic cancer cells augments angiogenic function of endothelial progenitor cells. Cancer Sci 2008;99(6):1131–8.

105. Hegde GV, Peterson KJ, Emanuel K, et al. Hedgehog-induced survival of B-cell chronic lymphocytic leukemia cells in a stromal cell microenvironment: a potential new therapeutic target. Mol Cancer Res 2008;6(12):1928–36.

106. Desch P, Asslaber D, Kern D, et al. Inhibition of GLI, but not Smoothened, induces apoptosis in chronic lymphocytic leukemia cells. Oncogene 2010; 29(35):4885–95.

107. Berlin JD, Bendell J, Hart L, et al. A phase 2, randomized, double-blind, placebo-controlled study of hedgehog pathway inhibitor (HPI) GDC-0449 in patients with previously untreated metastatic colorectal cancer (mCRC) [abstract LBA21]. Ann Oncol 2010;21(Suppl 8):viii10.

108. Chen W, Tang T, Eastham-Anderson J, et al. Canonical hedgehog signaling augments tumor angiogenesis by induction of VEGF-A in stromal perivascular cells. Proc Natl Acad Sci U S A 2011;108(23):9589–94.

109. Kaye SB, Fehrenbacher L, Holloway R, et al. A phase 2, randomized, placebo-controlled study of hedgehog (HH) pathway inhibitor GDC-0449 as maintenance

therapy in patients with ovarian cancer in 2nd or 3rd complete remission. Ann Oncol 2010;21(Suppl 8).

110. Metcalfe C, de Sauvage FJ. Hedgehog fights back: mechanisms of acquired resistance against Smoothened antagonists. Cancer Res 2011;71(15):5057–61.

111. Ji Z, Mei FC, Xie J, et al. Oncogenic KRAS activates hedgehog signaling pathway in pancreatic cancer cells. J Biol Chem 2007;282(19):14048–55.

112. Laner-Plamberger S, Kaser A, Paulischta M, et al. Cooperation between GLI and JUN enhances transcription of JUN and selected GLI target genes. Oncogene 2009;28(13):1639–51.

113. Stecca B, Ruiz I, Altaba A. A GLI1-p53 inhibitory loop controls neural stem cell and tumour cell numbers. EMBO J 2009;28(6):663–76.

114. Buonamici S, Williams J, Morrissey M, et al. Interfering with resistance to smoothened antagonists by inhibition of the PI3K pathway in medulloblastoma. Sci Transl Med 2010;2(51):51ra70.

Tyrosine Kinase Inhibitors in Lung Cancer

Anish Thomas, MD, Arun Rajan, MD, Giuseppe Giaccone, MD, PhD*

KEYWORDS

- Non–small cell lung cancer • Tyrosine kinase inhibitor
- Epidermal growth factor receptor • Anaplastic lymphoma kinase translocation
- Vascular endothelial growth factor

KEY POINTS

- Erlotinib is approved for use as monotherapy in locally advanced or metastatic non–small cell lung cancer (NSCLC) after failure of at least one prior chemotherapy and as maintenance for patients whose disease has not progressed after 4 cycles of platinum-based first-line chemotherapy.
- Presence of epidermal growth factor receptor (EGFR)-activating mutation is the strongest predictor of response rates and progression-free survival in patients with NSCLC treated with EGFR–tyrosine kinase inhibitors (TKIs), and it is recommended that all patients who are considered for first-line therapy with an EGFR-TKI undergo tumor testing for presence of EGFR mutations.
- The most common adverse reactions with EGFR-TKI are rashlike events and diarrhea, although uncommonly, life-threatening events like interstitial lung disease are observed.
- Crizotinib is approved for treatment of patients with locally advanced or metastatic anaplastic lymphoma kinase translocation (ALK)-positive NSCLC.
- The most commonly reported adverse events with crizotinib are nausea, diarrhea, vomiting, edema, and constipation.
- Clinical development of other growth-related protein kinase inhibitors and efforts to understand the biology of resistance to EGFR and ALK tyrosine kinase inhibition and strategies to overcome resistance are ongoing.

Lung cancer accounts for more deaths than does any other cancer in both men and women in the United States and worldwide.[1,2] Non–small cell lung cancer (NSCLC) constitutes approximately 85% of all lung cancers, and 40% of patients with newly diagnosed NSCLC have metastatic disease.[1] In patients with advanced NSCLC, as well as those who relapse after initial definitive therapy, platinum-based systemic

Financial disclosure and conflict of interest: None.
Funding support: Intramural Research Program, National Cancer Institute.
Medical Oncology Branch, National Cancer Institution, Room 12N226, 10 Center Drive, Bethesda, MD 20892, USA
* Corresponding author.
E-mail address: giacconeg@mail.nih.gov

Hematol Oncol Clin N Am 26 (2012) 589–605
doi:10.1016/j.hoc.2012.02.001
0889-8588/12/$ – see front matter Published by Elsevier Inc.

chemotherapy improves survival, quality of life, and symptom control compared with supportive care.[3] However, despite the addition of new therapies, the median overall survival (OS) of patients with advanced NSCLC is approximately 1 year and only 3.5% of patients survive 5 years after diagnosis.[4]

Protein kinases play a crucial role in signal transduction, cellular proliferation, differentiation, and other regulatory mechanisms. The identification of growth-related protein kinases, especially tyrosine kinases, as a therapeutic target for cancer and adenosine triphosphate (ATP)-binding domain of tyrosine kinases as an attractive target for drug design have led to clinical development of an array of tyrosine kinase inhibitors (TKIs) in various malignancies, including lung cancer. In recent years, clinical application of these agents, coupled with understanding of NSCLC as a heterogeneous disease with several genetic subsets, has led to median survival extending to beyond 30 months in selected patients with advanced NSCLC.[5] This review discusses TKIs in lung cancer, focusing on clinical evidence supporting the use and practical aspects of management of patients using inhibitors of 2 of the most extensively studied tyrosine kinases in the recent past: epidermal growth factor receptor (EGFR) and anaplastic lymphoma kinase (ALK).

EPIDERMAL GROWTH FACTOR RECEPTOR TYROSINE KINASE INHIBITORS

EGFR (HER1, ErbB1) is a member of a family of transmembrane glycoprotein receptors that also includes HER2, HER3, and HER4 (also known as ERBB2, ERBB3, and ERBB4, respectively). In normal cells, ligand binding to the extracellular domain of EGFR induces receptor homodimerization and heterodimerization, which leads to conformational changes in EGFR, activation of the intracellular tyrosine kinase domain, phosphorylation of specific tyrosine residues, and recruitment of a range of proteins, which activates downstream signaling pathways including mitogen-activated protein kinase (MAPK), phosphatidylinositol-3-OH kinase (PI3K/Akt), and the signal transducer and activator of transcription (STAT)-mediated pathways. In NSCLC, EGFR protein is expressed in 50% to 90% of cases, and EGFR-associated signaling pathways are frequently dysregulated.[6,7] The 2 major approaches to EGFR inhibition are the use of small-molecule inhibitors of intracellular tyrosine kinase domain and monoclonal antibodies, which block the extracellular domain of the receptor. Gefitinib and erlotinib are orally administered EGFR-TKIs, which compete with ATP for binding to the tyrosine kinase domain.

Clinical Trials of EGFR-TKIs in Lung Cancer

Results of initial phase II studies of EGFR-TKIs in previously treated patients with advanced NSCLC of all histologies appeared very promising. IDEAL 1 and IDEAL 2, both randomized, double-blind, phase II, multicenter trials, which evaluated 250 mg or 500 mg of continuous oral gefitinib in more than 400 patients, demonstrated a tumor objective response rate (ORR) of 9% to 19%, median survival of 6 to 8 months, and improvement in lung cancer symptoms.[8,9] There was no difference in ORR, time to progression, and median survival between the 2 doses, and the 500-mg dose level was associated with more adverse events. In May 2003, based on data from IDEAL 2 trial, gefitinib (250 mg) received accelerated approval by the US Food and Drug Administration (FDA) for monotherapy for patients with advanced NSCLC after failure of both platinum-based chemotherapy and docetaxel. A smaller phase II trial of continuous oral erlotinib in 57 patients also showed response rates of 12.3%, median survival of 8.4 months, and tumor-related symptom improvement.[10]

However, in previously untreated patients with advanced NSCLC of all histologies, randomized trials of combination of EGFR-TKIs with conventional chemotherapy showed no improvements in OS over chemotherapy alone.[11–14] The INTACT 1 and INTACT 2 trials demonstrated no survival benefit of concurrent administration of gefitinib with either cisplatin/gemcitabine or carboplatin/paclitaxel, respectively, compared with chemotherapy alone.[11,12] Similarly, the TALENT and TRIBUTE trials, which combined erlotinib with cisplatin/gemcitabine or carboplatin/paclitaxel, respectively, showed no survival benefit compared with chemotherapy alone.[13,14]

In chemotherapy pretreated NSCLC patients, 2 large multicenter phase III trials that evaluated monotherapy with EGFR-TKIs yielded divergent results.[15,16] The BR.21 trial randomized 731 patients with all histologies of advanced NSCLC who had received 1 or 2 prior chemotherapy regimens in a 2:1 ratio to receive either erlotinib or placebo.[16] Despite a high proportion of patients who had received 2 or more prior chemotherapies (50%), OS, the primary end point of the study (6.7 months vs 4.7 months; hazard ratio [HR] 0.70; $P<.001$), ORR (8.9% vs <1%; $P<.001$), and improvements in symptoms favored the erlotinib group. By contrast, a similarly designed ISEL trial of 1692 patients found no significant survival advantage for gefitinib either in the overall population of NSCLC patients who had received 1 or 2 prior chemotherapy regimens or in the adenocarcinoma coprimary population.[15] Although the 2 trial populations were similar in many respects, a higher proportion of the ISEL trial population had not responded to prior chemotherapy regimen (38% vs 18%) and had progressive disease (45% vs 28%) compared with the BR.21 population. Another possible explanation of the discordant results was the relatively low drug dosing in the ISEL trial, which used one-third of the maximum tolerated dose (MTD) of gefitinib (250 mg) compared with the MTD of erlotinib (150 mg) used in the BR.21 trial. As a result of these postmarketing phase III results, in 2005 the FDA restricted the use of gefitinib to patients who are currently benefiting or have previously benefited from its use.

In selected chemo-naïve patients with advanced NSCLC, 5 phase III open-label, randomized trials in East Asian patients demonstrated superior ORR and progression-free survival (PFS) when gefitinib was compared with platinum-based chemotherapy.[5,17–20] The IPASS and First-SIGNAL trial populations were enriched to increase the likelihood of response based on clinicopathologic features, that is, never-smokers/former light smokers and adenocarcinoma histology.[17,19] The OPTIMAL, WJTOG3405, and NEJ002 trial populations were molecularly defined based on the presence of EGFR-activating mutations and additionally in the case of NEJ002, absence of a resistant mutation.[5,18,20] IPASS, which was the largest of these trials, was designed with PFS as the primary end point to assess the noninferiority of gefitinib compared with carboplatin/paclitaxel in 1217 patients.[17] The study met its primary objective of demonstrating noninferiority and showed superiority of gefitinib for PFS (HR 0.74, 95% confidence interval [CI] 0.65–0.85; $P<.001$), ORR (43% vs 32.2%; $P<.001$), and quality of life in the overall study population.[17] Recently reported updated survival results showed no significant difference in OS between the treatment arms in the intention-to-treat population (HR 0.90, 95% CI 0.79–1.02; $P = .109$) as well as in the mutation-positive and mutation-negative subgroups.[21] One of the factors that possibly contributed to the lack of survival benefit is the high proportion of patients in the chemotherapy arm (64.3%) who received gefitinib at progression. Results of EURTAC, a phase III randomized study that compared erlotinib with platinum-based chemotherapy in chemo-naïve Caucasian patients with EGFR-activating mutations, also reported a PFS (9.4 months vs 5.2 months; HR 0.42; $P<.0001$), but no OS benefit of erlotinib.[22]

In the maintenance setting, several phase III trials have demonstrated modest improvements in PFS, but no OS advantage with gefitinib[23,24] or erlotinib[25–27] after chemotherapy in unselected patients with advanced NSCLC. In the SATURN study

(N = 884), erlotinib prolonged PFS in patients who had nonprogressive disease after 4 cycles of first-line platinum-doublet chemotherapy in the overall population as well as in the EGFR immunohistochemistry-positive subgroups. After a median follow-up more than 11 months, median PFS was longer with erlotinib than with placebo (12·3 weeks vs 11·1 week [HR 0·71, 95% CI 0·62–0·82; P< ·0001]).[25] In a prospectively planned analysis of the SATURN study, OS was significantly prolonged with maintenance erlotinib, compared with placebo (HR 0.72, 95% CI 0.59–0.89; P = .0019; median OS 11.9 vs 9.6 months, respectively) in patients who had stable disease after the first-line chemotherapy (n = 487, 55%).[28] However, no significant difference in OS was observed in the patients who had complete/partial response (n = 394, 44%) (HR 0.94, 95% CI 0.74–1.20; P = .6181; median OS 12.5 vs 12.0 months in the erlotinib and placebo groups, respectively).[28] The ATLAS trial, which evaluated the benefit of addition of erlotinib to bevacizumab as maintenance therapy after first-line platinum-doublet chemotherapy plus bevacizumab, also met its primary end point of improving PFS (4.76 months vs 3.75 months [HR 0.72, P = .0012]).[26,27] The phase III SWOG-S0023 study, which prospectively evaluated maintenance gefitinib after chemoradiotherapy in unselected patients with locally advanced NSCLC, was suspended before completing its target accrual after an unplanned interim analysis showed inferior OS in the gefitinib arm compared with the placebo arm (HR 0.633, 95% CI 0.44–0.91; P = .013).[29]

Based on the results of BR.21 and SATURN trials, erlotinib (150 mg) was approved by the FDA as monotherapy in locally advanced or metastatic NSCLC after failure of at least 1 prior chemotherapy regimen and as maintenance therapy for patients whose disease had not progressed after 4 cycles of platinum-based first-line chemotherapy.

Predictors of Response to EGFR-TKIs

Early trials of EGFR-TKIs in NSCLC identified the factors female sex, adenocarcinoma histology, East Asian descent, and no prior history of smoking to correlate with response to treatment.[8,9,15,16] Since then, several EGFR-related biomarkers including EGFR mutation, gene copy number, and protein expression have been investigated in major clinical trials for their predictive value. EGFR-activating mutations, which are found more frequently in patients with these clinicopathologic features, have emerged as the strongest predictor of response rates and PFS in patients treated with EGFR-TKIs.[21,30–32] EGFR-activating mutations are found in the kinase domain of the EGFR gene and comprise mostly in-frame deletions of exon 19 and L858R substitution in exon 21.[30,31,33–35] In unselected NSCLC patients, EGFR mutations are found in about 10% of the population. In clinicopathologically selected patients, the incidence is about 60% in Asians and 40% in whites.

Despite the strong correlation of clinicopathologic criteria and EGFR mutations, several recent reports show that EGFR mutations rather than clinicopathologic criteria should be used to select chemo-naïve patients for EGFR-TKI use. In the IPASS trial, patients with EGFR mutations who were treated with gefitinib had remarkably high ORR (71.2%), PFS (HR 0.48, 95% CI 0.36–0.64; P<.001) and improvement in quality of life. By contrast, patients with wild-type EGFR (n = 176) treated with gefitinib had inferior ORR (1.1%), PFS (HR 2.85, 95% CI 2.05–3.98; P<.001) and OS (HR 1.38, 95% CI 0.92–2.09; not significant).[17] The OS disadvantage of EGFR wild-type patients who were treated with gefitinib, although not statistically significant, persisted in updated survival analysis and was also observed in the First-SIGNAL study (HR 1.199, 95% CI 0.570–2.521; P = .632).[19,21] A differential response to EGFR-TKIs based on the type of EGFR mutation was noted in some studies,[17,36] although this could not be confirmed in others.[18]

Practical Considerations

Toxicities

The most common adverse reactions with EGFR-TKIs are rashlike events and diarrhea.[37,38] Erlotinib and gefitinib have similar toxicity profiles, but erlotinib is more toxic because its recommended dose is closer to the MTD. In the BR.21 trial, grade 3/4 rash occurred in 9% patients with a median time to onset of 8 days.[16] A spectrum of skin, hair, and nail changes are known to occur, but the most common dermatologic manifestation is a papulopustular rash involving the face and/or upper trunk. On initiation of EGFR-TKI, all patients should be advised to use emollients, minimize sun exposure, and use sunscreens. Once skin toxicity is manifest, depending on the severity, topical or systemic glucocorticoids, antibiotics, and immunomodulators may be used.[39] Several expert groups have issued guidelines for the grading and management of skin changes related to EGFR inhibition.[40–42] In the BR.21 trial, grade 3/4 diarrhea occurred in 6% patients with a median time to onset of 12 days.[16] Diarrhea is often mild, and loperamide may be used for symptomatic management. Most cases of rash and diarrhea are best addressed by symptomatic management and do not necessitate alteration in the course of treatment. However, in case of severe symptoms, dose modifications or treatment interruption may be necessary. In the BR.21 study, 6% and 1% of patients needed dose reduction for rash and diarrhea, respectively, and each resulted in discontinuation of erlotinib in 1% of patients.[16]

Interstitial lung disease (ILD)-like events have been observed in patients receiving EGFR-TKIs, with an overall incidence of about 1% and a higher incidence in Japanese patients. A prospective study of Japanese patients receiving either gefitinib or chemotherapy identified older age ($\geq$55), poor performance status, smoking, short duration since diagnosis of NSCLC, reduced normal lung on computed tomography scan, preexisting chronic ILD, and concurrent cardiac disease as risk factors for the development of ILD.[43] Patients often present with acute onset of dyspnea, sometimes associated with cough or low-grade fever, often becoming severe within a short time. These symptoms warrant immediate interruption of EGFR-TKI and institution of supportive measures including oxygen, corticosteroids, or assisted ventilation.[37,38]

Dosing

Erlotinib is used at its MTD of 150 mg daily, on an empty stomach at least 1 hour before or 2 hours after the ingestion of food. When dose reduction is necessary, the erlotinib dose should be reduced in 50-mg decrements. Gefitinib is used at 250 mg per day with or without food, a dose lower than its MTD, based on phase II data that showed similar efficacy, but less toxicity with 250 mg.[37,38]

Interactions

Drugs that alter the pH of the upper gastrointestinal (GI) tract may alter the solubility of erlotinib and gefitinib, thus reducing their bioavailability. Coadministration with omeprazole, a proton-pump inhibitor, decreased erlotinib exposure by 46%. Because proton pump inhibitors affect the pH of the upper GI tract for an extended period, separation of doses may not eliminate the interaction and hence concomitant use of proton-pump inhibitors with erlotinib should be avoided, if possible. If patients need to be treated with an H2-receptor antagonist (eg, ranitidine), it should be used in a staggered manner: erlotinib must be taken 10 hours after and at least 2 hours before a dose of H2-receptor antagonist. Erlotinib and gefitinib undergo extensive hepatic metabolism, predominantly by cytochrome P (CYP) 3A4. Inhibitors (eg, ketoconazole) and inducers (eg, rifampicin) of CYP3A4 would be expected increase and decrease drug exposure, respectively.[37,38] Cigarette smoking, which is known to induce many hepatic CYP450 enzymes, reduces erlotinib exposure, and patients should be advised to stop smoking.[44]

Monitoring

Patients with hepatic impairment should be closely monitored during therapy with erlotinib and gefitinib. Dosing should be interrupted or discontinued if total bilirubin is greater than 3 times the upper limit of normal (ULN) and/or transaminases are greater than 5 times the ULN in the setting of normal pretreatment values.[37,38]

Duration

Treatment should continue until disease progression or unacceptable toxicity occurs. Although accelerated progression of disease after discontinuation of TKIs has been observed in some studies,[45,46] there is no evidence at this time that treatment beyond progression is beneficial.

Erlotinib versus gefitinib

As already discussed, erlotinib is dosed at its MTD whereas gefitinib is not, and the area under the curve (AUC) of erlotinib at the standard dose is 7 times larger than that of gefitinib. In trials comparing first-line conventional chemotherapy with EGFR-TKIs, the response rates of EGFR-mutation–positive patients range between 58% and 83%[20,22] and 62.1% and 73.7%,[5,17,18] respectively, for erlotinib and gefitinib. PFS ranges for the same patient subgroups are 9.7 to 14 months and 9.5 to 10.8 months, respectively. However, these trials differ in terms of populations studied and sensitivity of mutational testing used. At present, lack of direct comparisons between erlotinib and gefitinib in similar clinical scenarios preclude definitive determination of superiority of one agent over the other.

Regarding first-line versus second-line treatment, based on available data it is not entirely clear if the order of use of EGFR-TKIs is significant. In the NEJ002 trial, 95% of the patients who received first-line carboplatin–paclitaxel crossed over to gefitinib on progression. Response rates and median OS in these patients were worse than those in patients who received first-line gefitinib (58.5% vs 73.7% and 30.5 months vs 23.6 months, respectively), indicating that gefitinib may be more effective as first-line therapy than as second-line or later therapy.[5] However, a Spanish Lung Cancer Group study found no difference in OS between first-line and second-line treatments with erlotinib in patients with EGFR-mutant tumors.[30]

EGFR-TKI Resistance

NSCLC patients with sensitizing mutations of EGFR who initially respond to gefitinib or erlotinib ultimately relapse. Primary resistance to EGFR inhibition is caused by mutations of the ERBB family of genes that render them insensitive to EGFR–tyrosine kinase inhibition (eg, insertion mutations in exon 20 of EGFR and HER2)[47] or mutations in a non-ERBB gene (eg, PIK3CA, K-RAS),[48] which results in EGFR-independent activation of downstream signaling pathways. There are 2 main mechanisms of secondary resistance: secondary mutations and activation of parallel pathways resulting in alternative mechanisms of activation of downstream targets. The most common causes of secondary resistance are threonine-to-methionine amino acid change at position 790 (T790M) of the EGFR kinase domain (found in 50% of cases)[49,50] and MET amplification (found in up to 20% cases).[51,52] Other proposed mechanisms of EGFR-TKI resistance include signaling via redundant tyrosine kinase receptors (eg, IGF-1R),[53] constitutive activation of downstream mediators (eg, mutational loss of PTEN phosphatase function leading to Akt activation),[54] ligand-independent activation of

EGFR, bypassing cellular EGFR dependence through epithelial-to-mesenchymal–like transition,[55] altered receptor trafficking, and efflux of the drug from the cell.[56]

Commonly used strategies aimed at overcoming EGFR-TKI resistance are to: (1) irreversibly inhibit EGFR tyrosine kinase by covalent cross-linking of receptors; (2) broaden the receptor tyrosine kinase targets of the drug using multikinase inhibitors; (3) target downstream PI3K or STAT5 pathways; (4) target a combination of pathways; or (5) target mutant EGFR for degradation.[57]

Lapatinib is an oral, reversible TKI that targets HER2 in addition to EGFR. In a randomized, open-label, multicenter, phase II study, lapatinib showed minimal single-agent response rates in patients with locally advanced or metastatic NSCLC.[58] Pan-ERBB inhibitors improve the efficacy of ERBB-targeted therapies by interfering with the cooperation that exists between the receptors.[59] Dacomitinib (PF00299804) is an irreversible pan-ERBB inhibitor, which in preclinical studies was effective against NSCLCs harboring wild-type and mutant EGFR as well as EGFR T790M mutations.[60,61] In pretreated NSCLC patients, a phase II study demonstrated a significant PFS advantage of dacomitinib over erlotinib, with benefit extending to several subgroups including EGFR wild-type tumors.[62] In the first-line setting, a phase II study in patients clinically enriched for EGFR mutation or with an EGFR mutation reported an encouraging 85% of EGFR-mutated patients and 57% of all patients treated with dacomitinib remaining progression-free at 9 months. The disease control rate was 86% in the entire study group and 94% in patients with EGFR-mutant tumors.[63] Treatment-related adverse events commonly seen were diarrhea, acne, rash, and mucositis. Dacomitinib is being evaluated in a phase III trial in patients who have failed standard therapy, and also in several other trials across lines of therapies and a range of histologies and molecular subtypes.

Afatinib (BIBW 2992) is a highly selective, potent, and irreversible inhibitor of both EGFR and HER2 kinases, which overcame T790M-mediated resistance in preclinical lung cancer models.[64] A phase IIb/III trial (LUX-Lung 1 trial) failed to demonstrate improvement in OS (primary end point) with afatinib compared with placebo in more than 580 patients with advanced NSCLC who had disease progression after chemotherapy and a first-generation EGFR-TKI. However, in a subset of patients who were most likely to have an EGFR mutation based on clinical criteria, improvement in PFS was observed (4.4 months vs 1.0 month for placebo). Afatinib is being investigated in first-line therapy for EGFR-mutant NSCLC and after first-generation EGFR-TKI failure.

Focal EGFR T790M amplification, at least partly attributable to selection of a preexisting EGFR T790M-amplified clone, can lead to resistance to irreversible pan-ERBB inhibitors.[65] As with first-generation EGFR tyrosine kinase inhibition, T790M mutation may interfere with the efficacy of irreversible pan-ERBB inhibitors also by disrupting the initial reversible binding of these inhibitors to the ATP binding site, thus delaying covalent bond formation.[66] Moreover, irreversible EGFR inhibitors can overcome T790M resistance only at suprapharmacologic concentrations.[67] At such doses concurrent inhibition of wild-type EGFR results in rash and diarrhea, and limits the ability to achieve plasma concentrations sufficient to inhibit EGFR T790M.

ANAPLASTIC LYMPHOMA KINASE TYROSINE KINASE INHIBITORS

EML4-ALK translocation was first identified as a driver mutation of lung carcinogenesis in 2007.[68] ALK and EML4 are both located in the short arm of chromosome 2 separated by 12 Mb, and are oriented in opposite 5′-3′ directions. EML4-ALK translocation results from a small inversion within chromosome 2p [inv (2)(p21p23)], which leads to fusion of the N-terminal portion of the protein encoded by the echinoderm microtubule-associated protein–like 4 (EML4) gene with the intracellular signaling portion of the receptor tyrosine kinase encoded by the ALK gene. The chimeric protein, EML4-ALK, possesses potent oncogenic activity both in vitro and in vivo.[68–70] Inhibition of ALK leads to apoptosis in vitro, and decreased tumor burden and improved survival in a transgenic mouse model that expressed EML4-ALK in lung alveolar epithelial cells.[69,71]

Depending on patient ethnicity and the enrichment criteria used, the frequency of EML4-ALK in patients with NSCLC varies between 1% and 13%. The typical phenotype of a patient with EML4-ALK translocation is that of a young, never, or light (<10 pack-years) smoker. EML4-ALK–positive tumors are more likely advanced-stage adenocarcinomas, predominantly the signet-ring cell subtype in Western cohorts and acinar subtype in the Asian population. NSCLC patients with EML4-ALK translocations share several clinical characteristics with patients harboring EGFR-mutant tumors, including never/light smoking history and adenocarcinoma histology, but differ in its increased frequency in men, the younger age group involved, and histologic characteristics. However, there is a near complete lack of overlap of EML4-ALK translocation and EGFR mutation in the same tumor. Among patients with NSCLC who have clinical characteristics associated with EGFR mutation but no detectable EGFR mutation as many as one in 3 patients may harbor EML4-ALK.[68–70,72–74]

Multiple EML4-ALK variants result from fusion of the variably truncated EML4 to the ALK gene, starting at a portion encoded by exon 20. Most of the EML4-ALK variants retain the transforming potential, but clinical implications of the different variants are not known.[69,70,74] Translocations involving non-EML4 fusion partners (eg, TFG and KIF5B) have also been described. The non-EML4 fusion partners for ALK may have implications in the diagnostic modality used in detection of ALK-translocated NSCLC, but their functional significance is not defined.[70]

Clinical Trials of ALK-TKIs

Crizotinib is an orally bioavailable, selective small-molecule inhibitor of the catalytic activity of c-Met kinase and the ALK fusion protein.[75] In a phase I study, Kwak and colleagues[76] identified 82 patients with advanced NSCLC from approximately 1500 patients. After a mean treatment duration of 6.4 months, the overall response rate was 57% including one confirmed complete response. Thirty-three percent of patients had stable disease, and the estimated probability of 6-month PFS was 72%. Updated data with 199 patients showed a response rate of 61%.[77] The response to treatment was exclusive to patients with ALK translocations, as demonstrated by lack of response in patients without ALK translocation who were treated in the dose escalation phase.[76] In preliminary results of a phase III study (N = 136), comparing second-line crizotinib to chemotherapy (pemetrexed or doxetaxel) a response rate of 53% as seen in 76 evaluable patients.[78] In patients with ALK-translocation–positive NSCLC, treatment with crizotinib was associated with a higher OS than that of historical, crizotinib-naïve controls. One-year OS was 71% in patients who received crizotinib as second-line or third-line therapy in the phase I study, compared with 46% for those who did not.[79] Based on response rates observed in these 2 studies,[77,78] crizotinib was granted accelerated approval by the FDA for treatment of patients with locally advanced or metastatic NSCLC. Further well-controlled clinical trials are needed to verify and describe the clinical benefit. In ALK gene–rearranged NSCLC patients, ongoing phase III trials are evaluating crizotinib in the first line, where it is being compared with platinum-based chemotherapy (pemetrexed and cisplatin or carboplatin) and in the second line with pemetrexed or docetaxel.

Despite the initial responses, the median PFS of patients who received crizotinib in the phase I trial was limited to 10 months. In a model of acquired resistance to crizotinib, established by exposing a highly sensitive EML4-ALK-positive NSCLC cell line to increasing doses of crizotinib, cells resistant to intermediate doses of crizotinib developed amplification of the EML4-ALK gene. Cells resistant to higher doses of crizotinib also developed a gatekeeper mutation, L1196M, within the kinase domain, rendering EML4-ALK insensitive to crizotinib.[80] Other mechanisms of acquired resistance that have been described include concurrent coactivation of EGFR signaling.[80–82]

Practical Considerations

Testing technique
Concurrent with its approval of crizotinib, the FDA approved the Vysis ALK Break-Apart FISH Probe Kit (Abbott Molecular, Inc, Des Plaines, IL, USA) to detect ALK rearrangements. The Break-Apart FISH assay detects disruption of the ALK locus but does not confirm EML4 as the partner fusion gene.

Dosage and interactions
The recommended daily dose of crizotinib is 250 mg taken orally twice daily with or without food. Dosing interruption and/or dose reduction to 200 mg taken orally twice daily may be required based on individual safety and tolerability, then to 250 mg taken orally once daily if further reduction is necessary.[83] Crizotinib is predominantly metabolized by CYP3A4/5 and hence concurrent use of strong CYP3A inhibitors and inducers should be avoided.[83]

Toxicities
The most commonly reported adverse events with crizotinib are nausea, diarrhea, vomiting, edema, and constipation.[76,83] Visual disturbances, noticed especially during changes in ambient lighting from dark to light, were reported by 62% of patients in clinical trials.[83] The spectrum of disorders described includes visual impairment, photopsia, blurred vision, vitreous floaters, photophobia, and diplopia.[83] Visual symptoms usually started within 2 weeks of drug administration and improved with continued treatment. Ophthalmologic evaluation is recommended, particularly if patients experience photopsia or new or increased vitreous floaters. Grade 3 elevations in alanine aminotransferase and aspartate aminotransferase were observed in 5% and 6% of patients respectively, with onset during cycle 2. These changes were reversible with temporary interruption of crizotinib, and in most cases, restarting crizotinib at a lower dose was well tolerated. Severe, life-threatening treatment-related pneumonitis has been reported in 1.6% of patients treated with crizotinib in clinical trials, and close monitoring for pulmonary symptoms is recommended.[83] In patients who have a history of or predisposition for QTc prolongation, or who are taking medications that are known to prolong the QT interval, periodic monitoring with electrocardiograms and electrolytes should be considered.[83]

MET/HEPATOCYTE GROWTH FACTOR INHIBITORS

The c-Met gene located on chromosome 7 encodes a receptor tyrosine kinase, whose only known high-affinity ligand is hepatocyte growth factor (HGF). High levels of intratumoral c-Met expression in NSCLC have been identified as a poor prognostic indicator and have been implicated in poor response to upfront EGFR inhibition, EGFR tyrosine kinase resistance, and propensity for metastasis. In untreated NSCLC, c-Met amplification occurs in 3% cases, but is seen in up to 22% of EGFR-mutant tumors with acquired resistance to EGFR-TKIs.[51,52,84,85]

Table 1
Clinical trial data on multikinase angiogenesis inhibitors in metastatic non-small cell lung cancer

Study (Year Published) Authors	No. of Patients Primary End Point Phase	Patients	Drugs	RR (%)	PFS (mo)	OS (mo)	Comments
EGFR + VEGF Inhibitors							
Vandetanib							
ZEAL (2011) de Boer et al[89]	534 Phase III PFS	Second line All histologies	Vandetanib + pemetrexed Placebo + pemetrexed	19[a] 8	4.4 3	10.5 9.2	Significant delay in the time to worsening of lung cancer symptoms with vandetanib
ZEST (2011) Natale et al[90]	1240 Phase III PFS	1–2 prior treatments All histologies	Vandetanib Erlotinib	12 12	2.6 2.0	6.9 7.8	Overall incidence of AEs grade ≥ 3 were higher with vandetanib than erlotinib (50% vs 40%)
ZODIAC (2010) Herbst RS[91]	1391 Phase III PFS	Second line All histologies	Vandetanib + docetaxel Placebo + docetaxel	17[a] 10	4[a] 3.2	10.6 10	Significant delay in the time to worsening of lung cancer symptoms in vandetanib arm
ZEPHYR (2010) Lee et al[92]	924 Phase III OS	Failure of prior therapy with an EGFR-TKI All histologies	Vandetanib Placebo (2:1 randomization)	2.6[a] 0.7	1.9[a] 1.8	8.5 7.8	
VEGF+ PDGFR Inhibitors							
Sunitinib							
SUN 1087 (2010) Scagliotti[95]	960 Phase III OS	1–2 prior treatments All histologies	Sunitinib + erlotinib Placebo + Erlotinib	10.6[a] 6.9	3.9[a] 2.1	9.0 8.5	
Cediranib							
NCIC CTG BR.24 (2010) Goss et al[93]	296 Phase II/III PFS	First line All histologies	Carboplatin + paclitaxel + cediranib Carboplatin + paclitaxel + placebo	38[a] 16	5.6 5.0		Dose-dependent increase in toxicities grade ≥ 3 and fatal serious adverse events in cediranib group
Axitinib							
(2009) Schiller et al[94]	32 Phase II ORR	84% had received prior chemotherapy All histologies	Axitinib	9	4.9	14.8	

Abbreviations: AEs, adverse events; EGFR, endothelial growth factor receptor; PDGFR, platelet-derived growth factor receptor; ORR, objective response rate; OS, overall survival; PFS, progression-free survival; RR, response rate; TKI, tyrosine kinase inhibitor; VEGF, vascular endothelial growth factor.

[a] Statistically significant difference.

Therapeutic strategies used for targeted MET inhibition include small interfering RNA, small molecules, and specific monoclonal antibodies.[86] ARQ197, a highly selective, orally administered MET inhibitor, binds to a region of MET outside of the ATP binding site and impairs kinase activation allosterically. In a phase II study, ARQ197 in combination with erlotinib improved PFS (median 16.1 weeks vs 9.7 weeks: HR 0.81, 95% CI 0.57–1.15; $P = .23$) compared with erlotinib alone in second-line/third-line EGFR-inhibitor–naïve NSCLC.[87] A prespecified analysis adjusting for prognostic factors yielded PFS HR 0.68 (95% CI 0.47–0.98; $P<.05$), with improved benefit noted in subgroups of patients with nonsquamous histology, K-RAS mutations, and EGFR wild-type status.[87] An ongoing phase III trial is evaluating ARQ 197 with erlotinib in patients with advanced nonsquamous NSCLC who have received 1 or 2 prior lines of therapy. Cabozantinib (XL184) is an oral, ATP-competitive small-molecule inhibitor of multiple kinases, in particular MET and vascular endothelial growth factor receptor (VEGFR). Preliminary results from a randomized phase II discontinuation study suggest single-agent activity of XL184 in patients with advanced NSCLC who failed multiple prior systemic therapies, with an overall disease control rate of 50%.[88] XL184 is being evaluated in combination with erlotinib in NSCLC patients who have progressive disease after initial response to erlotinib. Crizotinib is also a potent inhibitor of MET.

VASCULAR ENDOTHELIAL GROWTH FACTOR RECEPTOR TYROSINE KINASE INHIBITORS

Vascular endothelial growth factor (VEGF), a mitogen specific for vascular endothelial cells, plays a key role in angiogenesis. VEGF-related angiogenic signal is mediated by kinase domain receptor (KDR) and Fms-like tyrosine kinase (Flt-1), which have intracellular tyrosine kinase activity. Vandetanib (targets VEGFR-2 and -3, RET and EGFR tyrosine kinases), sunitinib (targets VEGFR-1/-2/-3, Flt PDGFR-b, c-kit), cediranib (targets VEGFR-1/-2/-3, PDGFR-b, c-kit) and axitinib (targets VEGFR-1/-2/-3, PDGFR-a, c-kit) are orally active small-molecule inhibitors that target the VEGF family of tyrosine kinases and a wide spectrum of other tyrosine kinase receptors. **Table 1** summarizes important phase II/III clinical trial data on these multikinase inhibitors in NSCLC.[89–95] Despite strong preclinical rationale, the lack of reliable prognostic or predictive markers for selecting patients who would benefit from antiangiogenic therapy has hampered the clinical development of these agents. Although several potential angiogenic biomarkers (eg, microvessel density, VEGF, VEGFRs) have been extensively studied, no definitive marker has been identified to date. Hence, patient selection for angiogenesis inhibitors is currently limited to clinical and/or histologic features.[96]

SUMMARY

Identification of novel tyrosine kinase targets and clinical development of its inhibitors have ushered in an era of personalized care in NSCLC. The lessons learned in the development of first-generation EGFR-TKIs have led to shortening of time between understanding the biology and clinicopathologic features of the patients, development of diagnostic tests, drug development, and identification of resistance mechanisms.[97] Ongoing efforts are focused on overcoming resistance mechanisms of existing targets, and identification of novel targets and biomarkers.

REFERENCES

1. Goldstraw P, Crowley J, Chansky K, et al. The IASLC Lung Cancer Staging Project: proposals for the revision of the TNM stage groupings in the forthcoming

(seventh) edition of the TNM Classification of malignant tumours. J Thorac Oncol 2007;2(8):706–14.

2. Jemal A, Siegel R, Xu J, et al. Cancer statistics, 2010. CA Cancer J Clin 2010; 60(5):277–300.

3. Chemotherapy in non-small cell lung cancer: a meta-analysis using updated data on individual patients from 52 randomised clinical trials. Non-Small Cell Lung Cancer Collaborative Group. BMJ 1995;311(7010):899–909.

4. Cancer Incidence—Surveillance, Epidemiology, and End Results (SEER) Registries Research Data. April 15, 2011. Available at: http://seer.cancer.gov. Accessed September 21, 2011.

5. Maemondo M, Inoue A, Kobayashi K, et al. Gefitinib or chemotherapy for non-small-cell lung cancer with mutated EGFR. N Engl J Med 2010;362(25):2380–8.

6. Hynes NE, Lane HA. ERBB receptors and cancer: the complexity of targeted inhibitors. Nat Rev Cancer 2005;5(5):341–54.

7. Citri A, Yarden Y. EGF-ERBB signalling: towards the systems level. Nat Rev Mol Cell Biol 2006;7(7):505–16.

8. Kris MG, Natale RB, Herbst RS, et al. Efficacy of gefitinib, an inhibitor of the epidermal growth factor receptor tyrosine kinase, in symptomatic patients with non-small cell lung cancer: a randomized trial. JAMA 2003;290(16):2149–58.

9. Fukuoka M, Yano S, Giaccone G, et al. Multi-institutional randomized phase II trial of gefitinib for previously treated patients with advanced non-small-cell lung cancer (The IDEAL 1 Trial) [corrected]. J Clin Oncol 2003;21(12):2237–46.

10. Perez-Soler R. Phase II clinical trial data with the epidermal growth factor receptor tyrosine kinase inhibitor erlotinib (OSI-774) in non-small-cell lung cancer. Clin Lung Cancer 2004;6(Suppl 1):S20–3.

11. Giaccone G, Herbst RS, Manegold C, et al. Gefitinib in combination with gemcitabine and cisplatin in advanced non-small-cell lung cancer: a phase III trial—INTACT 1. J Clin Oncol 2004;22(5):777–84.

12. Herbst RS, Giaccone G, Schiller JH, et al. Gefitinib in combination with paclitaxel and carboplatin in advanced non-small-cell lung cancer: a phase III trial—INTACT 2. J Clin Oncol 2004;22(5):785–94.

13. Gatzemeier U, Pluzanska A, Szczesna A, et al. Phase III study of erlotinib in combination with cisplatin and gemcitabine in advanced non-small-cell lung cancer: the Tarceva Lung Cancer Investigation Trial. J Clin Oncol 2007;25(12):1545–52.

14. Herbst RS, Prager D, Hermann R, et al. TRIBUTE: a phase III trial of erlotinib hydrochloride (OSI-774) combined with carboplatin and paclitaxel chemotherapy in advanced non-small-cell lung cancer. J Clin Oncol 2005;23(25):5892–9.

15. Thatcher N, Chang A, Parikh P, et al. Gefitinib plus best supportive care in previously treated patients with refractory advanced non-small-cell lung cancer: results from a randomised, placebo-controlled, multicentre study (Iressa Survival Evaluation in Lung Cancer). Lancet 2005;366(9496):1527–37.

16. Shepherd FA, Rodrigues Pereira J, Ciuleanu T, et al. Erlotinib in previously treated non-small-cell lung cancer. N Engl J Med 2005;353(2):123–32.

17. Mok TS, Wu YL, Thongprasert S, et al. Gefitinib or carboplatin-paclitaxel in pulmonary adenocarcinoma. N Engl J Med 2009;361(10):947–57.

18. Mitsudomi T, Morita S, Yatabe Y, et al. Gefitinib versus cisplatin plus docetaxel in patients with non-small-cell lung cancer harbouring mutations of the epidermal growth factor receptor (WJTOG3405): an open label, randomised phase 3 trial. Lancet Oncol 2010;11(2):121–8.

19. Lee DH, Han JY, Yu SY, et al. A randomized phase III study of gefitinib (IRESSA) versus standard chemotherapy (gemcitabine plus cisplatin) as a first-line treatment

for never-smokers with advanced or metastatic adenocarcinoma of the lung. Presented at World Conference on Lung Cancer. San Francisco (CA), July 31 to August 4, 2009.

20. Zhou C, Wu YL, Chen G, et al. Erlotinib versus chemotherapy as first-line treatment for patients with advanced EGFR mutation-positive non-small-cell lung cancer (OPTIMAL, CTONG-0802): a multicentre, open-label, randomised, phase 3 study. Lancet Oncol 2011;12(8):735–42.

21. Fukuoka M, Wu YL, Thongprasert S, et al. Biomarker analyses and final overall survival results from a phase III, randomized, open-label, first-line study of gefitinib versus carboplatin/paclitaxel in clinically selected patients with advanced non-small-cell lung cancer in Asia (IPASS). J Clin Oncol 2011;29(21): 2866–74.

22. Rosell R, Gervais R, Vergnenegre A, et al. Erlotinib versus chemotherapy (CT) in advanced non-small cell lung cancer (NSCLC) patients (p) with epidermal growth factor receptor (EGFR) mutations: interim results of the European Erlotinib Versus Chemotherapy (EURTAC) phase III randomized trial. J Clin Oncol 2011; 29(Suppl):[abstract: 7503].

23. Takeda K, Hida T, Sato T, et al. Randomized phase III trial of platinum-doublet chemotherapy followed by gefitinib compared with continued platinum-doublet chemotherapy in Japanese patients with advanced non-small-cell lung cancer: results of a west Japan thoracic oncology group trial (WJTOG0203). J Clin Oncol 2010;28(5):753–60.

24. Gaafar RM, Surmont VF, Scagliotti G, et al. A double-blind, randomized, placebo-controlled phase III intergroup study of gefitinib (G) in patients (pts) with advanced NSCLC, non-progressing after first-line platinum-based chemotherapy (EORTC 08021-ILCP 01/03) [abstract 7518]. J Clin Oncol 2010;28(Suppl):15s.

25. Cappuzzo F, Ciuleanu T, Stelmakh L, et al. Erlotinib as maintenance treatment in advanced non-small-cell lung cancer: a multicentre, randomised, placebo-controlled phase 3 study. Lancet Oncol 2010;11(6):521–9.

26. Miller VA, O'Connor P, Soh C, et al. A randomized, double-blind, placebo-controlled, phase IIIb trial (ATLAS) comparing bevacizumab (B) therapy with or without erlotinib (E) after completion of chemotherapy with B for first-line treatment of locally advanced, recurrent, or metastatic non-small cell lung cancer (NSCLC) [abstract LBA8002]. J Clin Oncol 2009;27(Suppl):18s.

27. Kabbinavar FF, Miller VA, Johnson BE, et al. Overall survival (OS) in ATLAS, a phase IIIb trial comparing bevacizumab (B) therapy with or without erlotinib (E) after completion of chemotherapy (chemo) with B for first-line treatment of locally advanced, recurrent, or metastatic non-small cell lung cancer (NSCLC) [abstract 7526]. J Clin Oncol 2010;28(Suppl):15s.

28. Coudert B, Ciuleanu T, Park K, et al. Survival benefit with erlotinib maintenance therapy in patients with advanced non-small-cell lung cancer (NSCLC) according to response to first-line chemotherapy. Ann Oncol 2012;23(2):388–94.

29. Kelly K, Chansky K, Gaspar LE, et al. Phase III trial of maintenance gefitinib or placebo after concurrent chemoradiotherapy and docetaxel consolidation in inoperable stage III non-small-cell lung cancer: SWOG S0023. J Clin Oncol 2008;26(15):2450–6.

30. Rosell R, Moran T, Queralt C, et al. Screening for epidermal growth factor receptor mutations in lung cancer. N Engl J Med 2009;361(10):958–67.

31. Sequist LV, Martins RG, Spigel D, et al. First-line gefitinib in patients with advanced non-small-cell lung cancer harboring somatic EGFR mutations. J Clin Oncol 2008;26(15):2442–9.

32. Hirsch FR, Varella-Garcia M, Bunn PA Jr, et al. Molecular predictors of outcome with gefitinib in a phase III placebo-controlled study in advanced non-small-cell lung cancer. J Clin Oncol 2006;24(31):5034–42.

33. Lynch TJ, Bell DW, Sordella R, et al. Activating mutations in the epidermal growth factor receptor underlying responsiveness of non-small-cell lung cancer to gefitinib. N Engl J Med 2004;350(21):2129–39.

34. Paez JG, Janne PA, Lee JC, et al. EGFR mutations in lung cancer: correlation with clinical response to gefitinib therapy. Science 2004;304(5676):1497–500.

35. Pao W, Miller V, Zakowski M, et al. EGF receptor gene mutations are common in lung cancers from "never smokers" and are associated with sensitivity of tumors to gefitinib and erlotinib. Proc Natl Acad Sci U S A 2004;101(36): 13306–11.

36. Jackman DM, Miller VA, Cioffredi LA, et al. Impact of epidermal growth factor receptor and KRAS mutations on clinical outcomes in previously untreated non-small cell lung cancer patients: results of an online tumor registry of clinical trials. Clin Cancer Res 2009;15(16):5267–73.

37. Tarceva (erlotinib) [package insert]. South San Francisco, CA: Genentech. Available at: http://www.accessdata.fda.gov/drugsatfda_docs/label/2010/021743s14s16lbl. pdf. Accessed October 2, 2011.

38. Iressa (gefitinib) [package insert]. Wilmington, DE: AstraZeneca. Available at: http://www1.astrazeneca-us.com/pi/iressa.pdf. Accessed October 2, 2011.

39. Lynch TJ Jr, Kim ES, Eaby B, et al. Epidermal growth factor receptor inhibitor-associated cutaneous toxicities: an evolving paradigm in clinical management. Oncologist 2007;12(5):610–21.

40. Gridelli C, Maione P, Amoroso D, et al. Clinical significance and treatment of skin rash from erlotinib in non-small cell lung cancer patients: results of an Experts Panel Meeting. Crit Rev Oncol Hematol 2008;66(2):155–62.

41. Potthoff K, Hofheinz R, Hassel JC, et al. Interdisciplinary management of EGFR-inhibitor-induced skin reactions: a German expert opinion. Ann Oncol 2011;22(3): 524–35.

42. Lacouture ME, Maitland ML, Segaert S, et al. A proposed EGFR inhibitor dermatologic adverse event-specific grading scale from the MASCC skin toxicity study group. Support Care Cancer 2010;18(4):509–22.

43. Kudoh S, Kato H, Nishiwaki Y, et al. Interstitial lung disease in Japanese patients with lung cancer: a cohort and nested case-control study. Am J Respir Crit Care Med 2008;177(12):1348–57.

44. Li J, Zhao M, He P, et al. Differential metabolism of gefitinib and erlotinib by human cytochrome P450 enzymes. Clin Cancer Res 2007;13(12):3731–7.

45. Riely GJ, Kris MG, Zhao B, et al. Prospective assessment of discontinuation and reinitiation of erlotinib or gefitinib in patients with acquired resistance to erlotinib or gefitinib followed by the addition of everolimus. Clin Cancer Res 2007;13(17): 5150–5.

46. Chaft JE, Oxnard GR, Sima CS, et al. Disease flare after tyrosine kinase inhibitor discontinuation in patients with EGFR-mutant lung cancer and acquired resistance to erlotinib or gefitinib. Clin Cancer Res 2011;17(19):6298–303.

47. Greulich H, Chen TH, Feng W, et al. Oncogenic transformation by inhibitor-sensitive and -resistant EGFR mutants. PLoS Med 2005;2(11):e313.

48. Pao W, Wang TY, Riely GJ, et al. KRAS mutations and primary resistance of lung adenocarcinomas to gefitinib or erlotinib. PLoS Med 2005;2(1):e17.

49. Kobayashi S, Boggon TJ, Dayaram T, et al. EGFR mutation and resistance of non-small-cell lung cancer to gefitinib. N Engl J Med 2005;352(8):786–92.

50. Pao W, Miller VA, Politi KA, et al. Acquired resistance of lung adenocarcinomas to gefitinib or erlotinib is associated with a second mutation in the EGFR kinase domain. PLoS Med 2005;2(3):e73.
51. Bean J, Brennan C, Shih JY, et al. MET amplification occurs with or without T790M mutations in EGFR mutant lung tumors with acquired resistance to gefitinib or erlotinib. Proc Natl Acad Sci U S A 2007;104(52):20932–7.
52. Engelman JA, Zejnullahu K, Mitsudomi T, et al. MET amplification leads to gefitinib resistance in lung cancer by activating ERBB3 signaling. Science 2007; 316(5827):1039–43.
53. Gong Y, Yao E, Shen R, et al. High expression levels of total IGF-1R and sensitivity of NSCLC cells in vitro to an anti-IGF-1R antibody (R1507). PLoS One 2009;4(10): e7273.
54. Sos ML, Koker M, Weir BA, et al. PTEN loss contributes to erlotinib resistance in EGFR-mutant lung cancer by activation of Akt and EGFR. Cancer Res 2009; 69(8):3256–61.
55. Uramoto H, Iwata T, Onitsuka T, et al. Epithelial-mesenchymal transition in EGFR-TKI acquired resistant lung adenocarcinoma. Anticancer Res 2010; 30(7):2513–7.
56. Engelman JA, Settleman J. Acquired resistance to tyrosine kinase inhibitors during cancer therapy. Curr Opin Genet Dev 2008;18(1):73–9.
57. Rubin BP, Duensing A. Mechanisms of resistance to small molecule kinase inhibition in the treatment of solid tumors. Lab Invest 2006;86(10):981–6.
58. Ross HJ, Blumenschein GR Jr, Aisner J, et al. Randomized phase II multicenter trial of two schedules of lapatinib as first- or second-line monotherapy in patients with advanced or metastatic non-small cell lung cancer. Clin Cancer Res 2010; 16(6):1938–49.
59. Britten CD. Targeting ErbB receptor signaling: a pan-ErbB approach to cancer. Mol Cancer Ther 2004;3(10):1335–42.
60. Engelman JA, Zejnullahu K, Gale CM, et al. PF00299804, an irreversible pan-ERBB inhibitor, is effective in lung cancer models with EGFR and ERBB2 mutations that are resistant to gefitinib. Cancer Res 2007;67(24):11924–32.
61. Gonzales AJ, Hook KE, Althaus IW, et al. Antitumor activity and pharmacokinetic properties of PF-00299804, a second-generation irreversible pan-erbB receptor tyrosine kinase inhibitor. Mol Cancer Ther 2008;7(7):1880–9.
62. Boyer MJ, Blackhall FH, Park K, et al. Efficacy and safety of PF299804 versus erlotinib (E): a global, randomized phase II trial in patients (pts) with advanced non-small cell lung cancer (NSCLC) after failure of chemotherapy (CT) [abstract LBA7523]. J Clin Oncol 2010;28(Suppl):18s.
63. Mok T, Spigel DR, Park K, et al. Efficacy and safety of PF-00299804 (PF299), an oral, irreversible, pan-human epidermal growth factor receptor (pan-HER) tyrosine kinase inhibitor (TKI), as first-line treatment (tx) of selected patients (pts) with advanced (adv) non-small cell lung cancer (NSCLC) [abstract LBA7537]. J Clin Oncol 2010;28(Suppl):15s.
64. Li D, Ambrogio L, Shimamura T, et al. BIBW2992, an irreversible EGFR/HER2 inhibitor highly effective in preclinical lung cancer models. Oncogene 2008; 27(34):4702–11.
65. Ercan D, Zejnullahu K, Yonesaka K, et al. Amplification of EGFR T790M causes resistance to an irreversible EGFR inhibitor. Oncogene 2010;29(16):2346–56.
66. Rauh D, Sos ML, Rode HB, et al. Chemogenomic profiling provides insights into the limited activity of irreversible EGFR inhibitors in tumor cells expressing the T790M EGFR resistance mutation. Cancer Res 2010;70(3):868–74.

67. Haber DA, Godin-Heymann N, Lllkus L, et al. The T790M "gatekeeper" mutation in EGFR mediates resistance to low concentrations of an irreversible EGFR inhibitor. Mol Cancer Ther 2008;7(4):874–9.

68. Soda M, Choi YL, Enomoto M, et al. Identification of the transforming EML4-ALK fusion gene in non-small-cell lung cancer. Nature 2007;448(7153):561–6.

69. Koivunen JP, Mermel C, Zejnullahu K, et al. EML4-ALK fusion gene and efficacy of an ALK kinase inhibitor in lung cancer. Clin Cancer Res 2008;14(13):4275–83.

70. Takeuchi K, Choi YL, Soda M, et al. Multiplex reverse transcription-PCR screening for EML4-ALK fusion transcripts. Clin Cancer Res 2008;14(20):6618–24.

71. Mano H, Soda M, Takada S, et al. A mouse model for EML4-ALK-positive lung cancer. Proc Natl Acad Sci U S A 2008;105(50):19893–7.

72. Shaw AT, Yeap BY, Mino-Kenudson M, et al. Clinical features and outcome of patients with non-small-cell lung cancer who harbor EML4-ALK. J Clin Oncol 2009;27(26):4247–53.

73. Rodig SJ, Mino-Kenudson M, Dacic S, et al. Unique clinicopathologic features characterize ALK-rearranged lung adenocarcinoma in the western population. Clin Cancer Res 2009;15(16):5216–23.

74. Sasaki T, Rodig SJ, Chirieac LR, et al. The biology and treatment of EML4-ALK non-small cell lung cancer. Eur J Cancer 2010;46(10):1773–80.

75. Christensen JG, Zou HY, Arango ME, et al. Cytoreductive antitumor activity of PF-2341066, a novel inhibitor of anaplastic lymphoma kinase and c-Met, in experimental models of anaplastic large-cell lymphoma. Mol Cancer Ther 2007; 6(12 Pt 1):3314–22.

76. Kwak EL, Bang YJ, Camidge DR, et al. Anaplastic lymphoma kinase inhibition in non-small-cell lung cancer. N Engl J Med 2010;363(18):1693–703.

77. Camidge DR, Bang Y, Kwak EL, et al. Progression-free survival (PFS) from a phase I study of crizotinib (PF-02341066) in patients with ALK-positive non small cell lung cancer (NSCLC). J Clin Oncol 2011;29(Suppl):[abstract 2501].

78. Crinò L, Kim D, Riely GJ, et al. Initial phase II results with crizotinib in advanced ALK-positive non-small cell lung cancer (NSCLC): PROFILE 1005. J Clin Oncol 2011;29(Suppl):[abstract 7514].

79. Shaw AT, Yeap BY, Solomon BJ, et al. Effect of crizotinib on overall survival in patients with advanced non-small-cell lung cancer harbouring ALK gene rearrangement: a retrospective analysis. Lancet Oncol 2011;12(11):1004–12.

80. Katayama R, Khan TM, Benes C, et al. Therapeutic strategies to overcome crizotinib resistance in non-small cell lung cancers harboring the fusion oncogene EML4-ALK. Proc Natl Acad Sci U S A 2011;108(18):7535–40.

81. Sasaki T, Koivunen J, Ogino A, et al. A novel ALK secondary mutation and EGFR signaling cause resistance to ALK kinase inhibitors. Cancer Res 2011;71(18): 6051–60.

82. Choi YL, Soda M, Yamashita Y, et al. EML4-ALK mutations in lung cancer that confer resistance to ALK inhibitors. N Engl J Med 2010;363(18):1734–9.

83. Xalkori (crizotinib) [package insert]. San Diego (CA): Pfizer. Available at: http://www.accessdata.fda.gov/drugsatfda_docs/appletter/2011/202570s000ltr.pdf. Accessed October 2, 2011.

84. Benedettini E, Sholl LM, Peyton M, et al. Met activation in non-small cell lung cancer is associated with de novo resistance to EGFR inhibitors and the development of brain metastasis. Am J Pathol 2010;177(1):415–23.

85. Comoglio PM, Giordano S, Trusolino L. Drug development of MET inhibitors: targeting oncogene addiction and expedience. Nat Rev Drug Discov 2008;7(6): 504–16.

86. Salgia R, Cipriani NA, Abidoye OO, et al. MET as a target for treatment of chest tumors. Lung Cancer 2009;63(2):169–79.
87. Schiller JH, Akerley WL, Brugger W, et al. Results from ARQ 197-209: a global randomized placebo-controlled phase II clinical trial of erlotinib plus ARQ 197 versus erlotinib plus placebo in previously treated EGFR inhibitor-naive patients with locally advanced or metastatic non-small cell lung cancer (NSCLC) [abstract LBA7502]. J Clin Oncol 2010;28(Suppl):18s.
88. Yasenchak C, Nackaerts K, Awada A, et al. Phase 2 results of XL184 in a cohort of patients (pts) with advanced non-small cell lung cancer (NSCLC). EJC Suppl 2010;8(7):126.
89. de Boer RH, Arrieta O, Yang CH, et al. Vandetanib plus pemetrexed for the second-line treatment of advanced non-small-cell lung cancer: a randomized, double-blind phase III trial. J Clin Oncol 2011;29(8):1067–74.
90. Natale RB, Thongprasert S, Greco FA, et al. Phase III trial of vandetanib compared with erlotinib in patients with previously treated advanced non-small-cell lung cancer. J Clin Oncol 2011;29(8):1059–66.
91. Herbst RS, Sun Y, Eberhardt WE, et al. Vandetanib plus docetaxel versus docetaxel as second-line treatment for patients with advanced non-small-cell lung cancer (ZODIAC): a double-blind, randomised, phase 3 trial. Lancet Oncol 2010;11(7):619–26.
92. Lee J, Hirsh V, Park K, et al. Vandetanib versus placebo in patients with advanced non-small cell lung cancer (NSCLC) after prior therapy with an EGFR tyrosine kinase inhibitor (TKI): a randomized, double-blind phase III trial (ZEPHYR) [abstract 7525]. J Clin Oncol 2010;28(Suppl):15s.
93. Goss GD, Arnold A, Shepherd FA, et al. Randomized, double-blind trial of carboplatin and paclitaxel with either daily oral cediranib or placebo in advanced non-small-cell lung cancer: NCIC Clinical Trials Group BR24 study. J Clin Oncol 2010; 28(1):49–55.
94. Schiller JH, Larson T, Ou SH, et al. Efficacy and safety of axitinib in patients with advanced non-small-cell lung cancer: results from a phase II study. J Clin Oncol 2009;27(23):3836–41.
95. Scagliotti G, Krzakowski M, Szczesna A, et al. Sunitinib (SU) in combination with erlotinib (E) for the treatment of advanced/metastatic non-small cell lung cancer (NSCLC): a phase III study (LBA 6). 35th European Society for Medical Oncology (ESMO) Congress. Milan (Italy), October 8-12, 2010.
96. Salgia R. Prognostic significance of angiogenesis and angiogenic growth factors in nonsmall cell lung cancer. Cancer 2011;117(17):3889–99.
97. Gerber DE, Minna JD. ALK inhibition for non-small cell lung cancer: from discovery to therapy in record time. Cancer Cell 2010;18(6):548–51.

Antimitotic Inhibitors

Susana M. Campos, MD, MPH[a], Don S. Dizon, MD[b],*

KEYWORDS

- Microtubule-targeting agents • Microtubule resistance • Epothilones • Eribulin
- Cabazitaxel • Aurora kinase inhibitors • PLK inhibitors • KSP inhibitors

KEY POINTS

- Microtubulin stabilizers have an important and established role in the treatment of solid tumors.
- Novel agents that approach the mitotics spindle are undergoing evaluation. These agents include aurora kinase inhibitors, kinesin spindle inhibitors, and pololike kinase inhibitors.
- Novel cytotoxics that are directed against the microtubular apparatus (eribulin and ixabepilone) have been approved for use in metastatic breast cancer.

The phrase *Omnis cellula e cellula* ("Every cell originates from another existing cell like it") was coined by Robert Virchow in 1858. Despite the simplicity of this phrase, the biologic process on which it is based (mitosis) is a tightly engineered event composed of canonical morphologic stages that ensure the integrity of the developing organism.

In the last several years, research dedicated to carcinogenesis has focused on the therapeutic exploitation of signal transduction pathways. Among these, a classic and attractive target for the development of antineoplastic agents is centered on the basic backbone of the cell: the cytoskeleton.

Microtubules are integral components of the cytoskeleton. They function in multiple capacities (ie, in the maintenance of cell shape and polarity, intracellular transport, and in the formation and dynamics of the mitotic spindle).[1] They represent a validated target for cytotoxic agents. In addition to modulators of microtubule dynamics, a body of literature shows the pivotal and integrative role of both tubulin-binding and nontubulin-binding agents. The kinesinlike proteins and the mitotic kinesins play a critical role in function of the mitotic spindle, chromosome segregation, mitotic checkpoint control, and cytokinesis, and represent druggable protein targets.[2]

This article reviews the development of novel antimitotic targets and their small molecules.

---

[a] Program in Gynecologic Oncology, Department of Medical Oncology, Dana-Farber Cancer Institute, Harvard Medical School, 450 Brookline Avenue, Boston, MA 02215, USA
[b] Warren Alpert Medical School of Brown University, Medical Oncology, Program in Women's Oncology, Women & Infants' Hospital, 101 Dudley Street, Providence, RI 02905, USA
* Corresponding author.
E-mail address: ddizon@wihri.org

Hematol Oncol Clin N Am 26 (2012) 607–628
doi:10.1016/j.hoc.2012.01.007
0889-8588/12/$ – see front matter © 2012 Elsevier Inc. All rights reserved.

MICROTUBULE STRUCTURE

Microtubules are hollow filaments that result from the polymerization α-tubulin and β-tubulin. They consist of a parallel arrangement of 13 protofilaments arranged in a head to tail order. One end is composed of α-tubulin (negative end) and the other end of β-tubulin (positive end), resulting in a polarized helix.[3] Microtubules are anchored at the negative end to a network of microtubule-associated proteins, leaving the positive end disposed to the cell periphery.[4,5] As a result of noncovalent association and disassociation of α and β heterodimers, microtubules oscillate between a state of polymerization and depolymerization. Two behaviors are shown by the microtubules: dynamic instability and treadmilling, both of which are dependent on the state of guanosine triphosphate (GTP).[6] Dynamic instability refers to switching of microtubules between periods of slow growth and rapid shortening, whereas treadmilling is characterized by the net addition of a tubulin subunit to the positive end and the parallel loss at the negative end.[6–9]

This engineered dynamic process is vital for the proper spindle function and subsequent alignment and segregation of chromosomes. Disruption of this process results in aberrant mitosis and prevents cell cycle progression, resulting in cell death.[10]

MICROTUBULE-TARGETING AGENTS

Microtubule-targeting agents either inhibit microtubule polymerization, resulting in decreased microtubule polymer mass, or promote microtubule polymerization, resulting in increased microtubule polymer mass and stabilization.[11] These compounds are characterized either as microtubule-stabilizing agents such as the taxanes and the epothilones or microtubule-destabilizing agents such as the vinca alkaloids and colchicines.

Microtubule-targeting agents bind to distinct binding sites on the β-tubulin.[12] The vinca domain is located adjacent to the GTP binding site in the β-tubulin.[13,14] The taxane site is located within the hydrophobic pocket between adjacent protofilaments in the lumen of the microtubule, whereas the colchicine site is located at the intradimer interface between the α- and β-tubulin.[15–17]

The oldest classes of cytotoxic agents that interfere with microtubules are the vinca alkaloids. These agents (vincristine, vinblastine, vindesine, vinorelbine, and vinflunine) were extracted from the leaves of the Madagascar periwinkle *Catharanthus roseus*.[18] They have been widely used in the management of both hematological and solid tumors. Current research has expanded the available compounds that bind to the vinca domain on the β-tubulin. These compounds include the halichondrins, which are isolated from the marine sponges.[19] These compounds block mitotic progression and induce apoptosis in cancer cells. They are at various stages of clinical development for the treatments of multiple disciplines.

Isolated in the 1960s from the bark of a yew tree (*Taxus brevifolia*), paclitaxel has revolutionized the management of multiple oncologic disciplines (ie, ovarian, breast, lung bladder cancer, and prostate cancer). A semisynthetic analogue, docetaxel, was isolated from the needles of the European yew (*Taxus baccata*), and is equally as instrumental in the disciplines listed earlier. Novel formulations of taxanes engineered to circumvent common toxicities are in clinical practice.[20] The epothilones and their analogues bind to the taxane site yet retain a unique mechanism of action. These agents are currently used in patients who are taxane refractory.

Historically, agents that bind to the colchicine site have not been targeted for anticancer development. However, recent interest has surfaced in the combretastatins, compounds isolated from the South African willow (*Combretum caffrum*).[21,22] These agents bind to tubulin and show potent anticancer activity by inhibiting cell cycle progression inhibiting mitosis, thereby triggering apoptosis.

Collectively, these agents are referred to as modulators of microtubule dynamics and have been the mainstay in the treatment of both solid and hematological tumors for several decades.

LIMITATIONS IN THE CLINICAL USE OF MICROTUBULE-TARGETING AGENTS
Drug Resistance

Intrinsic or acquired drug resistance is a limiting factor in the clinical applicability of microtubule-targeting agents. Several mechanisms of tubulin-binding agent resistance have been described.[23–25] One such mechanism is the result of deceased cellular drug accumulation caused by the overexpression of membrane-bound drug efflux proteins such as the *P*-glycoprotein. These proteins are a family of adenosine triphosphate (ATP)-dependent transporter proteins located in the cell membrane that are overexpressed in many tumors cell lines and effectively decrease the intracellular concentration of drug levels. Other mechanisms include direct alteration in tubulin-binding site and altered expression of tubulin isotypes (βI-tubulin, βIII-tubulin).[24] Altered expression of tubulin isotypes has been reported to have an impact on microtubule dynamics, for example the expression of βIII-tubulin results in resistance to taxanes and vinorelbine.[26–28] In addition to the mechanisms of resistance alterations in the levels mentioned earlier, intracellular location, posttranslational modifications, and function of microtubule-regulating proteins (tau, MAP2, MAP4) can influence the sensitivity to microtubule agents.[29] High expression of tau has been associated with breast neoplasms that are less responsive to paclitaxel.[30–32] Stathmin is a microtubule-sequestering protein that regulates the mitotic spindle by binding to tubulin heterodimers and inducing microtubule destabilization.[24] Investigators have reported that overexpression of stathmin decreases breast cell sensitivity to paclitaxel and vinblastine.[33–35] Changes to the microtubules induced by interactions with other cytoskeletal proteins are yet another mechanism of resistance.[36] The human pregnane X receptor is known to be a master switch in drug resistance. Activation of this pathway leads to enhanced expression of cytochrome CYP3A4, which enhances metabolic degradation of drugs, resulting in drug resistance.[37] This effect has been seen with epothilones as well as with taxanes.[37]

Side Effect Profile of Microtubule-Targeted Agents

One significant hurdle in the use of taxanes is their poor solubility, necessitating the use of solvents as vehicles. For example, paclitaxel is highly insoluble in water and requires emulsification with solvents, such as polyoxyethylated castor oil (Cremophor EL) and ethanol to allow intravenous administration. These formulations have the potential to cause severe toxicities such as hypersensitivity reactions and sensory and motor neuropathy. In addition, Cremophor can entrap paclitaxel and result in reduced drug clearance and nonlinear pharmacokinetics.[38,39]

Given the limitations of the current microtubule inhibitors, novel microtubule inhibitors are being investigated to circumvent resistance and toxicity and to deliver effective therapeutic choices.

Novel Microtubule-Targeted Agents

Novel taxanes
Novel formulations of paclitaxel have been introduced in to clinical care, including both ABI-007 (Abraxane), CT-2103 (Xytotax), and Cabazitaxel (Jevtana), which is a novel

taxane characterized by decreased propensity for *P*-glycoprotein–mediated drug resistance.[40]

ABI-007 (Abraxane) is an albumin-bound paclitaxel that is solvent free, reversibly binds paclitaxel, transports it across the endothelial cell, and concentrates in the vicinity of the neoplasm. This agent can be administered without the common predications. Preclinical data have suggested that this agent achieves higher antitumor activity and higher intracellular concentrations of active drug when compared with paclitaxel.[41] ABI-007 was compared with polyethylated castor oil-based standard paclitaxel in patients with metastatic breast cancer.[42] Patients (n = 454) were randomized to either ABI-007 260 mg/m^2 or paclitaxel 175 mg/m^2. Significantly higher response rates and longer time to tumor progression were reported with ABI-007 (23.0 vs 16.9 weeks, respectively; hazard ratio [HR] = 0.75; *P* = .006). Grade 3 sensory neuropathy was more common in the ABI-007 arm than in the standard paclitaxel arm. No hypersensitivity reactions occurred with ABI-007 despite the absence of premedication and shorter administration time. A randomized phase II study compared ABI-007 administered triweekly and weekly with triweekly docetaxel as first-line treatment of metastatic breast cancer.[43] A total of 302 patients were randomized to either 300 mg/m^2 of ABI-007 every 3 weeks, 100 mg/m^2 weekly for 3 of 4 weeks, 150 mg/m^2 weekly for 3 of 4 weeks, or docetaxel 100 mg/m^2 every 3 weeks. The investigators reported that ABI-007, regardless of dose, showed a greater overall response rate than docetaxel. This agent has been further explored in other disciplines such as gynecologic malignancies. Coleman and colleagues[44] reported a phase II evaluation of ABI-007 in the treatment of recurrent or persistent platinum-resistant ovarian, fallopian tube, or primary peritoneal cancer. Eligible patients were defined by persistent or progressive disease after primary chemotherapy or recurrence within 6 months of treatment completion. Treatment consisted of ABI-007 100 mg/m^2 days 1, 8, and 15 on a 28-day schedule. Of the 47 evaluable patients, the investigators reported 1 complete and 10 partial responses (23%), whereas 17 patients (36%) had stable disease. The median progression-free survival (PFS) was 4.5 months (95% confidence interval [CI]: 2.2–6.7), whereas the overall survival (OS) was 17.4 months (95% CI: 13.2–20.8). Seventeen patients (36%) had PFS greater than 6 months.

CT-2103 (Xyotax) (paclitaxel poliglumex [PPX]), is a conjugate of α-poly-L-glutamic acid and paclitaxel.[45] Like ABI-007, this macromolecular drug conjugate eliminates the need for Cremophor. PPX has been studied in recurrent or persistent ovarian or primary peritoneal cancer.[46] In one phase II study, patients received PPX at 235 mg/m^2 every 21 days or 175 mg/m^2.[47] The investigators reported that 16% and 41% of patients had a partial response or experienced stable disease, respectively. The median PFS was 2.8 months (95% CI 1.48–4.8 months) and median OS was 15.4 months. The most frequent grade 3 or 4 toxicities were neutropenia, constitutional symptoms, gastrointestinal symptoms, and neuropathy. This agent is being explored as maintenance therapy in ovarian cancer (clinical trial GOG 212).

In a phase II study conducted by Lin and colleagues,[48] an unexpected incidence of hypersensitivity reactions was noted with CT-2103 in patients with metastatic breast cancer. The investigators reported that CT-2103 had activity in this small study (response rate of 17%); however, neurotoxicity and hypersensitivity reactions were more frequent in this patient population than expected, and led to early termination of the trial. Grade 3 or 4 hypersensitivity reactions were observed in 4 patients; none occurred before cycle 4 of therapy. Given the delayed incidence of hypersensitivity reactions, it was suggested that these reactions were a true drug allergy, distinct from the hypersensitivity reactions seen with standard paclitaxel. Cabazitaxel (Jevtana) is a new taxane characterized by a favorable pharmacokinetic profile and a decreased propensity for P-glycoprotein–mediated drug resistance.[40] In June 2010, it was approved for the management of metastatic hormone-resistant prostate cancer. The approval of cabazitaxel was based primarily on the TROPIC (Treatment of Hormone-Refractory Metastatic Prostate Cancer Previously Treated with a Taxotere-Containing Regimen) trial. De Bono and colleagues[49] reported the results of a phase III trial in patients with metastatic castration-resistant prostate cancer who had received previous hormone therapy, but whose disease had progressed during or after treatment with a docetaxel-containing regimen. Patients received prednisone daily, and were randomly assigned to receive either 12 mg/m^2 mitoxantrone or 25 mg/m^2 cabazitaxel every 3 weeks. The primary end point was OS. Secondary end points included PFS and safety. The investigators reported that the median survival was 15.1 months (95% CI 14.1–16.3) in the cabazitaxel group and 12.7 months (11.6–13.7) in the mitoxantrone group. The HR for death of men treated with cabazitaxel compared with those taking mitoxantrone was 0.70 (95% CI 0.59–0.83, $P<.0001$). Median PFS was 2.8 months (95% CI 2.4–3.0) in the cabazitaxel group and 1.4 months (1.4–1.7) in the mitoxantrone group (HR 0.74, 0.64–0.86, $P<.0001$). The most common clinically significant grade 3 or higher adverse events were neutropenia, febrile neutropenia, and gastrointestinal events. This agent has provided a new avenue for patients with advanced prostate cancer.

The Epothilones

Epothilones are macrolide antibiotics that represent a unique class of antimicrotubule-targeting agents. Their mechanisms of action are similar to that of taxanes yet they show more potent activity and have the potential to evade the known mechanisms of taxane resistance, such as P-glycoprotein overexpression or the acquisition of mutations at β-tubulin-binding sites.[25,50–52] Naturally occurring epothilones are classified as epoxides (A, B, E, and F) or olefins (C and D).[53]

Epothilones A and B were isolated from the myxobacterium *Sorangium cellulosum*.[54] The epothilones disrupt microtubule dynamics by binding to the β-tubulin subunit of the α-β-tubulin dimer. They stabilize microtubules and result in the induction of mitotic arrest and apoptosis.[53] The binding site of epothilones overlaps with that of the taxanes on the β subunit of tubulin, but there is evidence that the 2 agents bind to tubulin differently.[55,56] The epothilones are more potent than both paclitaxel or docetaxel, with mean inhibitory concentration values in the nanomolar range.[57,58]

Epothilones A and B show modest in vivo activity. Early use of these agents was hampered by metabolic instability and a narrow therapeutic window. To improve antitumor efficacy, epothilone analogues have been synthesized.

Patupilone EPO906

Patupilone is the unmodified product of epothilone B. Phase I studies have explored several schedules of administration and have suggested that unlike the other microtubule agents diarrhea is prevalent with this agent.[59–61] Patupilone has been studied in several disciplines, including ovarian, colorectal, nonsmall lung cancer, gastric, prostate, and renal cell tumors.[62–64] Chi and colleagues[65] reported a phase II study of patupilone in patients with metastatic castration-resistant prostate cancer previously treated with docetaxel. Eighty-three patients were enrolled. A prostate-specific antigen (PSA) decline of 50% or greater occurred in 47% of patients. A partial response occurred in 24% of patients. Median time to PSA progression was 6.1 months (95% CI, 4.7–8.0) and median OS was 11.3 months (95% CI, 9.8–15.4). A phase I trial in patients with ovarian cancer (n = 45) reported an overall response rate of 19.5%, with a median duration of disease control of 15.8 months.[66] This agent has also been studied in combination studies with carboplatin (area under curve, 5–6 every 3 weeks). The overall response rate was 62%, whereas 14% of patients achieved stable disease.[67]

The phase II results have led to a randomized phase III trial comparing patupilone with pegylated liposomal doxorubicin (PLD). This recent phase III study (n = 829) included platinum-resistant and taxane-resistant patients with ovarian cancer and reported a significantly higher response rate than PLD (15.5 vs 7.9%), yet no OS benefit was appreciated (13.2 months for patupilone and 12.7 months for PLD).[68]

One intriguing aspect of this agent lies in its ability to penetrate the central nervous system (CNS). In addition, patupilone is reported to have radiosensitizing properties. A recent phase I trial reported the combined therapeutic approach of concurrent cranial irradiation and patupilone (given every week and every 3 weeks) in patients with primary or secondary CNS malignancies.[69] Primary CNS malignancies received radiotherapy (RT) to a median dose of 60 Gy. CNS metastases received whole-brain RT to a median dose of 37.4 Gy, and patients with recurrent gliomas underwent stereotactic RT to a median dose of 37.5 Gy. The investigators reported that when patupilone was combined with a variety of radiation doses and fractionation schedules, concurrent patupilone was well tolerated and safe, with a maximal tolerated dose of 8 mg/m^2 every 3 weeks.

Ixabepilone

Ixabepilone (BMS 247,550), a semisynthetic derivative of epothilone B, is the most widely investigated epothilone. In vitro studies have shown that the cytotoxicity of ixabepilone is 2.5 times that of paclitaxel.[58] Several dosing schedules in phase I studies have led to the recommended phase II dose of 40 mg/m^2.[70,71] Common side effects reported in all studies included neutropenia, hepatic enzyme dysfunction, alopecia, and neuropathy and hypersensitivity reactions.

Ixabepilone was approved in 2007 by the US Food and Drug Administration for the treatment of metastatic breast cancer. Thomas and colleagues[72] reported the results of 752 patients randomized to either ixabepilone 40 mg/m^2 plus capecitabine 2000 mg/m^2 on days 1 to 14 of a 21-day cycle, or capecitabine alone 2500 mg/m^2. The primary end point was PFS. Ixabepilone plus capecitabine prolonged PFS relative to capecitabine (median, 5.8 vs 4.2 months; HR, 0.75; 95% CI, 0.64–0.88; P = .0003) and yielded increased objective response rates (ORRs) (35% vs 14%; P<.0001). Grade 3 to 4 treatment-related sensory neuropathy, fatigue, and neutropenia were more frequent with combination therapy, as was the rate of death as a result of toxicity with patients with liver dysfunction. The investigators concluded that ixabepilone plus capecitabine showed superior efficacy to capecitabine alone in patients with metastatic breast cancer pretreated or resistant to anthracyclines and resistant to taxanes.

Jassem and colleagues[73] reported the results of a pooled analysis on a prespecified subset of patients whose disease relapsed within 12 months after adjuvant anthracyclines and taxanes. Patients received ixabepilone plus capecitabine (n = 149) or capecitabine alone (n = 144) as first-line chemotherapy for metastatic breast cancer. Analysis included PFS, OS, ORR, and toxicity. In 293 patients, ixabepilone plus capecitabine increased PFS (median: 5.6 months vs 2.8 months; HR, 0.58; P<.0001), overall response rate (46% vs 24%), and OS (median: 15.1 months vs 12.5 months; HR, 0.84; P = .208). Major toxicities of this regimen included neuropathy, neutropenia, and hand-foot syndrome.

The efficacy of ixabepilone has also been shown in other subsets, including patients with triple-negative disease. Perez and colleagues[74] analyzed the efficacy and safety data of ixabepilone in women with triple-negative breast disease from several studies. Of 2261 patients evaluated in these trials, 556 (24.5%) had triple-negative tumors. In the neoadjuvant setting, ixabepilone produced a pathologic complete response rate in the breast of 26% in triple-negative patients (vs 15% in the nontriple-negative population). In patients with metastatic breast cancer, the overall response rates in the phase II ixabepilone monotherapy trials ranged from 6% to 55%, comparable with rates seen in patients with nontriple-negative tumors. The combination of ixabepilone and capecitabine in the phase II study resulted in an overall response rate of 23% in triple-negative patients. A similar overall response rate (31%) was observed for a pre-planned pooled analysis of triple-negative patients in the phase III trials of ixabepilone plus capecitabine. The median PFS was significantly longer for triple-negative patients treated with ixabepilone plus capecitabine (4.2 months) compared with treatment with capecitabine alone (1.7 months). The overall consensus was that ixabepilone seems to offer an alternative chemotherapeutic agent for patients with triple-negative breast cancer.

Ixabepilone: Prostate Cancer

Despite the recent approval of docetaxel for the treatment of hormone-refractory prostate cancer, additional novel agents that can further improve patient outcomes are warranted. The epothilones have shown potent antitumor activity in vitro and in experimental animal models of prostate cancer. Studies of single-agent ixabepilone in patients with hormone-refractory prostate cancer have reported a confirmed PSA response rate.[75] Rosenberg and colleagues[76] recently reported a phase I study of ixabepilone, mitoxantrone, and prednisone in patients with metastatic castration-resistant prostate cancer previously treated with docetaxel-based therapy. Thirty-one percent of patients experienced PSA declines of 50% or greater, and 2 experienced objective responses. Of 21 patients treated with mitoxantrone 12 mg/m^2 plus ixabepilone 30 mg/m^2 or greater, 9 (43%) patients experienced PSA declines of 50% or greater (95% CI, 22%–66%).

Ixabepilone: Gynecologic Malignancies

A recent multi-institutional phase II trial of ixabepilone (20 mg/m^2, days 1, 8, and 15 on a 28-day cycle) in platinum-resistant and taxane-resistant ovarian cancer has been reported.[77] The overall response rate in 49 patients was 18.4%. Stable disease was the best response in 40.8% of the patients. The median PFS and OS were 4.4 and 14.8 months, respectively. These results are similar to other single-agent cytotoxics commonly used in this setting.[31–33]

Dizon and colleagues[78] conducted a phase II study to determine the response rate of ixabepilone in patients with persistent or recurrent endometrial cancer who had progressed despite standard therapy. Patients received ixabepilone 40 mg/m^2 as a 3-hour infusion on day 1 of a 21-day cycle. Fifty-two patients were entered on the study and 50 of these were eligible. The overall response rate was 12%; 1 patient achieved a complete remission (2%), and 5 achieved partial remission (10%). Stable disease for at least 8 weeks was noted in 30 patients (60%). The median PFS was 2.9 months, and the 6-month PFS was 20%. Major grade 3 toxicities were neutropenia, leukopenia, gastrointestinal, neurologic, constitutional, infection, and anemia. The investigators concluded that in a cohort of women with advanced or recurrent endometrial cancer who were previously treated with paclitaxel, ixabepilone showed modest activity of limited duration as a second-line agent.

EPOTHILONE B ANALOGUE: SAGOPILONE (ZK-EPO)

Sagopilone is a novel, fully synthetic epothilone currently being investigated. Morrow and colleagues[79] reported the results of a phase II study in women with metastatic breast cancer. Patients received sagopilone 16 or 22 mg/m² as 3-hour intravenous infusion every 21 days. Among the 65 patients who were evaluable for efficacy, there were 3 confirmed responses, yet OS was not reached. The main treatment-related adverse events were sensory neuropathy and fatigue.

Studies have reported that sagopilone crosses the blood-brain barrier. Freedman and colleagues[80] reported a phase II study of sagopilone (ZK 219,477; ZK-EPO) in patients with breast cancer with CNS metastasis. The primary end point was CNS ORR. Secondary end points included toxicity, PFS, and OS. Fifteen women, all of whom had progressive CNS disease despite whole-brain RT, were enrolled. Two patients achieved a partial response (ORR, 13.3%) and remained in the study for 6 cycles. Median PFS and OS were 1.4 months and 5.3 months, respectively. The most common grade 3 toxicities were lymphopenia and fatigue.

EPOTHILONE D ANALOGUES: KOS-862 AND KOS-1584

Two epothilone D agents, KOS-862, and KOS-1584, are undergoing clinical investigation.[81,82] Konner and colleagues[83] conducted a phase I trial to determine the maximum tolerated dose (MTD) of KOS-862. Thirty-two patients were enrolled. KOS-862 was well tolerated, with manageable toxicity, favorable pharmacologic profile, and the suggestion of clinical activity. Buzdar and colleagues[84] conducted a phase II trial of KOS-862 in patients with metastatic breast cancer. Fourteen percent of women had a partial response; however, there was a high incidence of grade 3 neurotoxicity (18.5%). Lam and colleagues[85] recently reported the results of a phase I study of KOS-1584 in patients with advanced solid tumors. Sixty-six patients were accrued. Diarrhea, arthralgias, and encephalopathy were dose-limiting toxicities. Two patients achieved partial responses, whereas 24 patients had stable disease. Further data on either agent are pending.

Microtubule-Destabilizing Agents

Vinca alkaloids

The vinca alkaloids are agents classified as destabilizing agents that cause microtubule polymerization, suppress treadmilling/dynamic instability, inhibit mitosis, and result in apoptosis.[86] Vinca alkaloids have a well-established role both in solid and hematological malignancies. Vincristine is well established as a therapeutic agent in the treatment of leukemias, lymphomas, and sarcomas. Vinblastine is an integral agent in the management of patients with testicular cancer Hodgkin disease and lymphoma, whereas vinorelbine is used in the management of nonsmall cell lung cancer. Although vinorelbine was never approved for the management of patients with breast cancer, there is significant activity as a single agent as well as in combination with trastuzumab.[87,88] Vindesine is being explored as a potential option in the management of acute lymphocytic leukemia.[89]

Vinflunine

Vinflunine is a novel vinca alkaloid that destabilizes microtubules and decreases microtubule growth rate.[11,90] Studies have reported a differential affinity for tubulin, a superior in vivo activity when compared with other vinca alkaloids, and a slow rate of resistance. This agent is water soluble, thereby obviating solvent vehicles.[91–93]

Clinical studies have focused on transitional cell carcinoma of the genitourinary tract, nonsmall cell lung cancer, and mesothelioma.[94–96] A dosing regimen of vinflunine of 280 to 350 mg/m^2 intravenously once every 21 days has been used in most trials. Neutropenia was the prominent toxicity observed in most studies. A phase II trial in breast cancer yielded encouraging results in that 18 of 60 patients experienced an objective response.[97] This agent has also been combined with trastuzumab and has yielded responses: 8 of 17 patients experienced a partial response.[98] The adverse side effects of this agent include neutropenia, fatigue, and constipation.

HALICHONDRIN B ANALOGUE: ERIBULIN MESYLATE

Eribulin mesylate is a microtubule-targeting chemotherapeutic agent that is a synthetic analogue of the natural compound halichondrin B. It was initially isolated from the sea sponge (*Halichondria okadai*).[99] Eribulin targets microtubules and suppresses dynamic instability at microtubule positive ends through inhibition of microtubule growth, with little or no effect on shortening.[99]

Eribulin binds at or near the vinca domain, a region that is located at the interface of 2 tubulin heterodimers. This agent has been investigated in several tumor types and is approved for patients with metastatic breast cancer. Cortes and colleagues[100] recently reported the results of a phase III study (EMBRACE [Eribulin Monotherapy Versus Treatment of Physician's Choice in Patients with Metastatic Breast Cancer]). Patients (n = 762) were randomly allocated to either eribulin mesylate (1.4 mg/m^2) or treatment of physician's choice (TPC). Patients accrued to this study had received numerous previous lines of therapy. The investigators reported that OS was significantly improved in women assigned to eribulin (median 13.1 months, 95% CI, 11.8–14.3) compared with TPC (10.6 months, 9.3–12.5; HR, 0.81; 95% CI, 0.66–0.99; $P = 0.041$). The most common adverse events in both groups were asthenia or fatigue, and peripheral neuropathy.

Hensley and colleagues[101] recently reported the activity of this eribulin mesylate agent in patients with ovarian cancer. Patients with recurrent, measurable epithelial ovarian cancer who had received 2 or fewer previous cytotoxic regimens were enrolled into 2 cohorts: platinum-resistant patients and platinum-sensitive patients. In the platinum-resistant cohort, 37 patients enrolled, and 36 patients were evaluable for response and toxicity. Two patients achieved a partial response (5.5%), and 16 patients (44%) had stable disease as their best response. The median PFS was 1.8 months (95% CI, 1.4–2.8 months). In the platinum-sensitive cohort, 37 patients were evaluable for response. Seven patients achieved a partial response (19%). The median PFS was 4.1 months (95% CI, 2.8–5.8 months). The major toxicity was grade 3 or 4 neutropenia (42% of platinum-resistant patients; 54% of platinum-sensitive patients).

Colchicines

Colchicine, isolated from the meadow saffron (*Colchicum autumnale*), is one of the earliest microtubule-targeting agents identified.[6] As a microtubule-depolymerizing agent, it binds at the interface of the α- and β-tubulin heterodimers.[17] Colchicine causes microtubule depolymerization by inhibiting lateral contacts between the protofilaments.[102] Although colchicine has no clinical use in malignant disciplines, multiple agents that bind to the colchicines-binding site are undergoing investigation.

Combretastatin

Combretastatins were originally isolated Pettit and colleagues from the root bark of the *Combretum caffrum* tree have been shown to target the microtubule, inhibiting the polymerization of tubulin to microtubules.[103,104] These agents show potent antineo-plastic activity by inhibiting cell progression at mitosis and initiating apoptosis.[21] Com-bretastatin A4 phosphate (CA4P) is a simple derivative of the natural product that was prepared to increase water solubility. CA4P has also been shown to be a vascular-disrupting agent.[105] CA4P is in clinical trials for treatment of cervical, colorectal, non-small cell lung, prostate, ovarian, and thyroid cancers.

Panzem

Matei and colleagues[106] studied the role of 2-methoxyestradiol (Panzem), a metabolite of estradiol that destabilizes microtubules and exerts antiangiogenic properties, in eligible patients with ovarian cancer. The primary end point was ORR. Eighteen patients were enrolled. The most common adverse events were fatigue, nausea, diar-rhea, neuropathy, edema, and dyspnea (most being grade 1–2). There were no objec-tive responses, but 7 patients had stable disease. Of those 7 patients, 2 patients had stable disease for greater than 12 months. The rate of clinical benefit was 31%. This agent has also been explored in neuroendocrine tumors and prostate cancer.[107,108]

Maytansine analogues

Maytansine and its analogues (maytansinoids) are potent microtubule-targeted compounds that bind to tubulin at the vinca-binding site.[109,110] Similar to vinca alka-loids, maytansine can depolymerize microtubules and arrest cells in mitosis.[111–113] Maytansine shows greater cytotoxicity in cells than the vinca alkaloids; however, a limiting factor in the use of these agents is their narrow therapeutic window because of neurotoxicity and gastrointestinal effects.[114] An attractive approach involving vec-torization of microtubule-binding agents to the tumor cell using a monoclonal antibody has reintroduced these agents into clinical practice. Trials of trastuzumab-DM1 (T-DM1), a maytansinoid conjugated to the human epidermal growth factor receptor 2-specific therapeutic antibody trastuzumab, showed impressive efficacy in heavily pretreated patients with metastatic breast cancer.[115,116] Phase I and phase II clinical trials of T-DM1 as a single agent and in combination with paclitaxel, docetaxel, and pertuzumab have shown clinical activity and a favorable safety profile in patients with HER2-positive metastatic breast cancer. Two randomized phase III trials of T-DM1 are recruiting patients: EMILIA (Open-Label Study of Trastuzumab Emtansine (T-DM1) vs Capecitabine+Lapatinib in Patients With HER2-Positive Locally Advanced or Metastatic Breast Cancer) is evaluating T-DM1 compared with lapatinib plus cape-citabine, and MARIANNE (Study of Trastuzumab Emtansine [T-DM1] Plus Pertuzu-mab/Pertuzumab Placebo Versus Trastuzumab [Herceptin] Plus a Taxane in Patients With Metastatic Breast Cancer) is evaluating T-DM1 plus placebo versus T-DM1 plus pertuzumab versus trastuzumab plus a taxane.

Novel Targeted Agents

Given the clinical effectiveness of microtubule modulators in oncology, continued efforts to identify novel agents that target the mitotic spindle and regulate cellular progression through mitosis continue. Nontubulin (ie, the kinase inhibitors) are under investigation. Although the mechanisms involved are not straightforward, they may work in 1 of 3 possible mechanisms: (1) they result in prolonged mitotic arrest, signaling apoptosis, which is the mechanism of action of microtubule assembly inhib-itors such as the taxanes and eribulin; (2) they may cause mitotic delays in metaphase, resulting in cell death; or (3) they cause a transient mitotic delay that causes inappro-priate chromosomal segregation, which results in cell death after mitosis.[117] Several are in clinical development, including aurora kinase (AK), pololike kinase (PLK), and kinesin spindle protein (KSP) inhibitors. The preliminary data on these agents are reviewed here.

AK inhibitors

Aurora A and B are serine/threonine kinases essential for the formation of normal mitotic spindles and function of centrosomes.[118] Aurora A has been suggested to be an oncogene, but recent data suggest that although aurora A kinase amplification and overexpression are not sufficient to induce transformation, it creates the environment by which other cellular changes and genetic alterations occur to complete oncoplastic transformation.[119] In addition to their roles in mitosis, aurora A and B are known to interact with other cellular processes important in oncogenesis, including those involving NF-κ-B, p53, and N-myc.[119–121] They are also frequently overexpressed in human tumors and hence have been identified for further development in cancer treatment.[119] Inhibition of AK has been shown to result in inappropriate chromosomal segregation, believed to be the result of effects on spindle assembly.[122] Depletion of aurora A in vitro causes G2-M arrest, which results in apoptosis.[119] Aurora B kinase plays an important role in mitosis and functions in both chromosome attachment and orientation. It is part of a chromosome passenger complex that includes inner centromere protein, borealin, and surviving.[119]

Alisertib is an orally active AK inhibitor that preferentially inhibits aurora A kinase.[117] It is a potent inhibitor of cell division in vitro and shows growth inhibition in tumor xenografts using both solid malignancy and lymphoma models.[117] In 1 phase I trial, 61 patients were treated in 16 different cohorts evaluating daily dosing (7 days on/14 days off), divided dosing (4 times a day for 7 days followed by 14 days off), and divided dosing with the addition of methylphenidate or modafinil.[123] Most patients treated were men with a median age of 60 years. The most common malignancies were colorectal, lung, genitourinary, and sarcoma. Seventy-nine percent had received 3 or more previous treatment regimens. The major dose-limiting toxicity (DLT) was neurocognitive changes and somnolence, which was grade 3 in 18%. It was otherwise well tolerated up to 60 mg/d in divided doses. Dose escalation was otherwise halted because of somnolence, which persisted despite psychostimulants. No responses were seen, but 9 patients had stable disease for at least 4 cycles. In a second phase I study of 43 patients, dose escalation using intermittent dosing in a 28-day cycle was conducted.[124] The DLTs consisted of somnolence and transaminitis; however, it was deemed that treatment of 10 to 14 days of a 28-day cycle was feasible. MTD was established at 70 mg/d administered in 4 divided doses for 14 days of a 28-day cycle. Again, no clinical responses were observed.

MK-0457 was evaluated in a phase I study evaluating a 5-day continuous infusion schedule (doses 0.5–12 mg/m^2/h were tested).[125] A total of 16 patients participated in this trial and DLT (neutropenia) was observed at the 12 mg/m^2/h dose level. Three of 16 patients had stable disease.

MLN8237 is another AK A inhibitor that is available orally. It underwent phase I testing as a once-daily dose administered 7 of 21 days, with doses ranging from 5 to 150 mg/d tested.[126] The MTD was reached at 150 mg/d and consisted of neutropenia, mucositis, and somnolence. No responses were recorded, although 5 patients achieved disease stability. It continues in clinical trials as a single agent and with chemotherapy.

The selective AK B inhibitor barasetib (AZD1152) was evaluated at 2 different dosing schedules in advanced solid tumors in a European study that recruited 59 patients.[127] MTD was set at 200 mg when used as a 2-hour infusion weekly and at 450 mg when dosed every 2 weeks. The DLT was the same in both schedules and consisted of neutropenia, which occurred in 58% of patients. Although no responses were recorded, 25% achieved stable disease. Another phase I to II study was performed in newly diagnosed or relapsed acute myelogenous leukemia (AML).[128] The MTD determined in the phase I setting was 1200 mg, dosed as a continuous infusion for 7 days of a 21-day cycle. The overall hematologic response rate was 25%, with toxicity consisting of stomatitis as the primary DLT. The response rate was similar to that achieved in a Japanese phase I study in which a 19% response rate was noted in a population with advanced AML, although in this more advanced population the predominant toxicity was neutropenia.[129]

Danusertib (PHA-739,358) is an intravenous pan-AK inhibitor that underwent phase I evaluation in solid tumors using a 24-hour infusion schedule every 14 days.[130] Fifty-six patients were enrolled, with febrile neutropenia established as the DLT. The recommended phase II dose was established at 750 mg/m^2, with granulocyte colony-stimulating factor recommended. Two responses were seen in this phase I study: a patient with lung cancer had an objective response that lasted for 23 weeks and a patient with recurrent ovarian cancer had a 27% reduction in tumor dimensions and a 30% decline in her cancer antigen 125. A second phase I study in Europe evaluated danusertib on a weekly schedule (3 weeks on/1 week off).[131] Fifty-six patients underwent evaluation and, again, neutropenia proved to be dose-limiting. The MTD was established at 330 mg/m^2 when infused over 6 hours. Although no responses were recorded, 24% had stable disease and 5 patients remained progression free at 6 months. Danusertib continues in clinical evaluation, particularly in imatinib-resistant chronic myelogenous leukemia (CML) based on the finding that it inhibits the multidrug-resistant T315I mutant of Bcr-Abl, which is responsible for 25% or more of CML resistance to imatinib.[132]

Other agents in this class include AS703569, SNS-314, and AMG-900. Early clinical trials are ongoing, with no results yet published.

PLK inhibitors

PLKs are serine/threonine kinases that are also involved in checkpoint regulation in mitosis. As with the AKs, they are highly upregulated in human malignancies.[133] Depletion of PLKs in cancer cells results in decreased cell proliferation and viability by interruption of the spindle assembly, resulting in prolonged mitotic arrest and eventual apoptosis.[133] A summary of published clinical trials involving this class is discussed.

GSK461364 is a competitive inhibitor of Plk-1. Forty patients were enrolled in a phase I study of this agent that evaluated 2 different schedules: 3 weeks on/1 week off and a semicontinuous 28-day cycle (days 1, 2, 8, 9, 15, and 16).[134] The DLTs were grade 4 neutropenia, grade 3 to 4 thrombocytopenia, and thromboembolic events (which occurred in 20% of patients); MTD was established at 300 mg for weekly dosing and 225 mg for semicontinuous dosing. No responses were recorded. Fifteen percent achieved stable disease, including 4 patients with esophageal cancer. The investigators concluded that sufficient interest was seen, although they recommended prophylactic anticoagulation in subsequent studies.

BI 2536 is a small molecule Plk-1 inhibitor that underwent a phase I evaluation in patients with advanced solid tumors in which 25-mg to 250-mg doses were administered; patients showing clinical benefit were treated with additional courses.[135] The MTD was set at 200 mg, with DLT defined as neutropenia (56% had grade 3–4 severity). No responses were recorded, although 23% treated at or above the MTD had stable disease for at least 3 months. A subsequent open-label phase I evaluation was performed in 70 patients, which tested 2 schedules: 2 weeks on/1 week off as a 1-hour infusion or as a 24-hour continuous infusion on day 1 of a 21-day cycle.[136] The MTD with weekly dosing was established at 100 mg/dose. With the continuous infusion schedule, doses up to 225 mg were tolerated and an MTD was not reached. Both schedules were associated with significant neutropenia: grade 3 to 4 in 36% using weekly dosing and 50% with the 24-hour infusion. No responses were recorded; 32% had stable disease with weekly dosing.

An open-label randomized phase II study of BI 2536 was also conducted in patients with advanced nonsmall cell lung cancer.[137] Ninety-five patients received BI 2536 as an intravenous infusion on day 1 (200 mg) or from days 1 to 3 (50–60 mg) of a 21-day cycle, with interpatient dose escalation allowed based on patient tolerance. There were 4 responses (overall response rate, 4.2%), and median PFS was 2 months. The median OS was 7 months and there were no differences in outcomes associated with drug schedule. Thirty-seven percent of patients had grade 4 neutropenia, and 2 drug-related deaths (sepsis and pulmonary hemorrhage) occurred.

ON 01,910.Na regulates mitotic pathways, including Plk-1. A first-in-man study involving 20 patients evaluated this agent as a 2-hour infusion on days 1, 4, 8, 11, 15, and 18 of a 28-day cycle.[138] The MTD was established at 3120 mg/dose. The predominant toxicities were associated with skeletal and abdominal adverse events, as well as significant tumor pain. One objective response was recorded in a patient with recurrent ovarian cancer. It persisted for up to 24 months. A separate phase I study was performed in 13 patients with high-risk myelodysplastic syndrome.[139] All patients were reported to have a response, including 4 who had a complete marrow response.

KSP inhibitors

Kinesins are enzymes that use ATP to translocate along or destabilize microtubules, and are important for the process of cell division.[140] KSP is a specific kinesin expressed only in dividing cells and thus is critical to the organization of the mitotic spindle.[141] Subsequent inhibition of KSP results in apoptosis because of mitotic arrest.

Ispinesib (SB-715,992) underwent phase II evaluation in 17 patients with metastatic or recurrent malignant melanoma.[142] The dose and schedule used were 18 mg/m^2 as a 1-hour infusion on a 3-week cycle. Although no responses were observed, 35% had stable disease for a median of 3 months. Grade 3 adverse events were limited, but consisted of dizziness and blurry vision. Because of lack of activity, it was not recommended for further evaluation in this population.

MK-0371 is a C2-hydroxymethyl dihydropyrrole KSP inhibitor designed to circumvent *P*-glycoprotein efflux and optimized for antitumor properties by incorporation of fluorine.[141] In phase I testing that involved 35 patients with taxane-refractory cancers, MT-0371 was evaluated using a 24-hour infusion schedule dosed every 21 days. The MTD was established at 17 mg/m^2/d without evidence of myelosuppression. The DLT seen at higher doses consisted of prolonged grade 4 neutropenia. No responses were noted, but stable disease for at least 4 cycles was seen in 16 patients.[143]

SUMMARY

Microtubule assembly agents are a mainstay in the treatment of multiple solid tumor malignancies and efforts are under way to explore other mechanisms to inhibit mitosis and associated mechanisms. Novel microtubulin-targeted agents have been recently approved, including nAb-paclitaxel, ixabepilone, and eribulin.

Mitotic inhibitors that involve AKs, PLKs, and KSPs are in early clinical development. Although activity with these agents seems limited, some promising early results suggest that they may have a role in the treatment of cancer, either with optimal dosing or in combination with cytotoxics.

REFERENCES

1. Nogales E. Structural insight into microtubule function. Annu Rev Biophys Biomol Struct 2001;30:397–420.
2. Ivachtchenko AV, Kiselyov AS, Tkachenko SE, et al. Novel mitotic targets and their small-molecule inhibitors. Curr Cancer Drug Targets 2007;7(8): 766–84.
3. Amos L, Klug A. Arrangement of subunits in flagellar microtubules. J Cell Sci 1974;14(3):523–49.
4. Zhou J, Shu HB, Joshi HC. Regulation of tubulin synthesis and cell cycle progression in mammalian cells by gamma-tubulin-mediated microtubule nucleation. J Cell Biochem 2002;84(3):472–83.
5. Joshi HC, Zhou J. Gamma tubulin and microtubule nucleation in mammalian cells. Methods Cell Biol 2001;67:179–93.
6. Zhou J, Giannakakou P. Targeting microtubules for cancer chemotherapy. Curr Med Chem Anticancer Agents 2005;5(1):65–71.
7. Mitchison T, Kirschner M. Dynamic instability of microtubule growth. Nature 1984;312(5991):237–42.
8. Margolis RL, Wilson L. Opposite end assembly and disassembly of microtubules at steady state in vitro. Cell 1978;13(1):1–8.
9. Rodionov VI, Borisy GG. Microtubule treadmilling in vivo. Science 1997; 275(5297):215–8.
10. McGrogan BT, Gilmartin B, Carney DN, et al. Taxanes, microtubules and chemoresistant breast cancer. Biochim Biophys Acta 2008;1785(2):96–132.
11. Perez EA. Microtubule inhibitors: differentiating tubulin-inhibiting agents based on mechanisms of action, clinical activity, and resistance. Mol Cancer Ther 2009;8(8):2086–95.
12. Downing KH. Structural basis for the interaction of tubulin with proteins and drugs that affect microtubule dynamics. Annu Rev Cell Dev Biol 2000;16:89–111.
13. Jordan MA, Margolis RL, Himes RH, et al. Identification of a distinct class of vinblastine binding sites on microtubules. J Mol Biol 1986;187(1):61–73.
14. Rai SS, Wolff J. Localization of the vinblastine-binding site on beta-tubulin. J Biol Chem 1996;271(25):14707–11.
15. Snyder JP, Nettles JH, Cornett B, et al. The binding conformation of Taxol in beta-tubulin: a model based on electron crystallographic density. Proc Natl Acad Sci U S A 2001;98(9):5312–6.
16. Uppuluri S, Knipling L, Sackett DL, et al. Localization of the colchicine-binding site of tubulin. Proc Natl Acad Sci U S A 1993;90(24):11598–602.
17. Ravelli RB, Gigant B, Curmi PA, et al. Insight into tubulin regulation from a complex with colchicine and a stathmin-like domain. Nature 2004;428(6979): 198–202.
18. Cutts JH, Beer CT, Noble RL. Biological properties of Vincaleukoblastine, an alkaloid in *Vinca rosea* Linn, with reference to its antitumor action. Cancer Res 1960;20:1023–31.
19. Bai RL, Paull KD, Herald CL, et al. Halichondrin B and homohalichondrin B, marine natural products binding in the vinca domain of tubulin. Discovery of

tubulin-based mechanism of action by analysis of differential cytotoxicity data. J Biol Chem 1991;266(24):15882–9.

20. Jordan MA, Wilson L. Microtubules as a target for anticancer drugs. Nat Rev Cancer 2004;4(4):253–65.

21. Hamel E, Lin CM. Interactions of combretastatin, a new plant-derived antimitotic agent, with tubulin. Biochem Pharmacol 1983;32(24):3864–7.

22. Cirla A, Mann J. Combretastatins: from natural products to drug discovery. Nat Prod Rep 2003;20(6):558–64.

23. Gottesman MM. Mechanisms of cancer drug resistance. Annu Rev Med 2002; 53:615–27.

24. Kavallaris M. Microtubules and resistance to tubulin-binding agents. Nat Rev Cancer 2010;10(3):194–204.

25. Fojo AT, Menefee M. Microtubule targeting agents: basic mechanisms of multidrug resistance (MDR). Semin Oncol 2005;32(6 Suppl 7):S3–8.

26. Sève P, Dumontet C. Is class III beta-tubulin a predictive factor in patients receiving tubulin-binding agents? Lancet Oncol 2008;9(2):168–75.

27. Kamath K, Wilson L, Cabral F, et al. BetaIII-tubulin induces paclitaxel resistance in association with reduced effects on microtubule dynamic instability. J Biol Chem 2005;280(13):12902–7.

28. Mozzetti S, Ferlini C, Concolino P, et al. Class III beta-tubulin overexpression is a prominent mechanism of paclitaxel resistance in ovarian cancer patients. Clin Cancer Res 2005;11(1):298–305.

29. Zhang CC, Yang JM, White E, et al. The role of MAP4 expression in the sensitivity to paclitaxel and resistance to vinca alkaloids in p53 mutant cells. Oncogene 1998;16(12):1617–24.

30. Pusztai L. Markers predicting clinical benefit in breast cancer from microtubule-targeting agents. Ann. Oncol 2007;18(Suppl 12):xii15–20.

31. Rouzier R, Rajan R, Wagner P, et al. Microtubule-associated protein tau: a marker of paclitaxel sensitivity in breast cancer. Proc Natl Acad Sci U S A 2005;102(23):8315–20.

32. Tanaka S, Nohara T, Iwamoto M, et al. Tau expression and efficacy of paclitaxel treatment in metastatic breast cancer. Cancer Chemother Pharmacol 2009; 64(2):341–6.

33. Alli E, Yang JM, Ford JM, et al. Reversal of stathmin-mediated resistance to paclitaxel and vinblastine in human breast carcinoma cells. Mol Pharmacol 2007;71(5):1233–40.

34. Su D, Smith SM, Preti M, et al. Stathmin and tubulin expression and survival of ovarian cancer patients receiving platinum treatment with and without paclitaxel. Cancer 2009;115(11):2453–63.

35. Devred F, Tsvetkov PO, Barbier P, et al. Stathmin/Op18 is a novel mediator of vinblastine activity. FEBS Lett 2008;582(17):2484–8.

36. Dumontet C, Jordan MA. Microtubule-binding agents: a dynamic field of cancer therapeutics. Nat Rev Drug Discov 2010;9(10):790–803.

37. Mani S, Huang H, Sundarababu S, et al. Activation of the steroid and xenobiotic receptor (human pregnane X receptor) by nontaxane microtubule-stabilizing agents. Clin Cancer Res 2005;11(17):6359–69.

38. Gelderblom H, Verweij J, Nooter K, et al. The drawbacks and advantages of vehicle selection for drug formulation. Eur J Cancer 2001;37(13): 1590–8.

39. Dorr RT. Pharmacology and toxicology of Cremophor EL diluent. Ann Pharmacother 1994;28(Suppl 5):S11–4.

40. Paller CJ, Antonarakis ES. Cabazitaxel: a novel second-line treatment for metastatic castration-resistant prostate cancer. Drug Des Devel Ther 2011;5: 117–24.

41. Gradishar WJ. Albumin-bound paclitaxel: a next-generation taxane. Expert Opin Pharmacother 2006;7(8):1041–53.

42. Gradishar WJ, Tjulandin S, Davidson N, et al. Phase III trial of nanoparticle albumin-bound paclitaxel compared with polyethylated castor oil-based pacli-taxel in women with breast cancer. J Clin Oncol 2005;23(31):7794–803.

43. Gradishar WJ, Krasnojon D, Cheporov S, et al. Significantly longer progression-free survival with nab-paclitaxel compared with docetaxel as first-line therapy for metastatic breast cancer. J Clin Oncol 2009;27(22):3611–9.

44. Coleman RL, Brady WE, McMeekin DS, et al. A phase II evaluation of nanopar-ticle, albumin-bound (nab) paclitaxel in the treatment of recurrent or persistent platinum-resistant ovarian, fallopian tube, or primary peritoneal cancer: a Gyne-cologic Oncology Group study. Gynecol Oncol 2011;122(1):111–5.

45. Langer CJ. CT-2103: emerging utility and therapy for solid tumours. Expert Opin Investig Drugs 2004;13(11):1501–8.

46. Galic VL, Herzog TJ, Wright JD, et al. Paclitaxel poliglumex for ovarian cancer. Expert Opin Investig Drugs 2011;20(6):813–21.

47. Sabbatini P, Sill MW, O'Malley D, et al. A phase II trial of paclitaxel poliglumex in recurrent or persistent ovarian or primary peritoneal cancer (EOC): a Gyneco-logic Oncology Group Study. Gynecol Oncol 2008;111(3):455–60.

48. Lin NU, Parker LM, Come SE, et al. Phase II study of CT-2103 as first- or second-line chemotherapy in patients with metastatic breast cancer: unex-pected incidence of hypersensitivity reactions. Invest New Drugs 2007;25(4): 369–75.

49. de Bono JS, Oudard S, Ozguroglu M, et al. Prednisone plus cabazitaxel or mi-toxantrone for metastatic castration-resistant prostate cancer progressing after docetaxel treatment: a randomised open-label trial. Lancet 2010;376(9747): 1147–54.

50. Kowalski RJ, Giannakakou P, Hamel E. Activities of the microtubule-stabilizing agents epothilones A and B with purified tubulin and in cells resistant to pacli-taxel (Taxol(R)). J Biol Chem 1997;272(4):2534–41.

51. Kolman A. Activity of epothilones. Curr Opin Investig Drugs 2005;6(6):616–22.

52. Kamath K, Jordan MA. Suppression of microtubule dynamics by epothilone B is associated with mitotic arrest. Cancer Res 2003;63(18):6026–31.

53. Fumoleau P, Coudert B, Isambert N, et al. Novel tubulin-targeting agents: anti-cancer activity and pharmacologic profile of epothilones and related analogues. Ann Oncol 2007;18(Suppl 5):v9–15.

54. Gerth K, Bedorf N, Höfle G, et al. Epothilons A and B: antifungal and cytotoxic compounds from *Sorangium cellulosum* (Myxobacteria). Production, physico-chemical and biological properties. J Antibiot 1996;49(6):560–3.

55. Borzilleri R, Vite G. Epothilones: new tubulin polymerization agents in preclinical and clinical development. Drugs Future 2002;27:1149–63.

56. Giannakakou P, Gussio R, Nogales E, et al. A common pharmacophore for epothilone and taxanes: molecular basis for drug resistance conferred by tubulin mutations in human cancer cells. Proc Natl Acad Sci U S A 2000; 97(6):2904–9.

57. Bollag DM, McQueney PA, Zhu J, et al. Epothilones, a new class of microtubule-stabilizing agents with a taxol-like mechanism of action. Cancer Res 1995; 55(11):2325–33.

58. Lee FY, Borzilleri R, Fairchild CR, et al. BMS-247550: a novel epothilone analog with a mode of action similar to paclitaxel but possessing superior antitumor efficacy. Clin Cancer Res 2001;7(5):1429–37.
59. Calvert P, O'Neill V, Twelves C, et al. A phase I clinical and pharmacokinetic study of EPO906 (Epothilone B), given every three weeks, in patients with advanced solid tumors. Proc Am Soc Clin Oncol 2001;20:[abstract: 429].
60. Rubin EH, Rothermel J, Tesfaye F, et al. Phase I dose-finding study of weekly single-agent patupilone in patients with advanced solid tumors. J Clin Oncol 2005;23(36):9120–9.
61. Østerlind K, Sánchez J, Zatloukal J, et al. Phase I/II dose escalation trial of patupilone every 3 weeks in patients with non-small cell lung cancer. J Clin Oncol 2005;23(Suppl 16):7110.
62. Hsin K, Boyer M, Ducreux M, et al. Efficacy of patupilone in advanced local or metastatic gastric cancer: a phase IIa trial. J Clin Oncol 2006;24(Suppl 18): 4069.
63. Sánchez J, Mellemgaard A, Perry M, et al. Efficacy and safety of patupilone in non-small cell lung cancer (NSCLC): a phase I/II trial. J Clin Oncol 2006; 24(Suppl 18):7104.
64. Poplin E, Moore M, O'Dwyer P, et al. Safety and efficacy of EPO906 in patients with advanced colorectal cancer: a review of 2 phase II trials. Proc Am Soc Clin Oncol 2003;22:[abstract: 1135].
65. Chi KN, Beardsley E, Eigl BJ, et al. A phase 2 study of patupilone in patients with metastatic castration-resistant prostate cancer previously treated with docetaxel: Canadian Urologic Oncology Group study P07a. Ann Oncol 2012;23(1):53–8.
66. Ten Bokkel Huinink WW, Sufliarsky J, Smit WM, et al. Safety and efficacy of patupilone in patients with advanced ovarian, primary fallopian, or primary peritoneal cancer: a phase I, open-label, dose-escalation study. J Clin Oncol 2009; 27(19):3097–103.
67. Forster M, Kaye S, Oza A, et al. A phase Ib and pharmacokinetic trial of patupilone combined with carboplatin in patients with advanced cancer. Clin Cancer Res 2007;13(14):4178–84.
68. Colombo N, Schwartz P, Barnias A, et al. Results of a randomized, open-label, phase III trial of patupilone versus pegylated liposomal doxorubicin in taxane/ platinum refractory/resistant patients with recurrent ovarian, fallopian tube, or peritoneal cancer. Ann Oncol 2010;21(Suppl 8):LBA24.
69. Fogh S, Machtay M, Werner-Wasik M, et al. Phase I trial using patupilone (epothilone B) and concurrent radiotherapy for central nervous system malignancies. Int J Radiat Oncol Biol Phys 2010;77(4):1009–16.
70. Aghajanian C, Burris HA 3rd, Jones S, et al. Phase I study of the novel epothilone analog ixabepilone (BMS-247550) in patients with advanced solid tumors and lymphomas. J Clin Oncol 2007;25(9):1082–8.
71. Mani S, McDaid H, Hamilton A, et al. Phase I clinical and pharmacokinetic study of BMS-247550, a novel derivative of epothilone B, in solid tumors. Clin Cancer Res 2004;10(4):1289–98.
72. Thomas ES, Gomez HL, Li RK, et al. Ixabepilone plus capecitabine for metastatic breast cancer progressing after anthracycline and taxane treatment. J Clin Oncol 2007;25(33):5210–7.
73. Jassem J, Fein L, Karwal M, et al. Ixabepilone plus capecitabine in advanced breast cancer patients with early relapse after adjuvant anthracyclines and taxanes: a pooled subset analysis of two phase III studies. Breast (Edinburgh, Scotland) 2012;21(1):89–94.

74. Perez EA, Patel T, Moreno-Aspitia A. Efficacy of ixabepilone in ER/PR/HER2-negative (triple-negative) breast cancer. Breast Cancer Res Treat 2010;121(2):261–71.

75. Dorff TB, Gross ME. The epothilones: new therapeutic agents for castration-resistant prostate cancer. Oncologist 2011;16(10):1349–58.

76. Rosenberg JE, Ryan CJ, Weinberg VK, et al. Phase I study of ixabepilone, mitoxantrone, and prednisone in patients with metastatic castration-resistant prostate cancer previously treated with docetaxel-based therapy: a study of the department of defense prostate cancer clinical trials consortium. J Clin Oncol 2009;27(17):2772–8.

77. De Geest K, Blessing JA, Morris RT, et al. Phase II clinical trial of ixabepilone in patients with recurrent or persistent platinum- and taxane-resistant ovarian or primary peritoneal cancer: a gynecologic oncology group study. J Clin Oncol 2010;28(1):149–53.

78. Dizon DS, Blessing JA, McMeekin DS, et al. Phase II trial of ixabepilone as second-line treatment in advanced endometrial cancer: gynecologic oncology group trial 129-P. J Clin Oncol 2009;27(19):3104–8.

79. Morrow PK, Divers S, Provencher L, et al. Phase II study evaluating the efficacy and safety of sagopilone (ZK-EPO) in patients with metastatic breast cancer that has progressed following chemotherapy. Breast Cancer Res Treat 2010;123(3):837–42.

80. Freedman RA, Bullitt E, Sun L, et al. A phase II study of sagopilone (ZK 219477; ZK-EPO) in patients with breast cancer and brain metastases. Clin Breast Cancer 2011;11(6):376–83.

81. Spriggs DR, Dupont J, Pezzulli S, et al. KOS-862 (Epothilone D): phase 1 dose escalating and pharmacokinetic (PK) study in patients with advanced malignancies [abstract: 894]. J Clin Oncol 2003;22.

82. Piro L, Rosen S, Parson M, et al. KOS-862 (epothilone D): a comparison of two schedules in patients with advanced malignancies [abstract: 539]. Proc Am Soc Clin Oncol 2003;22.

83. Konner J, Grisham RN, Park J, et al. Phase I clinical, pharmacokinetic, and pharmacodynamic study of KOS-862 (Epothilone D) in patients with advanced solid tumors and lymphoma. Invest New Drugs 2011. Available at: http://www.ncbi.nlm.nih.gov/pubmed/22072399. Accessed November 21, 2011.

84. Buzdar A, Silverman P, Kaufman P. A phase II study of KOS-862 (epothilone D) in anthracycline and taxane pretreated metastatic breast cancer: updated results [abstract: 1087]. Breast Cancer Res Treat 2005;94(Suppl 1):S69.

85. Lam ET, Goel S, Schaaf LJ, et al. Phase I dose escalation study of KOS-1584, a novel epothilone, in patients with advanced solid tumors. Cancer Chemother Pharmacol 2012;69(2):523–31.

86. Risinger AL, Giles FJ, Mooberry SL. Microtubule dynamics as a target in oncology. Cancer Treat Rev 2009;35(3):255–61.

87. Burstein HJ, Harris LN, Marcom PK, et al. Trastuzumab and vinorelbine as first-line therapy for HER2-overexpressing metastatic breast cancer: multicenter phase II trial with clinical outcomes, analysis of serum tumor markers as predictive factors, and cardiac surveillance algorithm. J Clin Oncol 2003;21(15):2889–95.

88. Aapro M, Finek J. Oral vinorelbine in metastatic breast cancer: a review of current clinical trial results. Cancer Treat Rev 2012;38(2):120–6.

89. Li Y, Zou D, Zhao Y, et al. Clinical characteristics and treatment outcome of adult acute lymphoblastic leukemia with t(4;11)(q21;q23) using a modified hyper-CVAD regimen. Acta Haematol 2009;122(1):23–6.

90. Yun-San Yip A, Yuen-Yuen Ong E, Chow LW. Vinflunine: clinical perspectives of an emerging anticancer agent. Expert Opin Investig Drugs 2008;17(4):583–91.

91. Kruczynski A, Hill BT. Vinflunine, the latest Vinca alkaloid in clinical development. A review of its preclinical anticancer properties. Crit Rev Oncol Hematol 2001;40(2):159–73.

92. Bennouna J, Campone M, Delord JP, et al. Vinflunine: a novel antitubulin agent in solid malignancies. Expert Opin Investig Drugs 2005;14(10):1259–67.

93. Bennouna J, Delord JP, Campone M, et al. Vinflunine: a new microtubule inhibitor agent. Clin Cancer Res 2008;14(6):1625–32.

94. Culine S, Theodore C, De Santis M, et al. A phase II study of vinflunine in bladder cancer patients progressing after first-line platinum-containing regimen. Br J Cancer 2006;94(10):1395–401.

95. Talbot DC, Margery J, Dabouis G, et al. Phase II study of vinflunine in malignant pleural mesothelioma. J Clin Oncol 2007;25(30):4751–6.

96. Krzakowski M, Douillard J, Ramlau R, et al. Phase III study of vinflunine versus docetaxel in patients (pts) with advanced non-small cell lung cancer (NSCLC) previously treated with a platinum-containing regimen. J Clin Oncol 2007; 25(Suppl 18):7511.

97. Campone M, Cortes-Funes H, Vorobiof D, et al. Vinflunine: a new active drug for second-line treatment of advanced breast cancer. Results of a phase II and pharmacokinetic study in patients progressing after first-line anthracycline/taxane-based chemotherapy. Br J Cancer 2006;95(9):1161–6.

98. Peacock N, Spigel D, Mainwaring M, et al. Preliminary results of a multicenter phase II trial of vinflunine (with trastuzumab in HER2+ pts) as first-line treatment in metastatic breast cancer. J Clin Oncol 2007;25(Suppl 18):1043.

99. Jordan MA, Kamath K, Manna T, et al. The primary antimitotic mechanism of action of the synthetic halichondrin E7389 is suppression of microtubule growth. Mol Cancer Ther 2005;4(7):1086–95.

100. Cortes J, O'Shaughnessy J, Loesch D, et al. Eribulin monotherapy versus treatment of physician's choice in patients with metastatic breast cancer (EMBRACE): a phase 3 open-label randomised study. Lancet 2011;377(9769): 914–23.

101. Hensley ML, Kravetz S, Jia X, et al. Eribulin mesylate (halichondrin B analog E7389) in platinum-resistant and platinum-sensitive ovarian cancer: a 2-cohort, phase 2 study. Cancer 2011. Available at: http://www.ncbi.nlm.nih.gov/pubmed/21935916. Accessed November 21, 2011.

102. Bhattacharyya B, Panda D, Gupta S, et al. Anti-mitotic activity of colchicine and the structural basis for its interaction with tubulin. Med Res Rev 2008;28(1): 155–83.

103. Pettit GR, Singh SB, Hamel E, et al. Isolation and structure of the strong cell growth and tubulin inhibitor combretastatin A-4. Experientia 1989;45(2):209–11.

104. Pettit GR, Singh SB, Niven ML, et al. Isolation, structure, and synthesis of combretastatins A-1 and B-1, potent new inhibitors of microtubule assembly, derived from *Combretum caffrum*. J Nat Prod 1987;50(1):119–31.

105. Ding X, Zhang Z, Li S, et al. Combretastatin A4 phosphate induces programmed cell death in vascular endothelial cells. Oncol Res 2011;19(7):303–9.

106. Matei D, Schilder J, Sutton G, et al. Activity of 2 methoxyestradiol (Panzem NCD) in advanced, platinum-resistant ovarian cancer and primary peritoneal carcinomatosis: a Hoosier Oncology Group trial. Gynecol Oncol 2009;115(1):90–6.

107. Kulke MH, Chan JA, Meyerhardt JA, et al. A prospective phase II study of 2-methoxyestradiol administered in combination with bevacizumab in patients

with metastatic carcinoid tumors. Cancer Chemother Pharmacol 2011;68(2): 293–300.

108. Harrison MR, Hahn NM, Pili R, et al. A phase II study of 2-methoxyestradiol (2ME2) NanoCrystal® dispersion (NCD) in patients with taxane-refractory, metastatic castrate-resistant prostate cancer (CRPC). Invest New Drugs 2011;29(6): 1465–74.

109. Bhattacharyya B, Wolff J. Maytansine binding to the vinblastine sites of tubulin. FEBS Lett 1977;75(1):159–62.

110. Mandelbaum-Shavit F, Wolpert-DeFilippes MK, Johns DG. Binding of maytansine to rat brain tubulin. Biochem Biophys Res Commun 1976;72(1):47–54.

111. Sieber SM, Mead JA, Adamson RH. Pharmacology of antitumor agents from higher plants. Cancer Treat Rep 1976;60(8):1127–39.

112. Remillard S, Rebhun LI, Howie GA, et al. Antimitotic activity of the potent tumor inhibitor maytansine. Science 1975;189(4207):1002–5.

113. Oroudjev E, Lopus M, Wilson L, et al. Maytansinoid-antibody conjugates induce mitotic arrest by suppressing microtubule dynamic instability. Mol Cancer Ther 2010;9(10):2700–13.

114. Issell BF, Crooke ST. Maytansine. Cancer Treat Rev 1978;5(4):199–207.

115. Krop IE, Beeram M, Modi S, et al. Phase I study of trastuzumab-DM1, an HER2 antibody-drug conjugate, given every 3 weeks to patients with HER2-positive metastatic breast cancer. J Clin Oncol 2010;28(16):2698–704.

116. Burris HA 3rd, Rugo HS, Vukelja SJ, et al. Phase II study of the antibody drug conjugate trastuzumab-DM1 for the treatment of human epidermal growth factor receptor 2 (HER2)-positive breast cancer after prior HER2-directed therapy. J Clin Oncol 2011;29(4):398–405.

117. Manfredi MG, Ecsedy JA, Chakravarty A, et al. Characterization of Alisertib (MLN8237), an investigational small molecule inhibitor of aurora A kinase using novel in vivo pharmacodynamic assays. Clin Cancer Res 2011;17(24): 7614–24.

118. Barr AR, Gergely F. Aurora-A: the maker and breaker of spindle poles. J Cell Sci 2007;120(Pt 17):2987–96.

119. Kitzen JJ, de Jonge MJ, Verweij J. Aurora kinase inhibitors. Crit Rev Oncol Hematol 2010;73(2):99–110.

120. Otto T, Horn S, Brockmann M, et al. Stabilization of N-Myc is a critical function of Aurora A in human neuroblastoma. Cancer Cell 2009;15(1):67–78.

121. Wu L, Ma CA, Zhao Y, et al. Aurora B interacts with NIR-p53, leading to p53 phosphorylation in its DNA-binding domain and subsequent functional suppression. J Biol Chem 2011;286(3):2236–44.

122. Wysong DR, Chakravarty A, Hoar K, et al. The inhibition of Aurora A abrogates the mitotic delay induced by microtubule perturbing agents. Cell Cycle 2009; 8(6):876–88.

123. Dees EC, Infante JR, Cohen RB, et al. Phase 1 study of MLN8054, a selective inhibitor of Aurora A kinase in patients with advanced solid tumors. Cancer Chemother Pharmacol 2011;67(4):945–54.

124. Macarulla T, Cervantes A, Elez E, et al. Phase I study of the selective Aurora A kinase inhibitor MLN8054 in patients with advanced solid tumors: safety, pharmacokinetics, and pharmacodynamics. Mol Cancer Ther 2010;9(10): 2844–52.

125. Katayama H, Sasai K, Kawai H, et al. Phosphorylation by aurora kinase A induces Mdm2-mediated destabilization and inhibition of p53. Nat Genet 2004;36(1):55–62.

126. Infante JR, Dees EC, Cohen RB. Phase I study of the safety, pharmacokinetics (PK), and pharmacodynamics (PD) of MLN8237, a selective Aurora A kinase inhibitor, in the United States [abstract: 280]. Eur J Cancer Suppl 2008; 6(12).

127. Boss DS, Witteveen PO, van der Sar J, et al. Clinical evaluation of AZD1152, an i.v. inhibitor of Aurora B kinase, in patients with solid malignant tumors. Ann Oncol 2011;22(2):431–7.

128. Löwenberg B, Muus P, Ossenkoppele G, et al. Phase I/II study to assess the safety, efficacy, and pharmacokinetics of barasertib (AZD1152) in patients with advanced acute myeloid leukemia. Blood 2011. Available at: http://www.ncbi.nlm.nih.gov/pubmed/21976672. Accessed October 29, 2011.

129. Tsuboi K, Yokozawa T, Sakura T, et al. A Phase I study to assess the safety, pharmacokinetics and efficacy of barasertib (AZD1152), an Aurora B kinase inhibitor, in Japanese patients with advanced acute myeloid leukemia. Leuk Res 2011; 35(10):1384–9.

130. Cohen RB, Jones SF, Aggarwal C, et al. A phase I dose-escalation study of danusertib (PHA-739358) administered as a 24-hour infusion with and without granulocyte colony-stimulating factor in a 14-day cycle in patients with advanced solid tumors. Clin Cancer Res 2009;15(21):6694–701.

131. Steeghs N, Eskens FA, Gelderblom H, et al. Phase I pharmacokinetic and pharmacodynamic study of the aurora kinase inhibitor danusertib in patients with advanced or metastatic solid tumors. J Clin Oncol 2009;27(30):5094–101.

132. Gontarewicz A, Brümmendorf TH. Danusertib (formerly PHA-739358)–a novel combined pan-Aurora kinases and third generation Bcr-Abl tyrosine kinase inhibitor. Recent Results Cancer Res 2010;184:199–214.

133. Schöffski P. Polo-like kinase (PLK) inhibitors in preclinical and early clinical development in oncology. Oncologist 2009;14(6):559–70.

134. Olmos D, Barker D, Sharma R, et al. Phase I study of GSK461364, a specific and competitive Polo-like kinase 1 inhibitor, in patients with advanced solid malignancies. Clin Cancer Res 2011;17(10):3420–30.

135. Mross K, Frost A, Steinbild S, et al. Phase I dose escalation and pharmacokinetic study of BI 2536, a novel Polo-like kinase 1 inhibitor, in patients with advanced solid tumors. J Clin Oncol 2008;26(34):5511–7.

136. Hofheinz RD, Al-Batran SE, Hochhaus A, et al. An open-label, phase I study of the Polo-like kinase-1 inhibitor, BI 2536, in patients with advanced solid tumors. Clin Cancer Res 2010;16(18):4666–74.

137. Sebastian M, Reck M, Waller CF, et al. The efficacy and safety of BI 2536, a novel Plk-1 inhibitor, in patients with stage IIIB/IV non-small cell lung cancer who had relapsed after, or failed, chemotherapy: results from an open-label, randomized phase II clinical trial. J Thorac Oncol 2010;5(7):1060–7.

138. Jimeno A, Li J, Messersmith WA, et al. Phase I study of ON 01910.Na, a novel modulator of the Polo-like kinase 1 pathway, in adult patients with solid tumors. J Clin Oncol 2008;26(34):5504–10.

139. Seetharam M, Fan AC, Tran M, et al. Treatment of higher risk myelodysplastic syndrome patients unresponsive to hypomethylating agents with ON 01910.Na. Leuk Res 2012;36(1):98–103.

140. Bergnes G, Brejc K, Belmont L. Mitotic kinesins: prospects for antimitotic drug discovery. Curr Top Med Chem 2005;5(2):127–45.

141. Cox CD, Coleman PJ, Breslin MJ, et al. Kinesin spindle protein (KSP) inhibitors. 9. Discovery of (2S)-4-(2,5-difluorophenyl)-n-[(3R,4S)-3-fluoro-1-methylpiperidin-4-yl]-2-(hydroxymethyl)-N-methyl-2-phenyl-2,5-dihydro-1H-pyrrole-1-carboxamide

(MK-0731) for the treatment of taxane-refractory cancer. J Med Chem 2008; 51(14):4239–52.

142. Lee CW, Bélanger K, Rao SC, et al. A phase II study of ispinesib (SB-715992) in patients with metastatic or recurrent malignant melanoma: a National Cancer Institute of Canada Clinical Trials Group trial. Invest New Drugs 2008;26(3): 249–55.

143. Stein MN, Tan A, Taber K, et al. Phase I clinical and pharmacokinetic (PK) trial of the kinesin spindle protein (KSP) inhibitor MK-0731 in patients with solid tumors. 2007 ASCO Annual Meeting Proceedings Part I. J Clin Oncol 2007; 25(Suppl 18):2548 (June 20 Supplement).

The Antifolates

Michele Visentin, PhD[a,b], Rongbao Zhao, PhD[a,b],
I. David Goldman, MD[a,b],*

KEYWORDS

- Methotrexate • Pralatrexate • Pemetrexed
- Antifolates • Reduced folate carrier (RFC)
- Proton-coupled folate transporter (PCFT)
- Folate receptors • Folate receptor-mediated endocytosis

KEY POINTS

- Antifolates disrupt cellular proliferation by blocking folate-dependent one-carbon biosynthetic and methylation reactions.
- Antifolates form active polyglutamate derivatives that are retained in tumor cells and result in sustained inhibition of their target enzymes.
- Antifolates currently approved for cancer treatment include methotrexate and pralatrexate, inhibitors of dihydrofolate reductase, and pemetrexed, which, in its polyglutamate forms, targets thymidylate synthase and 5-aminoimidazole-4-carboxamide ribonucleotide (AICAR) transformylase.
- Novel folate analogues and conjugates, currently in clinical trial, use membrane folate receptors for transport into tumor cells by an endocytic mechanism.

The antifolates were the first class of antimetabolites to enter the clinics 65 years ago. These agents disrupt the metabolic pathways that require one-carbon moieties supplied by the B9 folate vitamins that they resemble. Although renewing tissues of the bone marrow and intestinal tract are also folate-dependent and are sites of antifolate toxicity, the clinical utility of antifolates was established with the identification of doses and schedules of administration that provided sufficient selectivity to make these drugs effective in the treatment of cancer and inflammatory disorders. Many of the early key preclinical studies that defined the pharmacologic properties of this class of drugs, and treatment strategies, were conducted in vitro and in vivo in mice using murine leukemia cell lines.[1,2]

[a] Department of Medicine and the Albert Einstein Cancer Center, The Albert Einstein College of Medicine, 1300 Morris Park Avenue, Bronx, NY 10461, USA
[b] Department of Molecular Pharmacology and the Albert Einstein Cancer Center, The Albert Einstein College of Medicine, 1300 Morris Park Avenue, Bronx, NY 10461, USA
* Corresponding author. Departments of Medicines, Molecular Pharmacology and the Albert Einstein Cancer Center, The Albert Einstein College of Medicine, 1300 Morris Park Avenue, Bronx, NY 10461.
E-mail address: l.david.goldman@einstein.yu.edu

Hematol Oncol Clin N Am 26 (2012) 629–648
doi:10.1016/j.hoc.2012.02.002
0889-8588/12/$ – see front matter © 2012 Elsevier Inc. All rights reserved.

The first antifolate in the clinic was aminopterin. Its introduction, as first reported in the *New England Journal of Medicine* in June 1948,[3] was greeted with great enthusiasm when this agent was shown to produce, for the first time, remissions in children with acute lymphoblastic leukemia. Although these remissions were short lived, the activity of this agent established that this disease was treatable and provided optimism that this and other malignant diseases would be conquerable with cancer chemotherapeutics in the future. For reasons not fully understood, but attributed to the unpredictable toxicity of aminopterin, this drug was replaced with methotrexate (MTX) in the early 1950s, an antifolate less potent than aminopterin but with what was considered to be a more favorable therapeutic index.[2]

Despite its early clinical success, an understanding of the mechanism of action of MTX evolved slowly over the ensuing decades. Likewise, the efficacy and selectivity of leucovorin rescue that allowed the safe administration of high doses of MTX was established entirely empirically and, even today, the basis for the selectivity of this regimen is not widely appreciated nor fully understood. The lack of a basic understanding of the biochemical and molecular pharmacology of MTX hampered efforts to develop subsequent generations of antifolates that would lead to the realization of the full clinical potential of this class of drugs. Hence, it was more than 50 years after the introduction of MTX that the second antifolate, pemetrexed, was approved in 2004 for the treatment of mesothelioma and subsequently non–small cell lung cancer. This was followed by the approval of pralatrexate in 2009 for the treatment of cutaneous T-cell lymphoma.

This article focuses on the cellular, biochemical, and molecular pharmacology of antifolates and how a basic understanding of the mechanism of action of MTX, its cytotoxic determinants, mechanisms of resistance, and transport into and out of cells has led to the development of a new generation of antifolates, a process that continues both in the laboratory and in the clinics. Finally, new approaches to folate-based cancer chemotherapy are described based on the targeted delivery of drugs to malignant cells. These approaches include (1) the development of folate analogues transported by routes selectively expressed or active in tumor cells and (2) the selective endocytosis of folic acid, linked to cytotoxics, into tumor cells that express folate receptors. The evolution of antifolates, folate receptor targeted drugs, and membrane transport of folates and antifolates have been the subject of recent reviews.[4–11]

ANTIFOLATES ACHIEVE THEIR PHARMACOLOGIC EFFECTS BY THEIR PERTURBATIONS OF FOLATE METABOLISM

The structures of the B9 vitamins in their oxidized and reduced forms are illustrated in **Fig. 1**. Folic acid is not a physiologic folate but is an important source of folates ingested because it is added as a supplement to foods and it is the predominant form of folate in vitamin supplements. The major dietary folate in nature, 5-methyltetrahydrofolate (5-methylTHF), is absorbed in the proximal small intestine by a highly specific transport mechanism, the proton-coupled folate transporter (PCFT, see later discussion), following which it is delivered to the liver via the hepatic portal vein.[6,12] There, large amounts of 5-methylTHF accumulate as polyglutamate derivatives (see later discussion). Following conversion back to the monoglutamate form, this folate exits hepatic cells to circulate in the blood for delivery via the reduced folate carrier (RFC, see later discussion) to peripheral tissues. There it provides its methyl group to homocysteine for the synthesis of methionine with the generation of a tetrahydrofolate moiety in a vitamin B12 requiring reaction mediated by the enzyme methionine synthase (**Fig. 2**). The tetrahydrofolate generated then proceeds, through a variety of reactions, to acquire another carbon at various oxidation states at the N^5, N^{10}, or

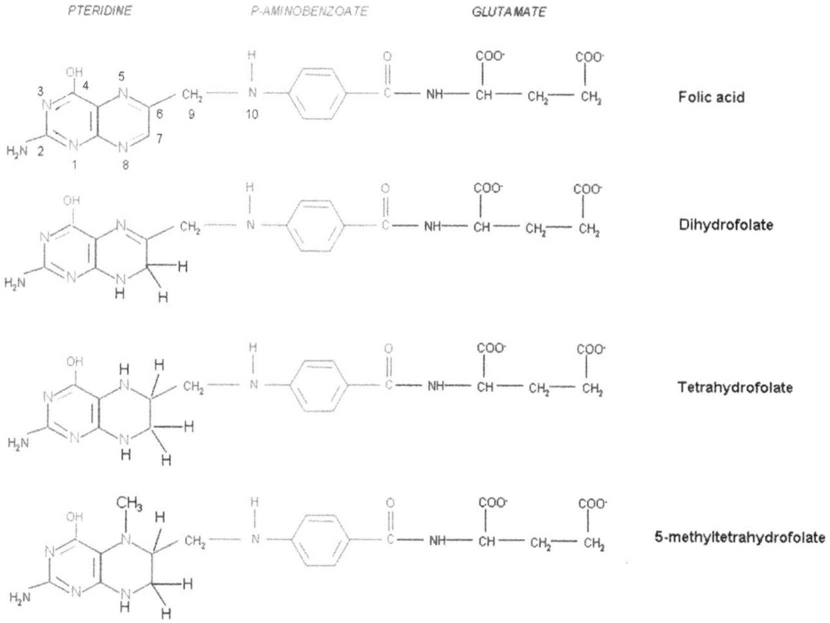

Fig. 1. The structures of folic acid, dihydrofolate, tetrahydrofolate, and 5-methyltetrahydrofolate. Folic acid is not a physiologic folate but is an important source of folate in foods and vitamins. Within cells, folic acid is reduced to dihydrofolate by dihydrofolate reductase (DHFR, see **Fig. 2**), albeit at a slow rate because it is a poor substrate for this enzyme. Dihydrofolate is the major oxidized form of folates within cells, and the preferred substrate for DHFR, mediating the formation of tetrahydrofolate that goes on to form a variety of tetrahydrofolate cofactors. Seen here is the major dietary folate and the major folate in the blood, 5-methyltetrahydrofolate.

shared between both positions, to form a family of tetrahydrofolate cofactors. These one-carbon derivatives sustain key biosynthetic reactions within cells, such as the addition of a single carbon in the synthesis of thymidylate and 2 carbons in the synthesis of purines, which are both required for the synthesis of DNA and RNA. Methionine goes on to form S-adenosyl methionine, which then mediates a variety of methylation reactions, including the methylation of cytosines within DNA, which is a key factor in the regulation of transcription and activities of oncogenes and tumor suppressor genes.[13] In the absence of vitamin B12, the use of 5-methylTHF cannot occur; 5-methylTHF is trapped so that neither its one-carbon nor tetrahydrofolate moieties are available for biosynthetic reactions.[14] Proliferating tissues, with a high requirement for folates, are the most susceptible to folate deficiency and to drugs that block these folate-dependent pathways.

In the synthesis of methionine and purines, the tetrahydrofolate molecule remains intact and another carbon moiety can be acquired to be used again in one-carbon reactions (see **Fig. 2**). However, in the synthesis of thymidylate from deoxyuridylate that requires 5,10-methylene tetrahydrofolate (5,10-methyleneTHF), tetrahydrofolate is oxidized to dihydrofolate. In proliferating cells, this reaction is so rapid that tetrahydrofolate cofactors would rapidly interconvert to 5,10-methyleneTHF, followed by oxidization to dihydrofolate, in minutes if it were not for the enzyme, dihydrofolate reductase (DHFR), which rapidly reduces dihydrofolate back to tetrahydrofolate to sustain the pool of tetrahydrofolate cofactors.

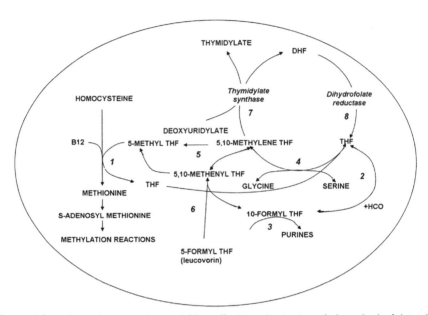

Fig. 2. Folate-dependent reactions within cells. Reaction1: 5-methyltetrahydrofolate (5-methylTHF) enters the folate cycle with the provision of its methyl group to homocysteine in the synthesis of methionine, a vitamin B12–dependent reaction mediated by methionine synthase. The tetrahydrofolate (THF) moiety can then acquire a carbon at various oxidation states. Reaction 2: Formate is added at the N^{10} position to form 10-formylTHF, which provides 2 carbons in reaction 3 for the synthesis of purines. Reaction 4: 5,10-methyleneTHF is formed from serine and THF in a reaction mediated by serine hydroxyl methyltransferase. Reaction 5: 5,10-methyleneTHF is reduced irreversibly to 5-methylTHF. Reaction 6: 5-formy-tetrahydrofolate dehydrase is the mechanism by which 5-formylTHF (leucovorin), enters these cyclical folate pathways. Reaction 7: The formation of thymidylate mediated by thymidylate synthase; the THF moiety is oxidized to dihydrofolate (DHF). Reaction 8: DHF is reduced to THF by dihydrofolate reductase. The latter is essential for maintaining THF cofactor pools within mammalian cells.

Fig. 3 illustrates the structures of aminopterin and MTX. The former differs from folic acid only in the substitution of an amino for a hydroxyl group at the N^4 position of the pteridine ring. MTX differs from aminopterin in having the addition of a methyl group at the N^{10} position in a bridge between the pteridine and p-amino-benzoic acid moieties. These structural differences from folic acid confer on these analogues an extremely high affinity for DHFR. The primary action of aminopterin and MTX, the classical anti-folates, is the inhibition of this enzyme. The 4-amino antifolates are among the most potent enzyme inhibitors known. When the interaction between the drug and its target enzyme is evaluated in cell-free systems, the inhibition constant is approximately 5 pM. This value is comparable to what can be achieved with inhibitors designed to bind within the transition state of the catalytic sites of enzymes.[15] However, micromolar levels of MTX are required to inhibit this enzyme within cells. There are 2 reasons for this discrepancy: (1) DHFR is present in cells in great excess so that inhibition of more than 95% of the enzyme is required to begin to suppress tetrahydrofolate synthesis and (2) as illustrated in **Fig. 4**, the substrate for this reaction, dihydrofolate, builds to high levels behind the block as tetrahydrofolate cofactors interconvert and cycle to 5,10-methyleneTHF, which is oxidized via thymidylate synthase. Dihydrofolate levels become so high that they compete with MTX for the small percentage of

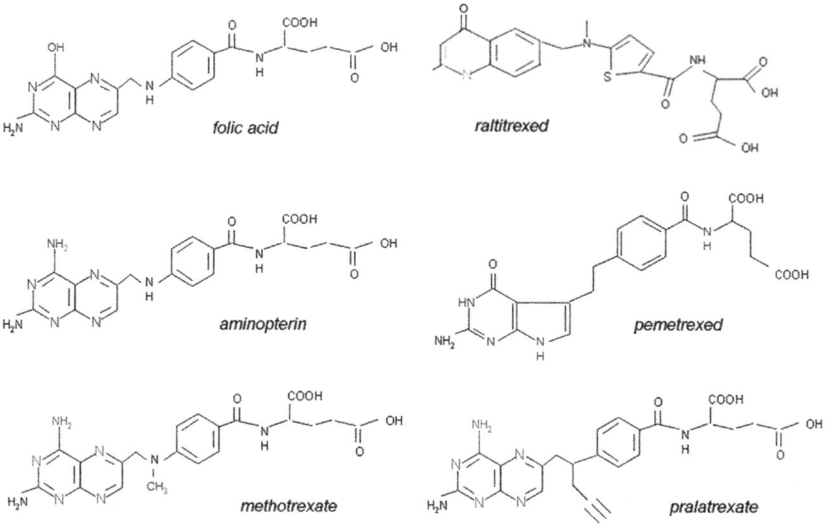

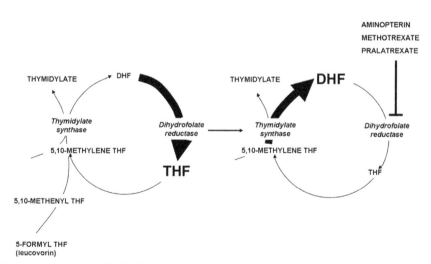

Fig. 3. The structures of folic acid and a group of antifolates. Except for aminopterin, all the antifolates are in clinical use in the United States and/or elsewhere.

Fig. 4. The impact of dihydrofolate reductase (DHFR) inhibitors on folate pools within cells. The left panel illustrates that under physiologic conditions dihydrofolate (DHF) produced during the synthesis of thymidylate mediated by thymidylate synthase is reduced to tetrahydrofolate (THF) so rapidly, because of the high levels of DHFR within cells, that the DHF level is trivial compared with the level of THF. The right panel illustrates the impact of suppression of DHFR by several 4-amino antifolates. High levels of DHF build up in cells by continued thymidylate synthase activity, interconversion of THF cofactors to 5,10-methyleneTHF, and oxidation to DHF. This leads to depletion of THF cofactor levels within cells and cessation of THF cofactor-dependent reactions. High DHF levels compete with MTX for the small percentage of enzyme sufficient to maintain THF cofactor pools within cells.

enzyme that is sufficient to support tetrahydrofolate synthesis. To overcome this inhibition and achieve saturation of the enzyme requires relatively high, micromolar, intracellular levels of MTX. Indeed, if after sufficient levels of MTX are present within the cell to completely block this reaction, cells are placed in an MTX-free environment, the drug rapidly leaves the cell, a small component of MTX bound to DHFR is displaced by the high levels of dihydrofolate, tetrahydrofolate synthesis resumes, tetrahydrofolate cofactors rapidly increase to normal levels, and dihydrofolate decreases to its usual very low levels leaving greater than 95% of the enzyme still associated with MTX. This sequence of events occurs within cancer cells as MTX blood levels increase and decrease after the administration of the drug. Hence, a potent inhibitor of DHFR in a cell-free system is a competitive and rapidly reversible inhibitor when interacting with its target enzyme within the dynamic environment of the cell where pools of substrate and products can undergo large changes when enzyme activities are perturbed.[16]

Based on this understanding of the critical elements of MTX interactions within cells, it becomes clear that a major determinant of the activity of this agent is the intracellular level achieved. There are 2 determinants of the cell antifolate level: (1) membrane transport and (2) metabolic conversion to derivatives that remain potent inhibitors of DHFR but are retained within the cell.

PHARMACOLOGIC CONSEQUENCES OF THE FORMATION OF METHOTREXATE POLYGLUTAMATE DERIVATIVES WITHIN CELLS

Physiologic folates form polyglutamate derivatives that are retained and build to high levels within cells; these are usually preferred substrates for tetrahydrofolate cofactor-requiring enzymes.[17,18] In a series of reactions, mediated by folylpolyglutamate synthetase (FPGS), glutamate molecules are added successively at the γ-carboxyl moiety to form a peptide chain of up to 6 to 8 glutamate residues. Antifolates undergo the same reaction and this has profound pharmacologic ramifications. The polyglutamation of antifolates (as seen for MTX in **Fig. 5**) converts these drugs from a form (monoglutamate) that is a good substrate for a variety of folate export processes, to forms that are not, leading to the retention and buildup of high levels of polyglutamate derivatives in tumor cells. In the case of MTX, these derivatives are at least as potent inhibitors of DHFR as the monoglutamate. The retention of MTX polyglutamate derivatives within cells, after antifolate blood levels decrease,

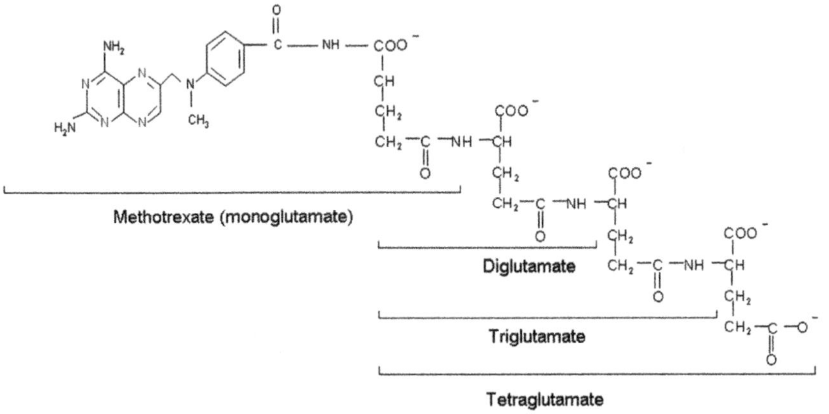

Fig. 5. The structure of the polyglutamate derivatives of MTX. Glutamates are progressively added to the γ-carboxyl of the MTX molecule and each successive polyglutamate derivative.

results in sustained inhibition of this enzyme for long intervals. In the case of pemetrexed, polyglutamation results in derivatives with a much higher affinity for its target enzymes than the monoglutamate and this, along with prolonged retention in tumor cells, allows regimens in which this agent can be administered every 3 weeks (see later discussion).

A key factor in the efficacy of any antineoplastic agent is its selectivity: the extent to which it kills malignant cells while sparing susceptible host tissues. In the case of MTX, the major toxicities are caused by its effects on intestinal and bone marrow cells. The basis for this selectivity seems to be due, at least in part, to the lesser accumulation of its polyglutamate derivatives in these normal replicating tissues in comparison with susceptible tumor cells.[19–22] Hence, when the drug is administered intravenously in a pulse, MTX is transported into tumor cells where polyglutamate derivatives are synthesized and accumulate. When the concentration of MTX in the blood decreases below a critical level, formation of polyglutamates cease but the polyglutamate derivatives already synthesized are retained and produce prolonged suppression of DHFR. On the other hand, while MTX monoglutamate builds within intestinal and bone marrow cells when the concentration of MTX in the blood is high, as the MTX blood level decreases, MTX monoglutamate exits the cells and, in the absence of polyglutamate derivatives, the small component of DHFR necessary to meet cellular demands for tetrahydrofolate is rapidly activated.[20–22] For a detailed analysis of the perturbations of cellular folate pools in response to 4-amino antifolates and the impact of the formation of polyglutamate derivatives, the reader is referred to an earlier review.[16]

THE MEMBRANE TRANSPORT OF ANTIFOLATES MEDIATED BY FACILITATIVE CARRIERS AND EXPORT PUMPS

The physiologic folates and most antifolates are bivalent anions that diffuse poorly across cell membranes, and only low levels of folates are present in the diet and in the blood. Hence, specific processes are required to achieve their efficient transport across the epithelia and into systemic cells (**Fig. 6**). Transport across the apical-brush border membrane of the duodenum and proximal jejunum is mediated by the PCFT, a process that functions optimally at the low pH found at the microenvironment of the surface of the villi of these tissues. Its critical role in this process was established with the demonstration that there are loss of function mutations in this gene in the autosomal hereditary disorder, hereditary folate malabsorption.[12,23,24] PCFT is expressed in many normal tissues but has limited function because of the ambient neutral pH. Besides the proximal small intestine, PCFT is highly expressed in the liver, choroid plexus, brush-border membrane of the proximal renal tubule, and in a broad spectrum of solid tumors.[25,26] Transport into systemic tissues is mediated by the RFC, a process that functions optimally at the neutral pH sustained in most tissues. RFC is expressed in all normal cells and is the major route of 5-methylTHF transport into these tissues. RFC is also a major route of transport of MTX and most other antifolates into tumor cells.[7,26]

MTX, raltitrexed, and pemetrexed share comparable affinities for RFC, with influx K_ms of approximately 5 to 7 μM at the optimal pH of this transporter, 7.4. The affinity of RFC for the natural isomer of 5-methylTHF is greater. The affinity of RFC for pralatrexate is 3 to 4 times greater than for MTX. The affinities and maximum transport velocities mediated by PCFT are highest at a pH of approximately 5.5 and decrease as the pH is increased. At its optimal low pH, the affinity of PCFT is greatest for pemetrexed ($K_m \sim 0.2$–0.5 μM) but still quite good for MTX ($K_m \sim 1.5$ μM). As the pH is increased, transport is much better preserved for pemetrexed than MTX or raltitrexed.[27,28]

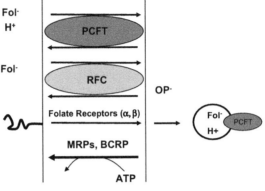

EXTRACELLULAR   **INTRACELLULAR**

Fig. 6. Folate-specific transporters in mammalian cells. There are 2 carrier mechanisms: RFC, an organic phosphate (OP⁻) antiporter, and PCFT, a proton-folate symporter. Both carriers transport folates and antifolates into cells against an electrochemical-potential gradient. Multidrug resistance–associated proteins (MRPs) and the breast cancer–resistance protein (BCRP) use the energy released in the hydrolysis of ATP to pump folate and antifolate mono-glutamates out of cells. BCRP and some MRPs can also export lower polyglutamates. Folate receptors transport folates into cells by an endocytic mechanism. Folate export from acidified endosomes is partly mediated by PCFT.

Both RFC and PCFT are facilitative carriers that mediate folate and antifolate entry (influx) and exit (efflux) from cells. The extent to which these processes are unequal will determine the final concentration gradient achieved across the cell membrane. PCFT contains 2 substrates binding sites: one for a proton the other for a folate/antifolate. This symporter uses the transmembrane proton gradient to achieve concentrative folate transport into cells. RFC contains only one substrate-binding site, which is for a folate/antifolate. However, a variety of structurally unrelated organic anions can compete for this site and can use this carrier, the most potent of which are the organic phosphates. This transporter uses the high concentration of organic phosphates within cells to achieve concentrative folate/antifolate transport into cells. Hence, although both transporters are bidirectional and are capable of transporting folates/antifolates into and out of cells, export mediated by PCFT is suppressed by the neutral pH within the intracellular compartment. Likewise, the high levels of organic phosphates within cells suppress the export mediated by RFC, an antiporter. These asymmetrical effects by protons and organic phosphates, respectively, result in concentrative (uphill) folate/antifolate transport into cells.

Antifolates are also substrates for members of the family of multidrug resistance–associated proteins (MRPs) and the breast cancer–resistance protein (BCRP).[29–31] These ATP-dependent exporters oppose the concentrative effects of RFC or PCFT to suppress the level of monoglutamate antifolates that accumulate within cells and thereby slow the formation of polyglutamate derivatives. When these exporters are inhibited, intracellular MTX levels increase. Once polyglutamate derivatives form, they are no longer substrates for most of these exporters. However, the lower polyglutamate derivatives of MTX are modest substrates for some MRPs and BCRP.[29,30] The level of monoglutamyl antifolates that accumulate within cells is determined by the net effect of the exporters and the carrier mediated concentrative transporters. Cumulatively, these factors influence the rate and extent of accumulation of antifolate polyglutamate derivatives within cells. Although overexpression of MRPs and BCRP can induce resistance to antifolates, it is unclear whether this contributes to resistance to these agents in the clinics.[31]

Membrane transport of MTX mediated by RFC is an important determinant of its cytotoxicity. The higher the affinity of RFC for this drug, the higher the free levels achieved within the intracellular water and the greater the rate and extent of formation of its polyglutamate derivatives. Impaired membrane transport mediated by RFC is an established mechanism of intrinsic and acquired resistance to MTX (see later discussion). In the absence of RFC function, the only way antifolate activity can be sustained is if the drug can enter tumor cells by passive diffusion or by another transport route. However, to achieve the former for a hydrophilic drug or the latter via PCFT, which operates inefficiently at neutral pH, requires high drug levels with a high potential for toxicity to normal tissues. The membrane transport of folates and antifolates has been the subject of recent reviews.[6,7,10,11]

HIGH-DOSE MTX WITH LEUCOVORIN RESCUE

With the recognition that MTX resistance in experimental tumor systems was often associated with impaired RFC-mediated transport across the cell membrane and with the assumption that delivery to cells within solid tumors is limited by a compromised vasculature, an approach was developed to circumvent these limitations that would permit the safe administration of high doses of MTX.[32–35]

The rationale for high-dose MTX is that high blood and extracellular drug levels facilitate diffusion of drug into the core of solid tumors and passive diffusion across the tumor cell membrane, where carrier-mediated transport might be compromised. Protection of normal tissues is achieved by the subsequent administration of low doses of 5-formyltetrahydrofolate (leucovorin) following treatment with MTX. Presumably, leucovorin has access to bone marrow and intestinal cells via an intact vascular supply to these normal tissues, and intact membrane transport, whereas delivery to tumor cells is limited by the low blood levels of the rescue agent, the compromised vascular supply, and impaired transport across the tumor cell membrane. Additionally, as the MTX blood level decreases, leucovorin concentrations in the blood are sufficiently high to competitively inhibit MTX transport into normal cells via RFC (a transport mechanism that MTX and leucovorin share), so that the MRP exporters pump the drug, unopposed, out of these cells. Although high-dose MTX regimens were implemented in the 1960s, these regimens remain part of the treatment arsenal for several malignancies (see later discussion).

A further understanding of the selectivity of high-dose MTX with leucovorin rescue emerged several decades after the introduction of this regimen and relates to the differential formation of MTX polyglutamate derivatives in tumors versus normal bone marrow and intestinal precursors.[19–22] This understanding was based on the revelation that polyglutamate derivatives of MTX are not only potent inhibitors of DHFR but also direct inhibitors of tetrahydrofolate-requiring enzymes: thymidylate synthase[36] and one of the enzymes required for the synthesis of purines, 5-aminoimidazole-4-carboxamide ribotide transformylase (AICAR transformylase).[37–39] These direct inhibitory effects block the use of the one-carbon moiety of leucovorin for thymidylate and purine synthesis in tumors; however, use is unimpeded in normal tissues that lack comparable levels of these derivatives.[40] An additional factor is the interconversion of leucovorin to other tetrahydrofolate cofactors and ultimately to dihydrofolate polyglutamates that displace MTX from, and thereby activate, DHFR in cells that do not contain MTX polyglutamate derivatives.[41]

There are a variety of ways of administering high doses of MTX, including pulses of the drug, or continuous infusions for up to 42 hours, following which low-dose leucovorin is begun. Specific regimens of administration have been developed and parameters have been designated to assure the safety of these protocols based on the expected renal excretion of MTX and the decline in the MTX blood level. Any compromise of renal function and glomerular filtration, which can occur after high-dose MTX, delays the clearance of the drug and requires prolongation of leucovorin rescue until the MTX concentration in the blood decreases to a safe level.[42,43]

CURRENT CLINICAL APPLICATIONS OF METHOTREXATE

MTX remains an important agent for the treatment of acute leukemia, lymphoma, osteosarcoma, and leptomeningeal metastases.[44–46] MTX continues to be used for the treatment of gestational trophoblast tumors[47] and in the cytoxan-MTX-fluorouracil regimen for the treatment of breast cancer.[48,49] This drug is also widely used for the treatment of rheumatoid arthritis, inflammatory bowel disease, psoriasis, and other inflammatory diseases.[50–55] Although introduced in the 1960s,[33,34] high-dose MTX regimens continue to have a role in the treatment of leukemia, lymphoma, and osteosarcoma.[46,56–58]

THE EMERGENCE OF A NEW-GENERATION 4-AMINO-ANTIFOLATE: PRALATREXATE

As an understanding of the pharmacologic properties of MTX emerged and its interaction with intact cells that were key determinants of its cytotoxicity were identified, a search was undertaken to create a structural analogue that would enhance its activity and its selectivity. The key parameters identified were membrane transport and polyglutamation. This finding led to the development of pralatrexate.[59,60] This antifolate differs from MTX in the substitution of a carbon for nitrogen at the N^{10} position and the substitution of a propargyl for the methyl group at that site (see **Fig. 3**). This drug has a much higher affinity for RFC and FPGS than MTX. This should lead to higher levels of the monoglutamate within cells, the substrate for FPGS and this, along with the much higher affinity for this enzyme, should result in a marked increase in the level of these active derivatives. The level of pralatrexate polyglutamate derivatives that form within cells or the extent to which they, like MTX, are direct inhibitors of thymidylate synthase and AICAR transformylase is unclear. Likewise, it is not yet established whether high doses of this drug can be administered safely within the context of a leucovorin rescue regimen.

Pralatrexate does seem to have enhanced selectivity because it can be administered at doses comparable to MTX, despite its enhanced properties that should lead to much higher levels in cells at comparable blood levels. The basis for this difference in selectivity is not clear. Pralatrexate appears to be more active in T-cell than B-cell leukemias and lymphomas; however, the basis for this difference has not been established. Pralatrexate is approved for treatment of cutaneous T-cell lymphoma with folate supplementation, which moderates toxicity to this agent.[61–63] Considerable additional information will be required about the cellular and biochemical pharmacologic properties of this drug before its full spectrum of clinical activities and utility can be realized.

THE EMERGENCE OF ANTIFOLATES THAT TARGET TETRAHYDROFOLATE-REQUIRING ENZYMES
Raltitrexed

The recognition that the polyglutamate derivatives of MTX have targets downstream of DHFR as direct inhibitors of thymidylate synthase and AICAR transformylase led to a drug development effort focused on the identification of antifolates, which, in their polyglutamate forms, are direct inhibitors of one or both of these enzymes. The first of these agents to be established in the clinic was raltitrexed (see **Fig. 3**).[64,65] In its poly-glutamate forms, this drug has a high affinity for thymidylate synthase. It is also a much better substrate than MTX for FPGS with comparable affinity for RFC. Raltitrexed has a low affinity for PCFT. This drug is used clinically primarily for the treatment of colo-rectal cancer in Europe and elsewhere; it is not approved for cancer treatment in the United States.[66–68]

Pemetrexed

The second inhibitor of tetrahydrofolate cofactor-requiring enzymes to enter the clinic and achieve approval in the United States was pemetrexed (see **Fig. 3**). In its polyglu-tamate forms, this drug is a potent inhibitor of thymidylate synthase. Initially it was considered to be an inhibitor of glycinamide ribonucleotide formyltransferase (GAR transformylase), which, like AICAR transformylase, is required for purine syn-thases.[69,70] However, recent studies indicates that the interruption of purine synthesis within cells is caused by inhibition of AICAR transformylase (see later discussion). Inhi-bition of thymidylate synthase occurs at extracellular levels of pemetrexed about 0.1 the concentration required for inhibition of purine synthesis. This drug is an excellent substrate for FPGS, 300 times more potent than MTX, and has comparable affinity for RFC.[64] What is of particular interest is that pemetrexed has a much higher affinity than MTX for PCFT both at acidic and neutral pH.[5,28,71] The high affinity for PCFT and delivery via this mechanism results in the preservation of pemetrexed activity even when transport mediated by RFC is abolished. Hence, tumor cells resistant to ralti-trexed or MTX because of impaired transport via RFC retain sensitivity to pemetrexed, which is a considerable advantage for this drug.[28,72]

Of recent particular interest are emerging data indicating that pemetrexed effects on purine synthesis in cells are caused by the suppression of AICAR transformylase resulting in the buildup of high cellular levels of ZMP, a purine precursor that activates AMP kinase which, in turn, results in inhibition of mTOR.[73,74] Hence, an antimetabolite that, on the one hand, has potent cytotoxic activity through its inhibition of thymidylate synthase can also inhibit a major signal transduction pathway, which cumulatively results in cell growth inhibition and cell death.

Pemetrexed is currently approved for the first- and second-line treatment of the nonsquamous histology of non–small cell lung cancer and mesothelioma, in combina-tion with cisplatin, and for maintenance therapy for lung cancer as a single agent.[75–78] The basis for the difference in activity between squamous and nonsquamous lung carcinomas is not clear. Ongoing clinical trials are evaluating pemetrexed efficacy in other malignancies. The development of pemetrexed and its cellular and biochemical properties is the subject of a recent review.[5]

THE IMPACT OF PHYSIOLOGIC FOLATES ON THE ANTITUMOR ACTIVITIES AND TOXICITY OF ANTIFOLATES

Drugs that require polyglutamation to achieve activity, in particular raltitrexed and pemetrexed, are generally sensitive to the level of physiologic folates with cells that are substrates for FPGS and compete with these antifolates for this enzyme.[79] Hence, the higher the folate levels in tumor cells, the poorer the activity of these agents.[80,81] On the other hand, folate sufficiency is also an important element in toxicity to patients receiving these drugs; the most sensitive indicator of B12 or folate deficiency is reflected in an elevated blood homocysteine level.[75,82] To avoid this toxicity, folic acid and vitamin B12 are coadministered with pemetrexed and pralatrexate in clinical regimens.[75,82,83] The strategy here is to provide sufficient folate supplementation to protect patients from serious toxicity while not substantially impairing the activity of the drug against the tumor. Accordingly, folic acid supplementation should be used at the lowest recommended dose and frequency of administration.

MECHANISMS OF RESISTANCE TO ANTIFOLATES

Mechanisms of resistance to MTX have been established by studies in tumor systems in vitro under conditions in which selective pressure has been applied by gradual exposure to increasing concentrations, or pulse exposures to high concentrations, of the drug. Chemical mutagenesis has also been used to accelerate and amplify mutational events contributing to resistance. All elements of the interaction of this drug with its cellular targets have been implicated in resistance. Membrane transport is a frequent mechanism of resistance due to the low expression or loss-of-function mutations, of RFC. Similar changes have been detected in human tumors as a basis for intrinsic or acquired resistance to MTX. Resistance has also developed because of loss-of-function mutations of FPGS resulting in impaired formation of MTX polygluta-mate derivatives. Finally, DHFR mutations resulting in a decreased affinity for the drug, or increased expression of the enzyme caused by a regulatory change or amplification of the gene, result in resistance. The pattern of resistance to pralatrexate is not yet known but is likely to be similar to that of MTX. The mechanisms of resistance to 4-amino-antifolates have been the subject of recent reviews.[16,84]

Resistance to pemetrexed acquired in tumor lines in vitro correlates best with increased levels of thymidylate synthase.[85] Based on studies on explanted human tumor specimens in vitro, low levels of thymidylate synthase, GAR transformylase, and MRP4 gene expression were associated with increased sensitivity to pemetrexed.[86] Decreased expression of FPGS leads to impaired formation of the active pemetrexed polyglutamate derivatives.[87] Resistance to pemetrexed in human solid tumors caused by impaired membrane transport has not been documented and is unlikely to occur because this drug can use both RFC and PCFT. Activity is retained with the loss of the former, because of transport mediated by the latter, and the accompanying contraction in tetrahydrofolate cofactor pools within the cells as a result of impaired uptake and accumulation of folates transported primarily by RFC.[28,72,88]

TARGETING DRUGS TO TUMOR CELLS VIA FOLATE TRANSPORTERS

A major emphasis of current drug-development efforts is generally directed to target-ing pathways or regulatory elements that drive the proliferation of malignant cells. Another approach is the development of cytotoxics and other agents that are selec-tively delivered to malignant cells via transporters that are selectively expressed or selectively active in malignant cells. These efforts have focused on 2 transporters: PCFT and folate receptors.

Folate Receptor-Targeted Drugs

There are 2 major folate receptor isotypes expressed on cell membranes with a binding constant for folic acid of 1 to 2 nM; the binding constant of the isolated protein is in the pM range. Folate receptor alpha (FRα) and folate receptor beta (FRβ) both transport folates and antifolates by a receptor-mediated endocytosis.[89,90] FRα is broadly expressed in epithelial tumors.[91] Its expression in normal tissues is restricted to certain epithelia (apical membrane of proximal renal tubular cells, retinal pigment epithelium, choroid plexus). FRβ is expressed in spleen, thymus, and late-stage myeloid cells but not CD34+ progenitors. It is highly expressed in hematopoietic malignancies[90] and also expressed on activated and tumor-associated macrophages.[92] These folate receptors are a component of an endocytic process in which folates bind to the receptor following which the surrounding membrane invaginates and forms an endosomal vesicle that buds off within the cytoplasm to circulate within the endosomal compartment where the endosomal pH decreases. The folate is then released from the receptor and is exported from the endosome into the cytosol in a process mediated in part by PCFT.

This endocytic mechanism has now been harnessed for the delivery of anticancer drugs.[9,90] In the most advanced application, directed to FRα, drugs are linked to folic acid via a spacer and another segment containing a cleavable disulfide bond (**Fig. 7**). The folic acid–drug complex binds to the receptor, is endocytosed, and when the reducing potential within the endosomes increases, the disulfide bond ruptures, the drug is released from folic acid, and exits the endosome. A requirement is that the drug must be sufficiently lipid soluble to freely diffuse across the endosomal membrane so that it can be available to interact with its intracellular targets. Another requirement is that the drug must be highly toxic because there are only a limited number of folate receptors on tumor cells with a limited capacity for delivery of the drug.

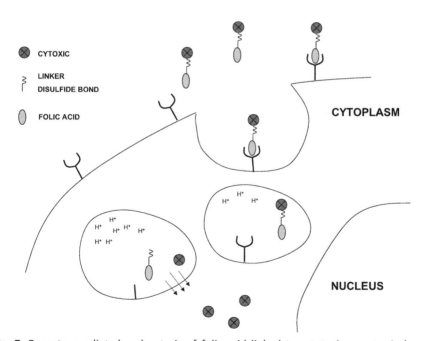

Fig. 7. Receptor-mediated endocytosis of folic acid linked to cytotoxic agents. A drug is coupled to folic acid via a hydrophilic linker molecule and a segment containing a cleavable disulfide bond. The complex binds to the folate receptor at the cell membrane, which invaginates and forms a vesicle that circulates within the endosomal compartment. As the vesicle matures, the reducing potential increases, rupturing the disulfide bond releasing the cytotoxic, which diffuses out of the endosome to reach its intracellular target. Folic acid can also be linked to technetium 99 to establish the presence of folate receptors and the competence of the endocytic mechanism before and after treatment with the cytotoxic conjugate.

The drug currently in clinical trials, that uses this technology, is folic acid linked to a highly potent vinca alkaloid, desacetylvinblastine.[93,94] The most advanced clinical trials to date have been focused on ovarian cancer, which, among cancers, has the highest expression of FRα.[95,96] Another disease in which this agent is being evaluated is lung cancer, where the expression of FRα is also prevalent. Complementing this therapeutic is a diagnostic reagent, folic acid linked to technetium 99, which allows scanning patients to establish the expression and function of folate receptors in the tumor.[97,98] Hence, only patients that express functional FRα would be expected to benefit from the drug. The diagnostic reagent also allows reevaluation of patients after they have failed one folic acid conjugate to determine whether the endocytic process remains intact. If that is the case, it would allow the administration of another conjugate in which folic acid is linked to a different cytotoxic. Another application of this technology is the linkage of folic acid to a fluorescent molecule for visual localization of the tumor in the intraoperative setting.[99] The status of these folic acid conjugates has been reviewed recently.[8,9]

Another class of drugs, in this case antifolates, is being developed that have high affinity for FRα but low affinity for RFC, which is the major route of delivery of antifolates to normal tissues. In this strategy, the drug is delivered exclusively via FRα, which is selectively expressed on tumors; there is limited or no transport mediated by RFC, thereby protected bone marrow and intestinal cells that express this carrier. One such antifolate, ONYX0801, a thymidylate synthase inhibitor, is currently in clinical development for the treatment of solid tumors.[100]

In another approach, antifolates are being developed with high affinity for PCFT but low affinity for RFC.[26,101,102] The strategy here, again, is to limit uptake into normal tissues via RFC. However, rather than targeting to folate receptors, the transport route targeted is PCFT. This transporter is widely expressed in solid tumors and, although also expressed in normal tissues, limited uptake is expected via this route under physiologic conditions. Hence, the compromised blood supply in solid tumors, resulting in local hypoxia, along with the release of lactate caused by the shift to anaerobic glycolysis inherent in malignant cells, should produce an acidic environment that favors PCFT-mediated transport.[103–105] On the other hand, PCFT-mediated transport should be negligible at the neutral pH of normal tissues with a physiologic blood supply and intact aerobic metabolism.

REFERENCES

1. Skipper HE, Perry S. Kinetics of normal and leukemic leukocyte populations and relevance to chemotherapy. Cancer Res 1970;30:1883–97.
2. Goldin A, Venditti JM, Humphreys SR, et al. A quantitative comparison of the antileukemic effectiveness of two folic acid antagonists in mice. J Natl Cancer Inst 1955;15:1657–64.
3. Farber S, Diamond LK, Mercer RD, et al. Temporary remission in acute leukemia in children produced by folic acid antagonist, 4-aminopteroyl glutamic acid (aminopterin). N Engl J Med 1948;238:787–93.
4. Goldman ID, Chattopadhyay S, Zhao R, et al. The antifolates: evolution, new agents in the clinic, and how targeting delivery via specific membrane transporters is driving the development of a next generation of folate analogs. Curr Opin Investig Drugs 2010;11:1409–23.
5. Chattopadhyay S, Moran RG, Goldman ID. Pemetrexed: biochemical and cellular pharmacology, mechanisms, and clinical applications. Mol Cancer Ther 2007;6:404–17.

6. Zhao R, Matherly LH, Goldman ID. Membrane transporters and folate homeostasis: intestinal absorption and transport into systemic compartments and tissues. Expert Rev Mol Med 2009;11:e4.
7. Matherly LH, Hou Z. Structure and function of the reduced folate carrier A paradigm of a major facilitator superfamily mammalian nutrient transporter. Vitam Horm 2008;79C:145–84.
8. Leamon CP, Jackman AL. Exploitation of the folate receptor in the management of cancer and inflammatory disease. Vitam Horm 2008;79:203–33.
9. Xia W, Low PS. Folate-targeted therapies for cancer. J Med Chem 2010;53: 6811–24.
10. Zhao R, Diop-Bove N, Visentin M, et al. Mechanisms of membrane transport of folates into cells and across epithelia. Annu Rev Nutr 2011;31:177–201.
11. Matherly LH, Hou Z, Deng Y. Human reduced folate carrier: translation of basic biology to cancer etiology and therapy. Cancer Metastasis Rev 2007;26:111–28.
12. Qiu A, Jansen M, Sakaris A, et al. Identification of an intestinal folate transporter and the molecular basis for hereditary folate malabsorption. Cell 2006;127: 917–28.
13. Stokstad EL. Historical perspective on key advances in the biochemistry and physiology of folates. In: Picciano MF, Stokstad EL, editors. Folic acid metabolism in health and disease. New York: Wiley-Liss; 1990. p. 1–21.
14. Fujii K, Nagasaki T, Huennekens FM. Accumulation of 5-methyltetrahydrofolate in cobalamin-deficient L1210 mouse leukemia cells. J Biol Chem 1982;257:2144–6.
15. Schramm VL. Enzymatic transition states, transition-state analogs, dynamics, thermodynamics, and lifetimes. Annu Rev Biochem 2011;80:703–32.
16. Zhao R, Goldman ID. Resistance to antifolates. Oncogene 2003;22:7431–57.
17. Lowe KE, Osborne CB, Lin BF, et al. Regulation of folate and one-carbon metabolism in mammalian cells. II. Effect of folylpoly-gamma-glutamate synthetase substrate specificity and level on folate metabolism and folylpoly-gamma-glutamate specificity of metabolic cycles of one-carbon metabolism. J Biol Chem 1993;268:21665–73.
18. Shane B. Folylpolyglutamate synthesis and role in the regulation of one-carbon metabolism. Vitam Horm 1989;45:263–335.
19. Koizumi S, Ueno Y, Ohno I, et al. Reversal of methotrexate cytotoxicity to human bone marrow cells and leukemic K562 cells by leucovorin: methotrexate polyglutamates formation as a possible important factor. Jpn J Cancer Res 1990; 81:1162–7.
20. Poser RG, Sirotnak FM, Chello PL. Differential synthesis of methotrexate polyglutamates in normal proliferative and neoplastic mouse tissues in vivo. Cancer Res 1981;41:4441–6.
21. Fry DW, Anderson LA, Borst M, et al. Analysis of the role of membrane transport and polyglutamylation of methotrexate in gut and Ehrlich tumor in vivo as factors in drug sensitivity and selectivity. Cancer Res 1983;43:1087–92.
22. Fabre I, Fabre G, Goldman ID. Polyglutamylation, an important element in methotrexate cytotoxicity and selectivity in tumor versus murine granulocytic progenitor cells in vitro. Cancer Res 1984;44:3190–5.
23. Zhao R, Min SH, Qiu A, et al. The spectrum of mutations in the PCFT gene, coding for an intestinal folate transporter, that are the basis for hereditary folate malabsorption. Blood 2007;110:1147–52.
24. Diop-Bove N, Kronn D, Goldman ID. Hereditary folate malabsorption [internet]. In: Pagon RA, Bird TD, Dolan CR, et al, editors. GeneReviews. Seattle (WA): University of Washington, Seattle 1993–2008.

25. Zhao R, Gao F, Hanscom M, et al. A prominent low-pH methotrexate transport activity in human solid tumor cells: contribution to the preservation of methotrexate pharmacological activity in HeLa cells lacking the reduced folate carrier. Clin Cancer Res 2004;10:718–27.

26. Desmoulin SK, Wang L, Hales E, et al. Therapeutic targeting of a novel 6-substituted pyrrolo[2,3-d]pyrimidine thienoyl antifolate to human solid tumors based on selective uptake by the proton-coupled folate transporter. Mol Pharmacol 2011;80:1096–107.

27. Zhao R, Qiu A, Tsai E, et al. The proton-coupled folate transporter (PCFT): impact on pemetrexed transport and on antifolate activities as compared to the reduced folate carrier. Mol Pharmacol 2008;74:854–62.

28. Zhao R, Hanscom M, Chattopadhyay S, et al. Selective preservation of pemetrexed pharmacological activity in HeLa cells lacking the reduced folate carrier; association with the presence of a secondary transport pathway. Cancer Res 2004;64:3313–9.

29. Volk EL, Schneider E. Wild-type breast cancer resistance protein (BCRP/ABCG2) is a methotrexate polyglutamate transporter. Cancer Res 2003;63:5538–43.

30. Kruh GD, Belinsky MG. The MRP family of drug efflux pumps. Oncogene 2003; 22:7537–52.

31. Assaraf YG. The role of multidrug resistance efflux transporters in antifolate resistance and folate homeostasis. Drug Resist Updat 2006;9:227–46.

32. Schoenbach EB, Greenspan EM, Colsky J. Reversal of aminopterin and amethopterin toxicity by citrovorum factor. J Am Med Assoc 1950;144:1558–60.

33. Djerassi I. Methotrexate infusions and intensive supportive care in the management of children with acute lymphocytic leukemia: follow-up report. Cancer Res 1967;27:2561–4.

34. Hryniuk WM, Bertino JR. Treatment of leukemia with large doses of methotrexate and folinic acid: clinical-biochemical correlates. J Clin Invest 1969;48:2140–55.

35. Pratt CB, Roberts D, Shanks EC, et al. Clinical trials and pharmacokinetics of intermittent high-dose methotrexate-"leucovorin rescue" for children with malignant tumors. Cancer Res 1974;34:3326–31.

36. Allegra CJ, Chabner BA, Drake JC, et al. Enhanced inhibition of thymidylate synthase by methotrexate polyglutamates. J Biol Chem 1985;260:9720–6.

37. Allegra CJ, Drake JC, Jolivet J, et al. Inhibition of phosphoribosylaminoimidazolecarboxamide transformylase by methotrexate and dihydrofolic acid polyglutamates. Proc Natl Acad Sci U S A 1985;82:4881–5.

38. Allegra CJ, Fine RL, Drake JC, et al. The effect of methotrexate on intracellular folate pools in human MCF-7 breast cancer cells. Evidence for direct inhibition of purine synthesis. J Biol Chem 1986;261:6478–85.

39. Baggott JE, Vaughn WH, Hudson BB. Inhibition of 5-aminoimidazole-4-carboxamide ribotide transformylase, adenosine deaminase and 5'-adenylate deaminase by polyglutamates of methotrexate and oxidized folates and by 5-aminoimidazole-4-carboxamide riboside and ribotide. Biochem J 1986;236: 193–200.

40. Matherly LH, Barlowe CK, Phillips VM, et al. The effects of 4-aminoantifolates on 5-formyltetrahydrofolate metabolism in L1210 cells. J Biol Chem 1987;262:710–7.

41. Matherly LH, Barlowe CK, Goldman ID. Antifolate polyglutamylation and competitive drug displacement at dihydrofolate reductase as important elements in leucovorin rescue in L1210 cells. Cancer Res 1986;46:588–93.

42. Treon SP, Chabner BA. Concepts in use of high-dose methotrexate therapy. Clin Chem 1996;42:1322–9.

43. Widemann BC, Adamson PC. Understanding and managing methotrexate nephrotoxicity. Oncologist 2006;11:694–703.
44. Gaynon PS, Angiolillo AL, Carroll WL, et al. Long-term results of the children's cancer group studies for childhood acute lymphoblastic leukemia 1983-2002: a Children's Oncology Group report. Leukemia 2010;24:285–97.
45. Chamberlain MC. Leptomeningeal metastasis. Semin Neurol 2010;30:236–44.
46. Jaffe N. Osteosarcoma: review of the past, impact on the future. The American experience. Cancer Treat Res 2009;152:239–62.
47. Savage P, Seckl M, Short D. Practical issues in the management of low-risk gestational trophoblast tumors. J Reprod Med 2008;53:774–80.
48. Colleoni M, Cole BF, Viale G, et al. Classical cyclophosphamide, methotrexate, and fluorouracil chemotherapy is more effective in triple-negative, node-negative breast cancer: results from two randomized trials of adjuvant chemoendocrine therapy for node-negative breast cancer. J Clin Oncol 2010;28:2966–73.
49. Gennari A, Sormani MP, Pronzato P, et al. HER2 status and efficacy of adjuvant anthracyclines in early breast cancer: a pooled analysis of randomized trials. J Natl Cancer Inst 2008;100:14–20.
50. Salliot C, van der HD. Long-term safety of methotrexate monotherapy in patients with rheumatoid arthritis: a systematic literature research. Ann Rheum Dis 2009; 68:1100–4.
51. Schwartz D, Ferguson JR. Current pharmacologic treatment paradigms for inflammatory bowel disease and the potential role of granulocyte/monocyte apheresis. Curr Med Res Opin 2007;23:2715–28.
52. Braus NA, Elliott DE. Advances in the pathogenesis and treatment of IBD. Clin Immunol 2009;132:1–9.
53. Kalb RE, Strober B, Weinstein G, et al. Methotrexate and psoriasis: 2009 National Psoriasis Foundation Consensus Conference. J Am Acad Dermatol 2009;60:824–37.
54. Chen M, Kallenberg CG. ANCA-associated vasculitides–advances in pathogenesis and treatment. Nat Rev Rheumatol 2010;6:653–64.
55. Sharaf PH, Yazici Y. Necrotizing vasculitis–a 2009 update. Bull NYU Hosp Jt Dis 2009;67:303–5.
56. Matloub Y, Bostrom BC, Hunger SP, et al. Escalating intravenous methotrexate improves event-free survival in children with standard-risk acute lymphoblastic leukemia: a report from the Children's Oncology Group. Blood 2011;118: 243–51.
57. Abramson JS, Hellmann M, Barnes JA, et al. Intravenous methotrexate as central nervous system (CNS) prophylaxis is associated with a low risk of CNS recurrence in high-risk patients with diffuse large B-cell lymphoma. Cancer 2010;116:4283–90.
58. Asselin BL, Devidas M, Wang C, et al. Effectiveness of high-dose methotrexate in T-cell lymphoblastic leukemia and advanced-stage lymphoblastic lymphoma: a randomized study by the Children's Oncology Group (POG 9404). Blood 2011;118:874–83.
59. DeGraw JI, Colwell WT, Piper JR, et al. Synthesis and antitumor activity of 10-propargyl-10-deazaaminopterin. J Med Chem 1993;36:2228–31.
60. Krug LM, Ng KK, Kris MG, et al. Phase I and pharmacokinetic study of 10-propargyl-10-deazaaminopterin, a new antifolate. Clin Cancer Res 2000;6: 3493–8.
61. Wang ES, O'Connor O, She Y, et al. Activity of a novel anti-folate (PDX, 10-propargyl 10-deazaaminopterin) against human lymphoma is superior to

methotrexate and correlates with tumor RFC-1 gene expression. Leuk Lymphoma 2003;44:1027–35.

62. O'Connor OA, Horwitz S, Hamlin P, et al. Phase II-I-II study of two different doses and schedules of pralatrexate, a high-affinity substrate for the reduced folate carrier, in patients with relapsed or refractory lymphoma reveals marked activity in T-cell malignancies. J Clin Oncol 2009;27:4357–64.

63. O'Connor OA, Hamlin PA, Portlock C, et al. Pralatrexate, a novel class of antifol with high affinity for the reduced folate carrier-type 1, produces marked complete and durable remissions in a diversity of chemotherapy refractory cases of T-cell lymphoma. Br J Haematol 2007;139:425–8.

64. Habeck LL, Mendelsohn LG, Shih C, et al. Substrate specificity of mammalian folylpolyglutamate synthetase for 5,10-dideazatetrahydrofolate analogs. Mol Pharmacol 1995;48:326–33.

65. Jackman AL, Taylor GA, Gibson W, et al. ICI D1694, a quinazoline antifolate thymidylate synthase inhibitor that is a potent inhibitor of L1210 tumor cell growth in vitro and in vivo: a new agent for clinical study. Cancer Res 1991;51: 5579–86.

66. Cocconi G, Cunningham D, Van Cutsem E, et al. Open, randomized, multicenter trial of raltitrexed versus fluorouracil plus high-dose leucovorin in patients with advanced colorectal cancer. Tomudex Colorectal Cancer Study Group. J Clin Oncol 1998;16:2943–52.

67. Popov I, Carrato A, Sobrero A, et al. Raltitrexed (Tomudex) versus standard leucovorin-modulated bolus 5-fluorouracil: results from the randomised phase III Pan-European Trial in Adjuvant Colon Cancer 01 (PETACC-1). Eur J Cancer 2008;44:2204–11.

68. Kempin S, Gutierrez J, Wilson E, et al. Raltitrexed (Tomudex): an alternative choice in patients intolerant to 5-fluorouracil. Cancer Invest 2002;20:992–5.

69. Shih C, Chen VJ, Gossett LS, et al. LY231514, a pyrrolo[2,3-d]pyrimidine-based antifolate that inhibits multiple folate-requiring enzymes. Cancer Res 1997;57: 1116–23.

70. Taylor EC, Kuhnt D, Shih C, et al. A dideazatetrahydrofolate analogue lacking a chiral center at C-6, N-[4-[2-(2-amino-3,4-dihydro-4-oxo-7H-pyrrolo[2, 3-d] pyrimidin-5-yl)ethyl]benzoyl]-L-glutamic acid, is an inhibitor of thymidylate synthase. J Med Chem 1992;35:4450–4.

71. Wang Y, Zhao R, Goldman ID. Characterization of a folate transporter in HeLa cells with a low pH optimum and high affinity for pemetrexed distinct from the reduced folate carrier. Clin Cancer Res 2004;10:6256–64.

72. Chattopadhyay S, Zhao R, Krupenko SA, et al. The inverse relationship between reduced folate carrier function and pemetrexed activity in a human colon cancer cell line. Mol Cancer Ther 2006;5:438–49.

73. Racanelli AC, Rothbart SB, Heyer CL, et al. Therapeutics by cytotoxic metabolite accumulation: pemetrexed causes ZMP accumulation, AMPK activation, and mammalian target of rapamycin inhibition. Cancer Res 2009;69:5467–74.

74. Rothbart SB, Racanelli AC, Moran RG. Pemetrexed indirectly activates the metabolic kinase AMPK in human carcinomas. Cancer Res 2010;70:10299–309.

75. Vogelzang NJ, Rusthoven JJ, Symanowski J, et al. Phase III study of pemetrexed in combination with cisplatin versus cisplatin alone in patients with malignant pleural mesothelioma. J Clin Oncol 2003;21:2636–44.

76. Hanna N, Shepherd FA, Fossella FV, et al. Randomized phase III trial of pemetrexed versus docetaxel in patients with non-small-cell lung cancer previously treated with chemotherapy. J Clin Oncol 2004;22:1589–97.

77. Scagliotti GV, Parikh P, Von Pawel J, et al. Phase III study comparing cisplatin plus gemcitabine with cisplatin plus pemetrexed in chemotherapy-naive patients with advanced-stage non-small-cell lung cancer. J Clin Oncol 2008; 26:3543–51.
78. Ciuleanu T, Brodowicz T, Zielinski C, et al. Maintenance pemetrexed plus best supportive care versus placebo plus best supportive care for non-small-cell lung cancer: a randomised, double-blind, phase 3 study. Lancet 2009;374:1432–40.
79. Andreassi JL, Moran RG. Mouse folylpoly-gamma-glutamate synthetase isoforms respond differently to feedback inhibition by folylpolyglutamate cofactors. Biochemistry 2002;41:226–35.
80. Zhao R, Gao F, Goldman ID. Marked suppression of the activity of some, but not all, antifolate compounds by augmentation of folate cofactor pools within tumor cells. Biochem Pharmacol 2001;61:857–65.
81. Chattopadhyay S, Tamari R, Min SH, et al. Commentary: a case for minimizing folate supplementation in clinical regimens with pemetrexed based on the marked sensitivity of the drug to folate availability. Oncologist 2007;12:808–15.
82. Niyikiza C, Baker SD, Seitz DE, et al. Homocysteine and methylmalonic acid: markers to predict and avoid toxicity from pemetrexed therapy. Mol Cancer Ther 2002;1:545–52.
83. Scagliotti GV, Shin DM, Kindler HL, et al. Phase II study of pemetrexed with and without folic acid and vitamin B12 as front-line therapy in malignant pleural mesothelioma. J Clin Oncol 2003;21:1556–61.
84. Assaraf YG. Molecular basis of antifolate resistance. Cancer Metastasis Rev 2007;26:153–81.
85. Zhang D, Ochi N, Takigawa N, et al. Establishment of pemetrexed-resistant non-small cell lung cancer cell lines. Cancer Lett 2011;309:228–35.
86. Hanauske AR, Eismann U, Oberschmidt O, et al. In vitro chemosensitivity of freshly explanted tumor cells to pemetrexed is correlated with target gene expression. Invest New Drugs 2007;25:417–23.
87. Mauritz R, Peters GJ, Priest DG, et al. Multiple mechanisms of resistance to methotrexate and novel antifolates in human CCRF-CEM leukemia cells and their implications for folate homeostasis. Biochem Pharmacol 2002;63: 105–15.
88. Zhao R, Zhang S, Hanscom M, et al. Loss of reduced folate carrier function and folate depletion result in enhanced pemetrexed inhibition of purine synthesis. Clin Cancer Res 2005;11:1294–301.
89. Kamen BA, Smith AK. A review of folate receptor alpha cycling and 5-methyltetrahydrofolate accumulation with an emphasis on cell models in vitro. Adv Drug Deliv Rev 2004;56:1085–97.
90. Salazar MD, Ratnam M. The folate receptor: what does it promise in tissue-targeted therapeutics? Cancer Metastasis Rev 2007;26:141–52.
91. Parker N, Turk MJ, Westrick E, et al. Folate receptor expression in carcinomas and normal tissues determined by a quantitative radioligand binding assay. Anal Biochem 2005;338:284–93.
92. Puig-Kroger A, Sierra-Filardi E, Dominguez-Soto A, et al. Folate receptor beta is expressed by tumor-associated macrophages and constitutes a marker for M2 anti-inflammatory/regulatory macrophages. Cancer Res 2009;69:9395–403.
93. Reddy JA, Dorton R, Westrick E, et al. Preclinical evaluation of EC145, a folate-vinca alkaloid conjugate. Cancer Res 2007;67:4434–42.
94. Leamon CP, Reddy JA, Vlahov IR, et al. Preclinical antitumor activity of a novel folate-targeted dual drug conjugate. Mol Pharm 2007;4:659–67.

95. Li J, Sausville EA, Klein PJ, et al. Clinical pharmacokinetics and exposure-toxicity relationship of a folate-vinca alkaloid conjugate EC145 in cancer patients. J Clin Pharmacol 2009;49:1467–76.

96. Dosio F, Milla P, Cattel L. EC-145, a folate-targeted vinca alkaloid conjugate for the potential treatment of folate receptor-expressing cancers. Curr Opin Investig Drugs 2010;11:1424–33.

97. Fisher RE, Siegel BA, Edell SL, et al. Exploratory study of 99mTc-EC20 imaging for identifying patients with folate receptor-positive solid tumors. J Nucl Med 2008;49:899–906.

98. Reddy JA, Xu LC, Parker N, et al. Preclinical evaluation of (99m)Tc-EC20 for imaging folate receptor-positive tumors. J Nucl Med 2004;45:857–66.

99. van Dam GM, Themelis G, Crane LM, et al. Intraoperative tumor-specific fluorescence imaging in ovarian cancer by folate receptor-alpha targeting: first in-human results. Nat Med 2011;17:1315–9.

100. Gibbs DD, Theti DS, Wood N, et al. BGC 945, a novel tumor-selective thymidylate synthase inhibitor targeted to alpha-folate receptor-overexpressing tumors. Cancer Res 2005;65:11721–8.

101. Desmoulin SK, Wang Y, Wu J, et al. Targeting the proton-coupled folate transporter for selective delivery of 6-substituted pyrrolo[2,3-d]pyrimidine antifolate inhibitors of de novo purine biosynthesis in the chemotherapy of solid tumors. Mol Pharmacol 2010;78:577–87.

102. Wang L, Desmoulin SK, Cherian C, et al. Synthesis, biological, and antitumor activity of a highly potent 6-substituted pyrrolo[2,3-d]pyrimidine thienoyl antifolate inhibitor with proton-coupled folate transporter and folate receptor selectivity over the reduced folate carrier that inhibits beta-glycinamide ribonucleotide formyltransferase. J Med Chem 2011;54:7150–64.

103. Helmlinger G, Yuan F, Dellian M, et al. Interstitial pH and pO2 gradients in solid tumors in vivo: high- resolution measurements reveal a lack of correlation. Nat Med 1997;3:177–82.

104. Stubbs M, Rodrigues L, Howe FA, et al. Metabolic consequences of a reversed pH gradient in rat tumors. Cancer Res 1994;54:4011–6.

105. Raghunand N, Altbach MI, van Sluis R, et al. Plasmalemmal pH-gradients in drug-sensitive and drug-resistant MCF-7 human breast carcinoma xenografts measured by 31P magnetic resonance spectroscopy. Biochem Pharmacol 1999;57:309–12.

Poly(Adenosine Diphosphate–Ribose) Polymerase Inhibitors in Cancer Treatment

Sook Ryun Park, MD, PhD[a], Alice Chen, MD[b],*

KEYWORDS

- Poly(ADP-ribose) polymerase • Inhibitor • Synthetic lethality • BRCA

KEY POINTS

- Many mechanisms are present in a cell to repair DNA damage, which when effective allow for cell survival. Understanding these mechanisms are important for both therapeutic treatment of cancer and overcoming resistance.
- The concept of synthetic lethality has be tested in treating patients with *BRCA* mutation with a PARP inhibitor. Initial results with olaparib was encouraging and supportive of synthetic lethality principle.
- The role of PARP inhibitor outside of *BRCA* mutation tumors await confirmation. Multiple studies are ongoing investigating PARP inhibitor with chemotherapy to see if inhibiting DNA repair will lead to tumor reduction and ultimately benefit to the patients.

Recently, the development of poly(adenosine diphosphate [ADP]-ribose) polymerase (PARP) inhibitors has brought a major breakthrough in the treatment of germline breast cancer susceptibility gene (*BRCA*)-mutant cancers.[1–4] These agents target a DNA repair pathway via a novel mechanism of action. A better understanding of DNA damage repair mechanisms can extend the therapeutic application of this novel drug class to a wide range of sporadic cancers. Early clinical success has accelerated the development of various PARP inhibitors that are being explored in many cancers with single agents or in combination with chemotherapy or radiotherapy. In this article, the authors review DNA repair mechanisms and the role of PARP as a therapeutic

Disclosure: The authors declared no conflicts of interest.
[a] Division of Cancer Treatment and Diagnosis, National Cancer Institute, 31 Center Drive, Room 3A44, Bethesda, MD 20892, USA
[b] Investigational Drug Branch, Cancer Therapy Evaluation Program, Division of Cancer Treatment and Diagnosis, National Cancer Institute, 6130 Executive Boulevard EPN 7131, Rockville, MD 20852, USA
* Corresponding author. 6130 Executive Boulevard EPN 7131, Rockville, MD 20852.
E-mail address: chenali@mail.nih.gov

target and summarize available PARP inhibitors, their clinical trials, biomarkers of PARP inhibitor sensitivity, and resistance mechanisms.

DNA DAMAGE AND REPAIR MECHANISMS

DNA damage is generated by a variety of factors, not only from external factors such as chemical agents, UV light, or ionizing radiation but also from internal factors such as reactive oxygen species or intrinsic DNA replication errors during cell division. DNA damages, if let unrepaired, can cause errors of DNA synthesis during replication, leading to cell death or irreversible mutations resulting in long-term oncogenesis. Thus, individuals with an inherited defect in the DNA repair system are often at an increased risk of cancer.[5] Common errors include (1) base modifications by frequently reactive oxygen species or chemical agents, such as loss of an amino group (deamination) or alkylation; (2) mismatch of nucleotide pairs by replication errors; (3) single-strand break (SSB) or double-strand break (DSB) by ionizing radiation; (4) failures in normal DNA metabolism by topoisomerases and nuclease; or (5) cross-links, covalent linkages between bases on intrastrand or interstrand. DSBs are the most critical form of DNA damage and can result in problems for transcription, replication, and chromosome segregation, eventually leading to apoptosis or carcinogenesis.[5]

To maintain genetic stability against constantly occurring DNA lesions, several strategies of DNA damage detection and repair have evolved. The principal and partly overlapping DNA repair pathways in humans can be largely divided into 2 groups: one is the repair pathway for DNA SSB and the other is for DNA DSB. The former can be subdivided into 3 different repair processes: (1) repair of base damage and SSBs by base excision repair (BER), (2) repair of bulky DNA adducts by nucleotide excision repair (NER), and (3) repair of mismatches and insertion/deletion loops by DNA mismatch repair (MMR). The DSB is repaired through (1) homologous recombination (HR) and (2) nonhomologous end joining (NHEJ).

Base Excision Repair

The BER pathway repairs damage to a single or a few bases caused by reactive oxygen species, alkylating agents, or ionizing radiation, such as oxidation, alkylation, hydrolysis, or deamination, that could cause mutations by incorrect base pairing or lead to breaks in DNA during replication if uncorrected (**Fig. 1A**).[5,6] PARP1 and PARP2 are recruited to the site of the SSB in this pathway.

Nucleotide Excision Repair

NER is used for the removal of large patches around DNA lesions that are bulky and/or alter the helical structure of the DNA molecule, including those caused by UV radiation, carcinogenic compounds, and cross-linking chemotherapeutic agents (see **Fig. 1B**).[7]

Mismatch Repair

MMR removes base mismatches by DNA polymerases and small insertion-deletion loops introduced during DNA replication and recombination (see **Fig. 1C**).[5] A variety of base pair abnormalities resulting from DNA damage are also subject to processing by MMR, which include base pairs containing O6-methylguanine, carcinogen adducts, UV photo products, and cisplatin adducts.[8] Defects in the MMR system dramatically increase mutation rates resulting in hereditary nonpolyposis colorectal cancer and some types of sporadic tumor.[9]

Nonhomologous End Joining

NHEJ can occur throughout the cell cycle, predominantly in the G1 phases. DNA break ends are directly ligated without the use of a homologous template, so NHEJ is prone to introducing errors ranging from small insertions and deletions at the break site to the joining of previously unlinked DNA ends (see **Fig. 1D**).[10]

Homologous Recombination

HR repairs DSB by using the undamaged sister chromatid or homologous chromosome, resulting in error-free repair, and occurs primarily during the S and G2 phases of the cell cycle. BRCA proteins are involved in this pathway (see **Fig. 1E**).

DNA REPAIR SYNTHETIC LETHALITY AS A THERAPEUTIC TARGET
PARP in DNA Repair

PARP is an abundant nuclear enzyme involved in several cellular processes involving mainly DNA repair and programmed cell death. PARP1 and PARP2 are the only members of the PARP family that are known to be involved in the DNA SSB repair via the BER pathway.[11,12] Once PARP detects an SSB, it binds to the sites of DNA damage through its DNA-binding domain and begins the synthesis of a poly(ADP-ribose) (PAR) chain from the substrate nicotinamide adenine dinucleotide (NAD^+) at sites of breakage. PARP induces poly(ADP-ribosyl)ation in PARP itself at the automodification domain and other proteins such as histone (H1 and H2B), which leads to chromatin decondensation to accommodate various DNA repair enzymes.[13] The auto-poly(ADP-ribosyl)ation of PARP1 mediates the recruitment of BER proteins such as DNA polymerase β, DNA ligase III, and scaffolding proteins such as x-ray repair cross-complementing 1 (XRCC1) heterodimer.[14] PARP1 then dissociates from the DNA because of its negative charge resulting from poly(ADP-ribosyl)ation, and the PAR chains are degraded by PAR glycohydrolase and possibly the ADP-ribose hydrolase ARH3 after repair of the DNA break.[15] Besides its firmly established role in BER and DNA SSB repair, PARP1 is involved in multiple types of other DNA damage repair processes, including the repair of DNA DSBs, DNA cross-links, and stalled replication forks. PARP1 promotes restart of stalled replication forks and HR by recruiting HR factors including ATM, MRE11, and NBS1.[16] Furthermore, PARP1 is recruited for DSB repair in the absence of essential components of the classical pathway of NHEJ such as Ku70.[17] Although PARP1 is the predominant enzyme that synthesizes PAR in response to DNA damage, PARP2 has been shown to interact with PARP1 and is also implicated in BER.[12] PARP2 is, however, unable to fully compensate for the loss of PARP1, accounting for approximately 10% of the total PARP activity of human cells.[11,18]

BRCA1 and BRCA2 in DNA Repair

BRCA1 plays a key role in the regulation of the cell cycle checkpoints and the HR-mediated DNA repair pathway. On DNA damage, *BRCA1* is rapidly phosphorylated and redistributes to sites of DNA breaks, where it interacts with RAD51 and other proteins involved in DNA DSB repair, such as MRN and CtIP.[19] Although *BRCA1* appears to function upstream of RAD51 filament polymerization, *BRCA2* directly binds to and translocates RAD51 to areas of DNA damage and stabilizes RAD51 filaments on DSB.[20] Absence of either factor causes DNA repair defect, primarily in HR, which contributes to tumorigenesis. Heterozygous germline mutations in *BRCA1* or *BRCA2* predispose to various type of cancers, especially breast and ovarian cancers. This HR deficiency also has a critical impact on chemosensitivity. *BRCA1*-mutated breast cancer cells are highly sensitive to DNA interstrand cross-linking–inducing agents such as cisplatin and mitomycin C because they disrupt replication forks during S phase, which requires HR-mediated DSB repair for S phase progression and cell survival.[21,22] Because of their heightened cytotoxicity in HR-defective cells, platinum agents have been extensively applied as chemotherapeutic drugs in *BRCA1*- or *BRCA2*-associated cancers with outcomes better than those of non-*BRCA*-associated cancers.[23,24]

Synthetic Lethality

The term synthetic lethality was coined in 1946. It describes a phenomenon in which 2 nonlethal mutations have no effect on cell viability in the presence of either

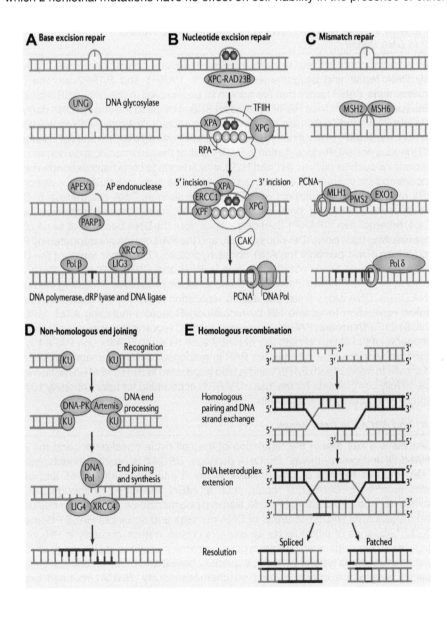

mutation alone but lead to cell death in combination.[25] This concept is now being exploited in cancer treatment. Because many cancer cells have cancer-relevant genetic lesions that are not present in normal cells, mimicking the effect of a second genetic mutation with a targeted agent should selectively kill only cancer cells with a large therapeutic window. To date, the most successful synthetic lethality relationship in DNA repair pathways for cancer treatment comes from PARP inhibition in BRCA-null tumors. Although PARP1 plays a critical role in DNA SSB repair, loss of PARP1 activity is not lethal in normal cells. When unrepaired DNA SSBs caused by the absence of PARP1 activity encounter DNA replication forks, they result in stalled replication forks that are subsequently converted to DNA DSBs. Although these DNA DSBs are effectively repaired by the HR pathway in normal cells,[5,26] cells that are defective in HR, such as BRCA1- or BRCA2-deficient cells, cannot repair them, resulting in cell death. Therefore, PARP inhibitors could be selectively lethal to cells lacking functional BRCA1 or BRCA2 with minimal toxicity to normal cells.

Synthetic lethality in BRCA1- and BRCA2-deficient cells when exposed to PARP inhibitors was confirmed in in vitro and in vivo mouse models.[27,28] Farmer and colleagues[27] showed that PARP1 depletion with RNA interference decreased clonogenic survival of BRCA1- and BRCA2-deficient embryonic stem cells compared with wild-type cells. Furthermore, clonogenic cell survival assays showed that BRCA1- or BRCA2-deficient cells were much more sensitive to the potent PARP inhibitors, KU0058684 and KU0058948, than heterozygous mutant or wild-type cells.[27] KU0058684 also blocked tumor growth in vivo in BRCA2-deficient cells. Similarly, Bryant and colleagues[28] demonstrated that BRCA2-deficient V-C8 cells were profoundly sensitive to the PARP inhibitors NU1025 and AG014361, as compared with the wild-type V79 cells. Human breast cancer cell lines MCF-7 and MDA-MB-231 also displayed a similar sensitivity to NU1025 on depletion of BRCA2 with RNA interference.[28]

Fig. 1. Major DNA damage repair mechanisms. (*A*) BER: a specific DNA glycosylase removes a damaged base, for example, uracil DNA glycosylase (UNG) for uracil. Subsequently, an apyrimidinic/apurinic (AP) site incision by an AP endonuclease 1 (APEX1) and the removal of 5'-deoxyribose-phosphate (dRP) residue by a dRP lyase occur followed by nucleotide gap filling by DNA polymerase β. (*B*) NER: after a DNA-distorting lesion is recognized with or without the xeroderma pigmentosum complementation group C (XPC)/Rad23 homolog B (RAD23B) protein complex, dual incisions on both sides of the lesion and excision of the damaged site occur by the general transcription factor TFIIH, XPG, and excision repair cross-complementation group 1 (ERCC1)/XPF complex. DNA polymerase fills the resulting nucleotide gap. (*C*) MMR: the mismatched bases are recognized by a heterodimer of MSH2/MSH6 and excised by exonuclease 1 (EXO1), which is recruited by a heterodimer of MLH1/PMS2. The resulting gap is filled by DNA polymerase δ along with proliferating cell nuclear antigen (PCNA) and replication protein A (RPA). (*D*) NHEJ: the 2 broken ends are processed and ligated directly by Ku70/Ku80 complex and the DNA-dependent protein kinase (DNA-PK) followed by DNA ligase IV (LIG4)/XRCC4. (*E*) HR: repair is initiated by resection of a DSB resulting in 3'single-stranded DNA overhangs, which invade into a homologous sequence followed by DNA synthesis at the invading end. Subsequently, the second 3'end is captured to form a Holliday junction. After gap-filling DNA synthesis and ligation, the structure is resolved at the Holliday junction in a crossover or noncrossover mode. (*Adapted from* Lange SS, Takata K, Wood RD. DNA polymerases and cancer. Nat Rev Cancer 2011;11:96–110; with permission. Copyright © 2011 Macmillan Publishers Ltd.)

BRCAness

The primary challenge to the promise of PARP inhibitors in the treatment of BRCA-mutant cancers is the low frequency of germline mutations in BRCA1 or BRCA2, only 10% to 15% of unselected ovarian cancers[29–31] and 5% to 10% of breast cancers.[32–34] In addition, BRCA1 and BRCA2 genes are infrequently mutated somatically in sporadic cancers, with 4% to 9% of unselected or sporadic ovarian cancers.[35–37] However, some sporadic cancers phenotypically behave like BRCA1/2-mutant cancers even though they do not have known BRCA mutations. These tumors may carry abnormalities in the expression or function of BRCA1 or BRCA2 or in other critical components of the HR DNA repair pathway. This phenomenon is called BRCAness and is characterized by defective HR.[38] One of the mechanisms of BRCAness is the silencing of BRCA1 or BRCA2 through the aberrant methylation of the promoter and has been reported in 11% to 14% of sporadic breast cancers[39–41] and 5% to 18% of ovarian cancers.[36,39,40,42] Preclinical studies have shown that tumor cell lines with decreased BRCA expression by mutation or epigenetic silencing responded equally well to the PARP inhibitor AG014699 that additionally inhibited the growth of epigenetically silenced BRCA1 xenograft tumors.[43] These suggest that PARP inhibitors may have a potential role in sporadic cancers as well as hereditary cancers. The amplification of the EMSY gene that encodes for EMSY protein that can interact with and silence the activation domain of BRCA2 has also been described as a potential mechanism of BRCA inactivation. The amplification of the EMSY gene was reported in 13% of sporadic breast cancers and 17% of high-grade serous ovarian cancers (HGSOCs).[44] Because Fanconi anemia proteins are involved in the HR pathway, the epigenetic silencing of Fanconi anemia complementation group F (FANCF) gene through promoter methylation is another potential mechanism of BRCAness.[45] The inhibition of the FANCF gene in ovarian cancer cell lines through promoter methylation was associated with enhanced sensitivity to DNA-damaging agents such as cisplatin; in reverse, demethylation of the FANCF promoter resulted in cisplatin resistance.[45] In addition to potential transcriptional and posttranslational abnormalities occurring in BRCA1 and BRCA2 pathways, deficiency of proteins involved in the HR pathway, such as RAD51, RAD54, DSS1, RPA1, NBS1, ATR, ATM, CHK1, or CHK2, can also induce sensitivity to PARP inhibitors.[46,47]

PARP INHIBITORS

The profound sensitivity of BRCA-mutant cells to PARP inhibition prompted the development of PARP inhibitors for cancer therapy (**Table 1**). At present, most PARP inhibitors in preclinical and clinical studies are third-generation PARP inhibitors and compete with the substrate NAD^+ for the catalytic domain of the PARP enzyme, leading to reversible inhibition of the enzyme. AZD2281/KU-0059436 (olaparib) and ABT-888 (veliparib) are the most common inhibitors assessed to date in clinical trials. Both drugs are administered orally and are potent inhibitors of PARP1 and PARP2, with a half maximal inhibitory concentration (IC_{50} or K_i) in the nanomolar range for 2 enzymes.[48,49] Preclinical activity of AG014361 has also been translated into the clinic as its clinical analogue CO338 (rucaparib, AG014699, PF-01367338) administered intravenously. It was initially tested in combination with temozolomide in melanoma.[50] Other PARP inhibitors under active clinical investigation include MK4827, BMN 673, CEP-9722, and E7016/GPI 21016 (see **Table 1**). Of note, BSI-201 (iniparib) was initially described as having PARP inhibitory activity, which proceeded into a phase 3 trial in triple-negative breast cancer (TNBC) in combination with carboplatin and paclitaxel,[51–53] but recent evidence suggests that iniparib does not seem to inhibit PARP1 and PARP2 at the clinical dose.[54,55]

Table 1
PARP inhibitors in active clinical investigation

Name	Route	Disease	Single/Combination Therapy	Phase of Clinical Development[a]	Company
Rucaparib (CO338, AGO 14699, PF-0367338)	IV	BRCA+ ovarian/breast cancer Melanoma	Single Temozolomide	2 2	Clovis Oncology (Boulder, CO, USA)
Olaparib (AZD2281)	Oral	BRCA+ ovarian cancer BRCA+ breast cancer High-grade SOC/TNBC Various solid tumors	Single agent Carboplatin, topotecan, paclitaxel, dacarbazine, or gemcitabine/cisplatin	2 1	AstraZeneca (London, UK)
Veliparib (ABT-888)	Oral	Melanoma Breast cancer Colorectal cancer Various solid tumors	Temozolomide Topotecan, irinotecan, cyclophosphamide, or doxorubicin/cyclophosphamide	2 1	Abbott (Abbott Park, IL, USA)
MK 4827	Oral	HGSOC enriched with BRCA+	Single	1	Merck (Whitehouse Station, NJ, USA)
BMN 673	Oral	Various solid tumors Hematologic malignancies	Single agent	1	Biomarin (Novato, CA, USA)
CEP-9722	Oral	Advanced solid tumor (phase 1)/cancer with defective DNA repair pathway (phase 2) Solid tumor	Single Temozolomide Gemcitabine/Cisplatin	1/2 1	Cephalon (Frazer, PA, USA)
E7016 (GPI 21016)	Oral	Solid tumor	Temozolomide	1	MGI Pharma/Eisai (Bloomington, MN, USA)

Abbreviations: BRCA, breast cancer susceptible gene; IV, intravenous; SOC, serous ovarian cancer; TNBC, triple-negative breast cancer.
[a] Indicates the most advanced phase in studies that have been published or presented. In CEP-9722 and E7016, ongoing trials are shown because there are no published studies.
Data from ClinicalTrials.gov, National Library of Medicine, Bethesda, MD.

MONOTHERAPY WITH PARP INHIBITORS IN *BRCA*-MUTANT CANCERS

On the basis of preclinical data showing hypersensitivity to PARP inhibitors in tumor cells lacking *BRCA1* or *BRCA2*, PARP inhibitor was used as a single agent in patients with *BRCA* mutation. The first landmark trial of PARP inhibitor as monotherapy was performed with olaparib enriched with *BRCA1/2* mutation carriers and limited to patients with *BRCA* mutation ovarian cancer in the expansion phase.[1] Olaparib was safe and well tolerated with no obvious differences in toxicities observed between *BRCA1* or *BRCA2* mutation carriers and noncarriers. The maximum tolerated dose (MTD) was 400 mg twice a day, and the dose-limiting toxicities (DLTs) included grade 3 mood alteration, fatigue, somnolence, and grade 4 thrombocytopenia. As expected, there was significant antitumor activity only in patients with *BRCA1*- or *BRCA2*-mutated cancers, including ovarian, breast, and prostate cancers, among whom 12 of 17 (63%) patients had clinical benefit and 9 of 19 (47%) patients achieved responses according to the Response Evaluation Criteria in Solid Tumors (RECIST). In the expansion cohort of 50 *BRCA* mutation carriers with ovarian, primary peritoneal, and fallopian tube cancers, 20 patients (40%) had a RECIST response, cancer antigen 125 responses, or both; 14 patients (28%) had RECIST responses.[2] Pharmacodynamic assay demonstrated that a dose of 60 mg or more twice daily reduced PARP activity in peripheral blood mononuclear cells (PBMCs) by more than 90% as compared with the value at baseline. Plucked eyebrow hair follicles were collected before treatment and again 6 hours after treatment, showing induction of γ-H2AX, which did not seem to increase further at doses greater than 100 mg twice daily, the lowest dose of this analysis. Based on these results, a dose of 100 mg twice daily may be adequate for PARP inhibitory effect; this dose was further studied in phase 2 studies along with a twice-daily dose of 400 mg, the MTD.

Subsequently, 2 proof-of-concept phase 2 studies with olaparib in patients with advanced or recurrent breast (International Collaborative Expertise for BRCA Education and Research through Genetics [ICEBERG]1) or ovarian cancer (ICEBERG2) who had *BRCA1* or *BRCA2* mutations have provided further support for synthetic lethal approach to cancer therapy.[3,4] Both studies recruited sequentially 2 dose cohorts treated with twice-daily doses of olaparib 400 mg (the established MTD) and then 100 mg (the lowest PARP inhibitory dose with clinical activity).[1,2] In ICEBERG1 trial, the objective response rate in breast cancer seemed to be higher in the 400-mg cohort (41%, 11/27) than in the 100-mg cohort (22%, 6/27), and median progression-free survival (PFS) also seemed to be longer in the 400-mg cohort (5.7 vs 3.8 months).[3] Similarly, ICEBERG2 trial in ovarian cancer showed that the high-dose cohort seemed to have better response rate (33% vs 13%) and median PFS (5.8 vs 1.9 months) than the low-dose cohort.[4] Overall, both trials confirmed the tolerability of olaparib in *BRCA 1/2* mutation carriers, with mainly grade 1 or 2 adverse events.

A subsequent randomized phase 2 study comparing the safety and efficacy of 2 doses of olaparib (200 or 400 mg twice daily continuously in 28-day cycles) with that of pegylated liposomal doxorubicin (PLD) (50 mg/m^2 every 4 weeks) was done in patients with *BRCA* mutation–associated ovarian cancer who had failed previous platinum-based chemotherapy.[56] A total of 97 patients were randomized into 3 groups. Although the 400-mg group had a numerically longer median PFS (8.8 vs 6.5 vs 7.1 months, respectively) and a higher response rate (25% vs 18% vs 31%, respectively) than the 200-mg or PLD groups, neither outcome reached statistical significance. These negative outcomes might be partially attributed to better PFS in the PLD group compared with historical cohorts. Regarding safety, both doses of olaparib were well tolerated with less toxicity compared with PLD. The PLD group had more grade 3 or 4 toxicities. Although the primary end point was not fulfilled, this study demonstrated the consistent efficacy with favorable safety of olaparib as monotherapy in *BRCA*-mutant ovarian cancer.

Another promising PARP inhibitor that has been studied in *BRCA1/2* mutation carriers is MK4827, a potent oral PARP1/2 inhibitor with an IC_{50} of 3.8 and 2.1 nM for PARP1 and PARP2, respectively.[57] A phase 1 study of MK4827 enriched with *BRCA1/2* mutation carriers had established MTD at a dose of 300 mg once daily.[58] DLTs included grade 3 fatigue and pneumonitis and grade 4 thrombocytopenia. Inhibition of PARP activity in PBMCs was demonstrated at doses of 80 mg or greater. The response rate was 37% (7/19) in patients with *BRCA*-mutated ovarian cancer and 20% (3/15) in patients with sporadic ovarian cancer. MK4827 was well tolerated with the most common toxicities of fatigue (52.5%), nausea (52.5%), vomiting (38.8%), diarrhea (21.3%), thrombocytopenia (33.8%), and neutropenia (21.3%), which were mostly graded 1 to 2 except for thrombocytopenia (grade 3/4, 15%).

Rucaparib was evaluated in a phase 2 study for *BRCA1/2*-mutated advanced ovarian and/or breast cancer in which 18 mg/m^2 of rucaparib was given on days 1 to 5 of a 21-day cycle.[59] PARP activity assessed in PBMC demonstrated a mean inhibition of 84% over baseline levels at 24 hours after a single dose of 18 mg/m^2 of AG014699. Although the overall response rate was 5% (2/38), 26% (10/38) achieved stable disease for 4 or more months. Rucaparib had an acceptable safety profile with drug-related toxicity, mainly grade 1 and 2; the most common toxicities were fatigue (39%), nausea (26.8%), diarrhea (19.5%), and dizziness (17.1%).

Overall, these data clearly provide clinical validation for single-agent PARP inhibitor activity in patients with *BRCA1/2* mutations.

MONOTHERAPY WITH PARP INHIBITORS IN SPORADIC CANCERS

The evidence of BRCAness has been shown particularly in a substantial proportion of sporadic ovarian cancer and TNBC or basal-like breast cancer. Overall, *BRCA1/2* deficiency as a result of germline or somatic *BRCA1/2* mutations, epigenetic loss of *BRCA1*, or expression loss by other mechanisms has been reported in 30% to 53% of ovarian cancers, which was associated with high-grade serous/undifferentiated tumor histology and improved PFS with chemotherapy.[36,37] TNBC overlaps substantially with basal-like breast cancer. *BRCA1*-associated cancers generally cluster with the basal-like subtype in gene expression profiling studies.[60] Most *BRCA1*-associated breast cancers share many phenotypic features with TNBC and basal-like breast cancer.[61] This notion of shared BRCAness is the rationale for testing PARP inhibition in sporadic TNBC or HGSOC because even without germline *BRCA1/2* mutations, these tumors may harbor other lesions that impair HR.

To address whether sporadic cancers with BRCAness would also be responsive to PARP inhibitors as are *BRCA*-mutant cancers, a phase 2 study of single-agent olaparib (400 mg twice daily continuously) in patients with HGSOC or undifferentiated ovarian cancer or TNBC was conducted in which patients were stratified according to whether they had a germline *BRCA1/2* mutation or not (or unknown *BRCA* mutation status).[62] Ninety patients (64 with ovarian cancer and 26 with breast cancer) received treatment with a median of 3 prior chemotherapy regimens. Although the breast cancer cohorts did not have any confirmed objective response, the ovarian cancer cohorts showed a response rate of 41% in patients with *BRCA* mutations and 24% in patients without mutations. The median PFSs were 221 days and 192 days, respectively. The most common adverse events were grade 1 or 2 fatigue, nausea, and vomiting. These results demonstrate the activity of a PARP inhibitor in patients with HGSOC without germline *BRCA1/2* mutations.

In addition, promising results of a randomized, double-blind, placebo-controlled phase 2 study of maintenance olaparib in patients with platinum-sensitive relapsed HGSOC independent of germline *BRCA* status were also recently reported.[63] Patients who had maintained an objective response following the last platinum-containing regimen were randomized to a twice-daily dose of 400 mg of olaparib (n = 136) or placebo (n = 129). The olaparib group had a significantly longer PFS, median 8.4 versus 4.8 months. Approximately 20% of patients in both groups had *BRCA1/2* mutations, and a preplanned subgroup analysis showed that the PFS benefit from olaparib was not restricted to patients with *BRCA* mutation–associated ovarian cancer. No unexpected toxicities were seen.

Overall, these data provide clinical evidence for single-agent PARP inhibitor activity in cancers with BRCAness phenotype even without *BRCA* mutations.

COMBINATION OF PARP INHIBITORS WITH CHEMOTHERAPY

Radiotherapy and chemotherapeutic agents such as platinum compounds confer their antitumor effects by inducing DNA damage, which, if not repaired, triggers cell death. As PARP inhibitors could impair DNA repair mechanisms, the potential of PARP inhibitors as a chemosensitizer or radiosensitizer has been raised. Consequently, preclinical studies have shown activity of a PARP inhibitor in combination with DNA-damaging agents such as alkylating agents (such as cyclophosphamide and temozolomide), type I topoisomerase inhibitors (such as irinotecan and topotecan), platinum agents (such as cisplatin and carboplatin), and anthracyclines. These combinations are being tested clinically with various PARP inhibitors as discussed later.

Rucaparib (CO338, AG014699, PF-01367338)

Rucaparib was the first PARP inhibitor to undergo a phase 1 trial as an enhancing agent for chemotherapy. A phase 1 study of the combination of AG014699 with temozolomide in unselected advanced solid tumors determined that the recommended phase 2 dose was intravenous rucaparib, 12 mg/m^2/d, and oral temozolomide, 200 mg/m^2/d, for 5 days every 28 days. At this dose, PARP was inhibited by more than 70% in PBMC. DLTs included myelosuppression at the dose level of 18 mg/m^2/d and temozolomide 200 mg/m^2/d.[50] A phase 2 study was conducted with rucaparib and temozolomide in untreated metastatic melanoma.[64] However, significantly more myelosuppression was observed than was predicted from the phase 1 study. Of 46 patients treated, grade 4 thrombocytopenia and neutropenia were seen in 30% and 41% of patients in cycle 1, respectively, resulting in 39% dose reduction and/or dose delay. Given that severe myelosuppression is uncommon with temozolomide monotherapy, it has been suggested that PARP inhibitors may inhibit the repair of DNA damage from temozolomide in bone marrow stem cells. Partial response was seen in 18% of the 40 evaluable patients.

Olaparib (AZD2281, KU-0059436)

Several phase 1 trials of olaparib combined with chemotherapy have been reported in *BRCA*-mutant cancer or sporadic cancer. A phase 1 study of olaparib combined with carboplatin in *BRCA1/2*-mutated ovarian or breast cancer initially evaluated the continuous schedule of olaparib, 100 or 200 mg twice daily, on days 1 to 21 plus carboplatin AUC 3 on days 1 or 2 every 3 weeks.[65] However, the schedule was changed to intermittent administration of olaparib (olaparib, 200 or 400 mg twice daily, on days 1 to 7 plus carboplatin AUC 3, 4, or 5 on days 1 or 2 every 3 weeks) because of thrombocytopenia and delayed recovery of neutropenia. The recommended dose was olaparib, 400 mg twice daily, on days 1 to 7 with carboplatin AUC 5 on days 1 or 2 every 3 weeks. Main toxicity was grade 3/4 marrow suppression. Of 27 evaluable patients, the response rate was 39% in ovarian cancer and 74% in breast cancer, and the clinical benefit rate was 83% and 100%, respectively. A phase 1 study of olaparib with topotecan in advanced solid tumors reported prolonged thrombocytopenia and neutropenia. Although the MTD was established as topotecan, 1.0 mg/m²/d, on days 1 to 3 plus olaparib, 100 mg twice daily, on days 1 to 21 every 3 weeks, no responses were seen. The investigators did not recommend further development of this combination. When olaparib was combined with weekly paclitaxel in patients with metastatic TNBC, significant myelosuppression required granulocyte colony–stimulating factor as secondary prophylaxis. The confirmed partial response rate was 37%. A phase 1 trial of the combination of olaparib and dacarbazine also showed higher incidence of neutropenia and delayed recovery than observed with single-agent dacarbazine.[66] The optimal tolerated dose was defined as olaparib, 100 mg twice daily, on days 1 to 7 and dacarbazine, 600 mg/m², on day 1 every 3 weeks. Although 2 patients with melanoma had partial responses in the initial dose escalation phase, there was no response in the dose confirmation cohort enrolling chemonaive patients with melanoma (overall response rate, 5%). In a phase 1 study of olaparib combined with gemcitabine/cisplatin, the MTD was olaparib, 100 mg once a day, on days 1 to 4; cisplatin, 50 mg/m², on day 3; and gemcitabine, 400 mg/m², on days 3 and 10 every 3 weeks or olaparib 100 mg twice daily on day 1, cisplatin 60 mg/m² on day 1, and gemcitabine 500 mg/m² on days 1 and 8 every 3 weeks.[67] However, these MTDs were still associated with the high incidence of grade 3/4 neutropenia (50%) and thrombocytopenia (17%–50%). Of 21 evaluable patients, 2 (9.5%) had partial responses. Ongoing clinical trials of olaparib in combination with chemotherapy are summarized in **Table 2**.

Veliparib (ABT-888)

Veliparib was initially evaluated in the first nontherapeutic phase 0 clinical trial in oncology that guided the design of subsequent phase 1 trials of veliparib in combination with chemotherapeutic agents.[68] This study suggested that an appropriate phase 1 starting dose of veliparib in combination with DNA-damaging agents is 10 mg twice daily, based on the measured levels of PARP inhibition between paired blood and tumor specimens. In a subsequent phase 1 study of veliparib combined with topotecan for refractory solid tumors and lymphomas, there were 3 DLTs in the 6 patients on dose level 1 (veliparib, 10 mg twice daily, on days 1–7; topotecan, 1.2 mg/m²/d, on days 1–5 in a 3-week cycle).[69] Further dose reduction of topotecan to 0.6 mg/m²/d showed no DLT in 6 patients that was defined as the MTD combined with veliparib, 10 mg twice daily, on days 1 to 5. There was no tumor response. A phase 1 study of the combination of veliparib and weekly irinotecan determined that the MTD was veliparib, 40 mg twice daily, on days 1 to 14 and irinotecan, 100 mg/m², on days 1 and 8 every 3 weeks with DLTs including grade 3/4 fatigue, leukopenia/neutropenia, and diarrhea.[70] Of 30 evaluable patients, 6 (20%) had partial responses and the clinical benefit rate was 63%. A phase 1 study of veliparib in combination with a fixed dosing of doxorubicin (60 mg/m²) and cyclophosphamide (600 mg/m²) for breast cancer and other solid tumors showed that the MTD was veliparib, 100 mg, twice daily on days 1 to 4 in a 3-week cycle.[71] The most common toxicities were fatigue and myelosuppression. There were 3 partial responses in 5 BRCA mutation carriers (60%), and 79% of the patients with breast cancer had clinical benefit.

In contrast, when veliparib was combined with metronomic oral cyclophosphamide in a phase 1 study for refractory solid tumor and lymphoma, myelosuppression was

Phase	Regimen	Disease	Study Designation
2	Olaparib	Advanced solid tumor with *BRCA1/2* mutation	NCT01078662
1	Olaparib + cisplatin	Advanced solid tumor	NCT00782574
1	Olaparib + gemcitabine	Advanced pancreatic cancer	NCT00515866
1	Olaparib + liposomal doxorubicin	Advanced solid tumor	NCT00819221
1	Olaparib + irinotecan	Advanced colorectal cancer	NCT00535353
1	Olaparib + paclitaxel vs olaparib + carboplatin vs olaparib + paclitaxel/carboplatin	Advanced TNBC or ovarian cancer	NCT00516724
1	Olaparib + temozolomide	Advanced glioblastoma	NCT01390571
1	Group 1: olaparib on days 1–7 + carboplatin on day 1 every 3 wk Group 2A: olaparib on days 1–7 + carboplatin on day 8 in cycle 1 followed by carboplatin on day 1 + olaparib on days 2–8 in cycle 2 Group 2B: reverse sequence	Refractory gynecologic cancers such as breast, ovarian, fallopian, primary peritoneal, uterine, cervical cancer, or malignant mixed müllerian tumors	NCT01237067
1/2	Phase 1: irinotecan/cisplatin/ mitomycin (ICM) Phase 2: IC/ICM ± olaparib	Advanced pancreatic cancer	NCT01296763
2	Olaparib + paclitaxel vs placebo + paclitaxel	Advanced gastric cancer	NCT01063517
2	Paclitaxel/carboplatin ± olaparib	Advanced ovarian cancer	NCT01081951

Table 2
Ongoing clinical trials of olaparib

Abbreviations: BRCA, breast cancer susceptible gene; TNBC, triple-negative breast cancer.
Data from ClinicalTrials.gov, National Library of Medicine, Bethesda, MD.

not prominent.[72] The MTD was veliparib, 60 mg, and cyclophosphamide, 50 mg, both given once a day. Confirmed partial responses were observed in 3 among 18 patients (17%); 2 *BRCA*-mutant ovarian cancers and 1 TNBC. At present, a phase 2 study of this regimen is ongoing in patients with *BRCA*-mutant ovarian cancer, HGSOC/ TNBC, or low-grade non-Hodgkin lymphoma. A phase 1 study of veliparib combined with intravenous cyclophosphamide for advanced solid tumor also showed a favorable toxicity profile.[73] DLTs included myelosuppression. The highest dose evaluated so far is 200 mg twice daily on days 1 to 4 with cyclophosphamide, 750 mg/m^2, on day 3 in a 3-week cycle. The most common toxicities were fatigue, anemia, and neutropenia. There was one partial response among 30 patients.

Two phase 2 trials of veliparib with temozolomide have been reported in metastatic breast cancer and colorectal cancer, respectively.[74,75] In both trials, treatment consisted of veliparib, 40 mg, twice daily on days 1 to 7 and temozolomide 150 mg/m^2/d on days 1 to 5 every 4 weeks.[74] The objective response rate was 4.1% and the disease control rate was 22% in these heavily treated patients with a median number of prior chemotherapeutic regimen of 3.5. The median duration of disease control was 22 weeks (range, 15–40 weeks). In the breast cancer study, frequent grade 4 thrombocytopenia led to general decrease of veliparib to 30 mg twice daily with better tolerability.[75] The objective response rate and clinical benefit rate was 37.5% and 62.5%, respectively, in *BRCA* mutation carriers (n = 8). The median PFS was 5.5 months (*BRCA* carriers) and 1.8 months (noncarriers) (*P* = .0042). Recently, a randomized phase 2 placebo-controlled study compared temozolomide (150 mg/m^2/d for 5 days) plus veliparib (20 or 40 mg twice daily on days 1-7) every 4 weeks versus temozolomide plus placebo in patients with advanced melanoma.[76] The primary end point of PFS showed 113 days in the 20-mg group versus 110 days in the 40-mg group versus 60 days in the placebo group; these trends were not significant. Grade 3/4 adverse events, mainly of hematological toxicities, were seen in 38% (placebo), 54% (veliparib 20 mg), and 57% (veliparib 40 mg) of patients. Ongoing clinical trials of veliparib in combination with chemotherapy or chemoradiotherapy are summarized in **Tables 3** and **4**.

MK4827

MK4827 had been combined with carboplatin with/without paclitaxel or PLD and temozolomide (**Table 4**).

BMN 673

Two single agent phase I trial in solid tumor and hematologic malignancies are ongoing at this time (see **Table 4**).

CEP-9722

Two phase 1 studies of CEP-9722 in combination with temozolomide and gemcitabine/cisplatin, respectively, in patients with advanced solid tumors are ongoing (see **Table 4**).

E7016/GPI 21016

A phase 1 study of E7016 combined with temozolomide in patients with advanced solid tumors is ongoing (see **Table 4**).

BIOMARKERS FOR EFFICACY OF PARP INHIBITORS
Biomarkers for PARP Inhibitor Sensitivity

Potential biomarkers of PARP inhibitor sensitivity in sporadic cancer include *BRCA1/2* somatic mutation, *BRCA1* promoter methylation, *BRCA1* suppression in the absence of methylation, phosphatase and tensin homolog (*PTEN*) deficiency, *ATM* mutation, *MRE11*-dominant negative mutations in MMR–deficient cancers, and *FANCF* promoter methylation. PTEN is a tumor suppressor gene that inactivates the PI3K/AKT survival pathway, and its loss of function is a frequent event in a variety of human cancers, occurring through mutations, deletions, or promoter hypermethylation.[77,78] Preclinical data have demonstrated that PTEN has a role in maintaining chromosomal stability and controlling DNA DSB repair by regulating the transcription of RAD51, and PTEN-deficient tumor cells are defective in HR repair and sensitive to PARP inhibitors such as olaparib and veliparib.[79–83] Of note, it was reported that a patient with PTEN-deficient endometrial adenocarcinoma without *BRCA1* or *BRCA2* mutations had a clear response to olaparib.[84] Future clinical trials are needed to confirm this promising finding.

In addition to these specific molecular defects, there has been an approach to identify unifying biomarkers of HR deficiency that all these diverse mechanisms share. One example is the potential signature of BRCAness that has been reported based on the differences in gene expression between hereditary *BRCA1/2*-related cancers and sporadic cancers.[85,86] These gene expression signatures were associated with responsiveness to DNA-damaging chemotherapy that provides interesting proofs of principle. The other example is to assess the HR pathway competency using

Table 3
Ongoing clinical trials of veliparib

Phase	Regimen	Disease	Study Designation
1	Veliparib	*BRCA1/2*-mutated cancer; platinum-refractory ovarian, fallopian tube, or primary peritoneal cancer; or basal-like breast cancer	NCT00892736
1	Veliparib ± mitomycin	Advanced solid tumor with a defective FA pathway	NCT01017640
1	Veliparib + PLD	Recurrent ovarian cancer, fallopian tube cancer, or primary peritoneal cancer or metastatic breast cancer	NCT01145430
1	Veliparib + gemcitabine	Advanced solid tumor	NCT01154426
1	Veliparib + gemcitabine + cisplatin	Advanced biliary, pancreatic, urothelial, or non–small cell lung cancer	NCT01282333
1	Veliparib + carboplatin	Advanced TNBC or estrogen receptor and/or progesterone receptor (+), HER2 (−) breast cancer with a defective FA pathway	NCT01251874
1	Veliparib + gemcitabine + carboplatin	Advanced solid tumor	NCT01063816
1	Veliparib + weekly paclitaxel + weekly carboplatin	Advanced solid tumors	NCT01281150
1	Veliparib + triweekly paclitaxel + triweekly carboplatin	Patients with hepatic or renal dysfunction and advanced solid tumors	NCT01366144
1	Veliparib + triweekly paclitaxel + triweekly carboplatin	Advanced solid cancer (stratum I), advanced solid cancer with a germline *BRCA1/2* mutation (stratum II)	NCT00535119
1	Veliparib + paclitaxel + carboplatin + bevacizumab	Newly diagnosed stage II–IV ovarian epithelial, fallopian tube, or primary peritoneal carcinoma	NCT00989651
1	Veliparib + cisplatin + vinorelbine	Advanced TNBC and/or *BRCA1/2*-mutant breast cancer	NCT01104259
1	Veliparib + temozolomide	Metastatic castration-resistant prostate cancer	NCT01085422
1	Veliparib + FOLFIRI (irinotecan 150 mg/m² or 180 mg/m²)	Escalation phase: advanced solid tumor / Expansion phase: advanced colorectal cancer	NCT01123876
1/2	Veliparib + triweekly paclitaxel + triweekly cisplatin	Stage IVB, recurrent, or persistent cervix cancer	NCT01281852

Phase	Intervention	Condition	NCT number
1/2	Veliparib + topotecan	Advanced solid tumors (phase 1), relapsed or refractory ovarian cancer or primary peritoneal cancer (phase 2)	NCT01012817
1/2	Veliparib + bendamustine + rituximab	Advanced lymphoma, multiple myeloma, or solid tumors	NCT01326702
2	Veliparib ± carboplatin	*BRCA1/2*-mutant advanced breast cancer	NCT01149083
2	Cyclophosphamide ± veliparib	Estrogen receptor and/or progesterone receptor (+) and HER2 (−) metastatic breast cancer	NCT01351909
2	Cyclophosphamide ± veliparib	*BRCA1/2*-mutant ovarian cancer, primary peritoneal or ovarian high-grade carcinoma, or fallopian tube cancer; TNBC (not responsive to hormone-related therapy); or low-grade non-Hodgkin lymphoma	NCT01306032
2	Veliparib + temozolomide	Advanced solid tumor	NCT01193140
2	Veliparib + temozolomide	Advanced hepatocellular carcinoma progressing following sorafenib or intolerant to sorafenib	NCT01205828
2	Veliparib + temozolomide vs PLD alone	Recurrent high-grade serous ovarian, fallopian tube, or primary peritoneal cancer	NCT01113957
2	Neratinib vs veliparib + carboplatin vs paclitaxel + trastuzumab followed by doxorubicin + cyclophosphamide vs AMG 386	Stage II or III or T4, any N, M0 breast cancer	NCT01042379
1	Veliparib + WBRT	Metastatic brain tumor	NCT00649207
1	Veliparib + LDFWAR	Advanced solid tumor with peritoneal carcinomatosis	NCT01264432
1/2	Veliparib + temozolomide + radiotherapy	Newly diagnosed glioblastoma multiforme	NCT00770471
1/2	Veliparib + chemoradiotherapy with paclitaxel + carboplatin	Unresectable stage III non-small cell lung cancer	NCT01386385

Abbreviations: BRCA, breast cancer susceptible gene; FA, Fanconi anemia; FOLFIRI, 5-fluorouracil/leucovorin/irinotecan; HER2, human epidermal growth factor receptor 2; LDFWAR, low-dose fractionated whole abdominal radiation therapy; PLD, pegylated liposomal doxorubicin; TNBC, triple-negative breast cancer; WBRT, whole brain radiation therapy.
Data from ClinicalTrials.gov, National Library of Medicine, Bethesda, MD.

Table 4
Ongoing clinical trials of MK4827, BMN 673, CEP-9722, or E7016

Phase	Regimen	Disease	Study Designation
1	MK4827	Advanced solid tumor	NCT01226901
1	MK4827	Dose escalation phase: advanced solid tumor (part A). Expansion phase: prostate, recurrent platinum-resistant HGSOC (part B); T-cell prolymphocytic leukemia or chronic lymphocytic leukemia (part C); advanced colorectal, endometrial, triple-negative or estrogen receptor–positive breast cancer, or partially platinum-sensitive epithelial ovarian cancer (part D)	NCT00749502
1	MK4827 + PLD	Advanced solid tumor (part A) and platinum-resistant/refractory HGSOC (part B)	NCT01227941
1	MK4827 + temozolomide	Advanced solid tumor (part A); advanced glioblastoma multiforme or melanoma (part B)	NCT01294735
1	BMN 673	Hematologic malignancies	NCT 01399840
1	BMN 673	Advanced solid tumor	NCT 01286987
1/2	CEP-9722	Advanced solid tumor	NCT01311713
1	CEP-9722 ± temozolomide	Advanced solid tumor	NCT00920595
1	CEP-9722 + gemcitabine + cisplatin	Advanced solid tumor	NCT01345357
1	E7016 + temozolomide	Advanced solid tumor (escalation phase) and glioma (expansion phase)	NCT01127178

Abbreviations: HGSOC, high-grade serous ovarian cancer; PLD, pegylated liposomal doxorubicin.
Data from ClinicalTrials.gov, National Library of Medicine, Bethesda, MD.

surrogate markers, such as RAD51 foci formation on DNA damage.[87] Although these approaches are promising, further assessment and validation is needed for use in the clinical setting.

Biomarkers for PAPR Inhibitor Resistance

Recently, genetic reversion of *BRCA1* or *BRCA2* mutations, which causes restoration of normal *BRCA1* or *BRCA2* protein function, was recognized as a mechanism of acquired resistance to both platinum and PARP inhibitors in *BRCA1*- or *BRCA2*-mutated tumor cells.[88–90] A recent study in 110 patients with ovarian cancer with a *BRCA1/2* mutation has shown that a secondary somatic *BRCA1/2* mutation was found more frequently in recurrent cancer than in primary cancer (28.3% vs 3.1%, $P = .0003$) and in platinum-resistant recurrences than in platinum-sensitive recurrences (46.2% vs 5.3%, $P = .003$).[91] In addition, 12 (92%) of 13 recurrent cancers with secondary mutations were platinum resistant, and 2 of 3 patients with platinum-resistant recurrent cancer with secondary mutations were also refractory to olaparib, although 1 patient responded to veliparib combined with carboplatin/gemcitabine. By contrast, all 3 patients with platinum-resistant recurrent cancer without secondary mutations achieved responses (2 complete responses, 1 partial response) to olaparib ± carboplatin. Larger studies are needed to reveal to what extent this mechanism will drive clinical resistance to

PARP inhibitors in patients with *BRCA1/2*-related cancers. In addition to genetic reversion, recent evidence also suggested a role for P-glycoprotein efflux pump in the development of resistance to olaparib.[92] Other potential resistance mechanisms include the p53 binding protein (53BP1) loss that partially rescues the HR defect in *BRCA1*-deficient cells and reverts their hypersensitivity to DNA-damaging agents.[93,94] Furthermore, 53BP1-deficient *BRCA1^Δ11/Δ11* cells were no longer sensitive to PARP inhibition.[93] The expression of 53BP1 was lost or reduced in subsets of *BRCA1/2*-associated and sporadic TNBC/basal-like breast cancers.[94]

SUMMARY

The use of PARP inhibitors to create synthetic lethality or modulate cytotoxicity may be one of the most exciting developments in cancer research in this decade. This new class of drugs shows promise as a treatment of a wide range of cancers, not just those associated with *BRCA1/2* genetic mutations. The evaluation of PARP inhibitors is being expanded to combined therapy with chemotherapy, radiotherapy, or other molecularly targeted agents and to a variety of treatment settings, including neoadjuvant, adjuvant, or prophylaxis setting. At the same time, many unanswered questions remain about the optimal use of PARP inhibitors. Could a single-agent PARP inhibitor be a possible alternative front-line treatment of *BRCA*-associated cancer or other HR-defective cancer? If PARP inhibitors are to be combined with chemotherapy or radiotherapy, what is the best administration schedule, dose, or chemotherapeutic partner to maximize efficacy while minimizing toxicity? What are robust predictive biomarkers of sensitivity and resistance to PARP inhibitors alone or combined with chemotherapy or radiotherapy? To what extent the PARP enzyme needs to be inhibited for the best efficacy? What creates the differences between the individual agents in the PAPR inhibitor class resulting in distinct toxicity and efficacy profiles? What are the consequences of long-term administration of PARP inhibitor? This question may be especially important because this class moves into the adjuvant setting or for long-term administration in prevention studies in *BRCA* mutation carriers. Carefully designed clinical trials incorporating translational end points are required to get answers about these important challenges.

REFERENCES

1. Fong PC, Boss DS, Yap TA, et al. Inhibition of poly(ADP-ribose) polymerase in tumors from BRCA mutation carriers. N Engl J Med 2009;361(2):123–34.
2. Fong PC, Yap TA, Boss DS, et al. Poly(ADP)-ribose polymerase inhibition: frequent durable responses in BRCA carrier ovarian cancer correlating with platinum-free interval. J Clin Oncol 2010;28(15):2512–9.
3. Tutt A, Robson M, Garber JE, et al. Oral poly(ADP-ribose) polymerase inhibitor olaparib in patients with BRCA1 or BRCA2 mutations and advanced breast cancer: a proof-of-concept trial. Lancet 2010;376(9737):235–44.
4. Audeh MW, Carmichael J, Penson RT, et al. Oral poly(ADP-ribose) polymerase inhibitor olaparib in patients with BRCA1 or BRCA2 mutations and recurrent ovarian cancer: a proof-of-concept trial. Lancet 2010;376(9737):245–51.
5. Hoeijmakers JH. Genome maintenance mechanisms for preventing cancer. Nature 2001;411(6835):366–74.
6. Chan KK, Zhang QM, Dianov GL. Base excision repair fidelity in normal and cancer cells. Mutagenesis 2006;21(3):173–8.
7. Muniandy PA, Liu J, Majumdar A, et al. DNA interstrand crosslink repair in mammalian cells: step by step. Crit Rev Biochem Mol Biol 2010;45(1):23–49.

8. Iyer RR, Pluciennik A, Burdett V, et al. DNA mismatch repair: functions and mechanisms. Chem Rev 2006;106(2):302–23.

9. Peltomaki P. Role of DNA mismatch repair defects in the pathogenesis of human cancer. J Clin Oncol 2003;21(6):1174–9.

10. Walker JR, Corpina RA, Goldberg J. Structure of the Ku heterodimer bound to DNA and its implications for double-strand break repair. Nature 2001;412(6847): 607–14.

11. Ame JC, Spenlehauer C, de Murcia G. The PARP superfamily. Bioessays 2004; 26(8):882–93.

12. Schreiber V, Ame JC, Dolle P, et al. Poly(ADP-ribose) polymerase-2 (PARP-2) is required for efficient base excision DNA repair in association with PARP-1 and XRCC1. J Biol Chem 2002;277(25):23028–36.

13. de Murcia G, Huletsky A, Lamarre D, et al. Modulation of chromatin superstructure induced by poly(ADP-ribose) synthesis and degradation. J Biol Chem 1986;261(15):7011–7.

14. El-Khamisy SF, Masutani M, Suzuki H, et al. A requirement for PARP-1 for the assembly or stability of XRCC1 nuclear foci at sites of oxidative DNA damage. Nucleic Acids Res 2003;31(19):5526–33.

15. Oka S, Kato J, Moss J. Identification and characterization of a mammalian 39-kDa poly(ADP-ribose) glycohydrolase. J Biol Chem 2006;281(2):705–13.

16. Haince JF, McDonald D, Rodrigue A, et al. PARP1-dependent kinetics of recruitment of MRE11 and NBS1 proteins to multiple DNA damage sites. J Biol Chem 2008;283(2):1197–208.

17. Wang M, Wu W, Rosidi B, et al. PARP-1 and Ku compete for repair of DNA double strand breaks by distinct NHEJ pathways. Nucleic Acids Res 2006;34(21): 6170–82.

18. Ame JC, Rolli V, Schreiber V, et al. PARP-2, a novel mammalian DNA damage-dependent poly(ADP-ribose) polymerase. J Biol Chem 1999;274(25):17860–8.

19. Scully R, Chen J, Ochs RL, et al. Dynamic changes of BRCA1 subnuclear location and phosphorylation state are initiated by DNA damage. Cell 1997;90(3):425–35.

20. Esashi F, Galkin VE, Yu X, et al. Stabilization of RAD51 nucleoprotein filaments by the C-terminal region of BRCA2. Nat Struct Mol Biol 2007;14(6):468–74.

21. Moynahan ME, Cui TY, Jasin M. Homology-directed DNA repair, mitomycin-C resistance, and chromosome stability is restored with correction of a BRCA1 mutation. Cancer Res 2001;61(12):4842–50.

22. Tassone P, Di Martino MT, Ventura M, et al. Loss of BRCA1 function increases the antitumor activity of cisplatin against human breast cancer xenografts in vivo. Cancer Biol Ther 2009;8(7):648–53.

23. Narod SA. BRCA mutations in the management of breast cancer: the state of the art. Nat Rev Clin Oncol 2010;7(12):702–7.

24. Tan DS, Rothermundt C, Thomas K, et al. "BRCAness" syndrome in ovarian cancer: a case-control study describing the clinical features and outcome of patients with epithelial ovarian cancer associated with BRCA1 and BRCA2 mutations. J Clin Oncol 2008;26(34):5530–6.

25. Dobzhansky T. Genetics of natural populations. Xiii. Recombination and variability in populations of Drosophila pseudoobscura. Genetics 1946;31(3):269–90.

26. Arnaudeau C, Lundin C, Helleday T. DNA double-strand breaks associated with replication forks are predominantly repaired by homologous recombination involving an exchange mechanism in mammalian cells. J Mol Biol 2001;307(5):1235–45.

27. Farmer H, McCabe N, Lord CJ, et al. Targeting the DNA repair defect in BRCA mutant cells as a therapeutic strategy. Nature 2005;434(7035):917–21.

28. Bryant HE, Schultz N, Thomas HD, et al. Specific killing of BRCA2-deficient tumours with inhibitors of poly(ADP-ribose) polymerase. Nature 2005;434(7035):913–7.

29. Risch HA, McLaughlin JR, Cole DE, et al. Prevalence and penetrance of germline BRCA1 and BRCA2 mutations in a population series of 649 women with ovarian cancer. Am J Hum Genet 2001;68(3):700–10.

30. Pal T, Permuth-Wey J, Betts JA, et al. BRCA1 and BRCA2 mutations account for a large proportion of ovarian carcinoma cases. Cancer 2005;104(12):2807–16.

31. Risch HA, McLaughlin JR, Cole DE, et al. Population BRCA1 and BRCA2 mutation frequencies and cancer penetrances: a kin-cohort study in Ontario, Canada. J Natl Cancer Inst 2006;98(23):1694–706.

32. Eeles RA. Screening for hereditary cancer and genetic testing, epitomized by breast cancer. Eur J Cancer 1999;35(14):1954–62.

33. Langston AA, Malone KE, Thompson JD, et al. BRCA1 mutations in a population-based sample of young women with breast cancer. N Engl J Med 1996;334(3):137–42.

34. Malone KE, Daling JR, Neal C, et al. Frequency of BRCA1/BRCA2 mutations in a population-based sample of young breast carcinoma cases. Cancer 2000;88(6):1393–402.

35. Merajver SD, Pham TM, Caduff RF, et al. Somatic mutations in the BRCA1 gene in sporadic ovarian tumours. Nat Genet 1995;9(4):439–43.

36. Press JZ, De Luca A, Boyd N, et al. Ovarian carcinomas with genetic and epigenetic BRCA1 loss have distinct molecular abnormalities. BMC Cancer 2008;8:17.

37. Hennessy BT, Timms KM, Carey MS, et al. Somatic mutations in BRCA1 and BRCA2 could expand the number of patients that benefit from poly (ADP ribose) polymerase inhibitors in ovarian cancer. J Clin Oncol 2010;28(22):3570–6.

38. Turner N, Tutt A, Ashworth A. Hallmarks of 'BRCAness' in sporadic cancers. Nat Rev Cancer 2004;4(10):814–9.

39. Catteau A, Harris WH, Xu CF, et al. Methylation of the BRCA1 promoter region in sporadic breast and ovarian cancer: correlation with disease characteristics. Oncogene 1999;18(11):1957–65.

40. Esteller M, Silva JM, Dominguez G, et al. Promoter hypermethylation and BRCA1 inactivation in sporadic breast and ovarian tumors. J Natl Cancer Inst 2000;92(7):564–9.

41. Rice JC, Ozcelik H, Maxeiner P, et al. Methylation of the BRCA1 promoter is associated with decreased BRCA1 mRNA levels in clinical breast cancer specimens. Carcinogenesis 2000;21(9):1761–5.

42. Baldwin RL, Nemeth E, Tran H, et al. BRCA1 promoter region hypermethylation in ovarian carcinoma: a population-based study. Cancer Res 2000;60(19):5329–33.

43. Drew Y, Mulligan EA, Vong WT, et al. Therapeutic potential of poly(ADP-ribose) polymerase inhibitor AG014699 in human cancers with mutated or methylated BRCA1 or BRCA2. J Natl Cancer Inst 2011;103(4):334–46.

44. Hughes-Davies L, Huntsman D, Ruas M, et al. EMSY links the BRCA2 pathway to sporadic breast and ovarian cancer. Cell 2003;115(5):523–35.

45. Taniguchi T, Tischkowitz M, Ameziane N, et al. Disruption of the Fanconi anemia-BRCA pathway in cisplatin-sensitive ovarian tumors. Nat Med 2003;9(5):568–74.

46. McCabe N, Turner NC, Lord CJ, et al. Deficiency in the repair of DNA damage by homologous recombination and sensitivity to poly(ADP-ribose) polymerase inhibition. Cancer Res 2006;66(16):8109–15.

47. Bryant HE, Helleday T. Inhibition of poly (ADP-ribose) polymerase activates ATM which is required for subsequent homologous recombination repair. Nucleic Acids Res 2006;34(6):1685–91.

48. Menear KA, Adcock C, Boulter R, et al. 4-[3-(4-cyclopropanecarbonylpiperazine-1-carbonyl)-4-fluorobenzyl]-2H-phthalazin-1-one: a novel bioavailable inhibitor of poly(ADP-ribose) polymerase-1. J Med Chem 2008;51(20):6581–91.

49. Penning TD, Zhu GD, Gandhi VB, et al. Discovery of the Poly(ADP-ribose) polymerase (PARP) inhibitor 2-[(R)-2-methylpyrrolidin-2-yl]-1H-benzimidazole-4-carboxamide (ABT-888) for the treatment of cancer. J Med Chem 2009;52(2):514–23.

50. Plummer R, Jones C, Middleton M, et al. Phase I study of the poly(ADP-ribose) polymerase inhibitor, AG014699, in combination with temozolomide in patients with advanced solid tumors. Clin Cancer Res 2008;14(23):7917–23.

51. Mendeleyev J, Kirsten E, Hakam A, et al. Potential chemotherapeutic activity of 4-iodo-3-nitrobenzamide. Metabolic reduction to the 3-nitroso derivative and induction of cell death in tumor cells in culture. Biochem Pharmacol 1995;50(5):705–14.

52. Bauer PI, Mendeleyeva J, Kirsten E, et al. Anti-cancer action of 4-iodo-3-nitrobenzamide in combination with buthionine sulfoximine: inactivation of poly(ADP-ribose) polymerase and tumor glycolysis and the appearance of a poly(ADP-ribose) polymerase protease. Biochem Pharmacol 2002;63(3):455–62.

53. O'Shaughnessy J, Schwartzberg LS, Danso MA, et al. A randomized phase III study of iniparib (BSI-201) in combination with gemcitabine/carboplatin (G/C) in metastatic triple-negative breast cancer (TNBC). J Clin Oncol 2011;29(Suppl 15) [abstract: 1007].

54. Ji J, Lee MP, Kadota M, et al. Pharmacodynamic and pathway analysis of three presumed inhibitors of poly (ADP-ribose) polymerase: ABT-888, AZD2281, and BSI201 [abstract 4527]. In: Programs and abstracts of the 102nd Annual Meeting of American Association for Cancer Research. Orlando, April 2–6, 2011.

55. Maegley KA, Bingham P, Tatlock JH, et al. All PARP inhibitors are not equal: an in vitro mechanistic comparison of PF-01367338 to iniparib. J Clin Oncol 2011;29(Suppl 15) [abstract: e13576].

56. Kaye S, Kaufman B, Lubinski J, et al. Phase II study of the oral PARP inhibitor olaparib (AZD2281) versus liposomal doxorubicin in ovarian cancer patients with BRCA1 and/or BRCA2 mutations. Ann Oncol 2010;21(Suppl 8):viii304 [abstract: 971O].

57. Jones P, Altamura S, Boueres J, et al. Discovery of 2-{4-[(3S)-piperidin-3-yl]phenyl}-2H-indazole-7-carboxamide (MK-4827): a novel oral poly(ADP-ribose) polymerase (PARP) inhibitor efficacious in BRCA-1 and -2 mutant tumors. J Med Chem 2009;52(22):7170–85.

58. Schelman WR, Sandhu SK, Moreno Garcia V, et al. First-in-human trial of a poly (ADP)-ribose polymerase (PARP) inhibitor MK-4827 in advanced cancer patients with antitumor activity in BRCA-deficient tumors and sporadic ovarian cancers. J Clin Oncol 2011;29(Suppl 15) [abstract: 3102].

59. Drew Y, Ledermann JA, Jones A, et al. Phase II trial of the poly(ADP-ribose) polymerase (PARP) inhibitor AG-014699 in BRCA 1 and 2-mutated, advanced ovarian and/or locally advanced or metastatic breast cancer. J Clin Oncol 2011;29(Suppl 15) [abstract: 3104].

60. Sorlie T, Tibshirani R, Parker J, et al. Repeated observation of breast tumor subtypes in independent gene expression data sets. Proc Natl Acad Sci U S A 2003;100(14):8418–23.

61. Foulkes WD, Smith IE, Reis-Filho JS. Triple-negative breast cancer. N Engl J Med 2010;363(20):1938–48.

62. Gelmon KA, Tischkowitz M, Mackay H, et al. Olaparib in patients with recurrent high-grade serous or poorly differentiated ovarian carcinoma or triple-negative

breast cancer: a phase 2, multicentre, open-label, non-randomised study. Lancet Oncol 2011;12(9):852–61.

63. Ledermann JA, Harter P, Gourley C, et al. Phase II randomized placebo-controlled study of olaparib (AZD2281) in patients with platinum-sensitive relapsed serous ovarian cancer (PSR SOC). J Clin Oncol 2011;29(Suppl 15) [abstract: 5003].

64. Plummer R, Lorigan P, Evans J, et al. First and final report of a phase II study of the poly(ADP-ribose) polymerase (PARP) inhibitor, AG014699, in combination with temozolomide (TMZ) in patients with metastatic malignant melanoma (MM). J Clin Oncol 2006;24(Suppl 18) [abstract: 8013].

65. Lee J, Annunziata CM, Minasian LM, et al. Phase I study of the PARP inhibitor olaparib (O) in combination with carboplatin (C) in BRCA1/2 mutation carriers with breast (Br) or ovarian (Ov) cancer (Ca). J Clin Oncol 2011;29(Suppl 15) [abstract: 2520].

66. Khan OA, Gore M, Lorigan P, et al. A phase I study of the safety and tolerability of olaparib (AZD2281, KU0059436) and dacarbazine in patients with advanced solid tumours. Br J Cancer 2011;104(5):750–5.

67. Giaccone G, Rajan A, Kelly RJ, et al. A phase I combination study of olaparib (AZD2281; KU-0059436) and cisplatin (C) plus gemcitabine (G) in adults with solid tumors. J Clin Oncol 2010;28(Suppl 15) [abstract: 3027].

68. Kummar S, Kinders R, Gutierrez ME, et al. Phase 0 clinical trial of the poly (ADP-ribose) polymerase inhibitor ABT-888 in patients with advanced malignancies. J Clin Oncol 2009;27(16):2705–11.

69. Kummar S, Chen A, Ji J, et al. Phase I study of PARP inhibitor ABT-888 in combination with topotecan in adults with refractory solid tumors and lymphomas. Cancer Res 2011;71(17):5626–34.

70. LoRusso P, Ji JJ, Li J, et al. Phase I study of the safety, pharmacokinetics (PK), and pharmacodynamics (PD) of the poly(ADP-ribose) polymerase (PARP) inhibitor veliparib (ABT-888; V) in combination with irinotecan (CPT-11; Ir) in patients (pts) with advanced solid tumors. J Clin Oncol 2011;29(Suppl 15) [abstract: 3000].

71. Tan AR, Toppmeyer D, Stein MN, et al. Phase I trial of veliparib, (ABT-888), a poly(ADP-ribose) polymerase (PARP) inhibitor, in combination with doxorubicin and cyclophosphamide in breast cancer and other solid tumors. J Clin Oncol 2011; 29(Suppl 15) [abstract: 3041].

72. Kummar S, Chen AP, Ji JJ, et al. A phase I study of ABT-888 (A) in combination with metronomic cyclophosphamide (C) in adults with refractory solid tumors and lymphomas. J Clin Oncol 2010;28(Suppl 15) [abstract: 2605].

73. Tan AR, Gibbon D, Stein MN, et al. Preliminary results of a phase I trial of ABT-888, a poly(ADP-ribose) polymerase (PARP) inhibitor, in combination with cyclophosphamide. J Clin Oncol 2010;28(Suppl 15) [abstract: 3000].

74. Pishvaian MJ, Slack R, Witkiewicz A, et al. A phase II study of the PARP inhibitor ABT-888 plus temozolomide in patients with heavily pretreated, metastatic colorectal cancer. J Clin Oncol 2011;29(Suppl 15) [abstract: 3502].

75. Isakoff SJ, Overmoyer B, Tung NM, et al. A phase II trial of the PARP inhibitor veliparib (ABT888) and temozolomide for metastatic breast cancer. J Clin Oncol 2010;28(Suppl 15) [abstract: 1019].

76. Middleton M, Friedlander P, Hamid O, et al. Efficacy of veliparib (ABT-888) plus temozolomide versus temozolomide alone: a randomized, double-blind, placebo-controlled trial in patients with metastatic melanoma [abstract: 13LBA]. In: Programs and abstracts of the 36th European Society for Medical Oncology Congress. Stockholm, September 23–27, 2011.

77. Li J, Yen C, Liaw D, et al. PTEN, a putative protein tyrosine phosphatase gene mutated in human brain, breast, and prostate cancer. Science 1997;275(5308):1943–7.
78. Keniry M, Parsons R. The role of PTEN signaling perturbations in cancer and in targeted therapy. Oncogene 2008;27(41):5477–85.
79. Shen WH, Balajee AS, Wang J, et al. Essential role for nuclear PTEN in maintaining chromosomal integrity. Cell 2007;128(1):157–70.
80. Gupta A, Yang Q, Pandita RK, et al. Cell cycle checkpoint defects contribute to genomic instability in PTEN deficient cells independent of DNA DSB repair. Cell Cycle 2009;8(14):2198–210.
81. Mendes-Pereira AM, Martin SA, Brough R, et al. Synthetic lethal targeting of PTEN mutant cells with PARP inhibitors. EMBO Mol Med 2009;1(6–7):315–22.
82. Dedes KJ, Wetterskog D, Mendes-Pereira AM, et al. PTEN deficiency in endometrioid endometrial adenocarcinomas predicts sensitivity to PARP inhibitors. Sci Transl Med 2010;2(53):53ra75.
83. McEllin B, Camacho CV, Mukherjee B, et al. PTEN loss compromises homologous recombination repair in astrocytes: implications for glioblastoma therapy with temozolomide or poly(ADP-ribose) polymerase inhibitors. Cancer Res 2010;70(13):5457–64.
84. Forster MD, Dedes KJ, Sandhu S, et al. Treatment with olaparib in a patient with PTEN-deficient endometrioid endometrial cancer. Nat Rev Clin Oncol 2011;8(5):302–6.
85. Konstantinopoulos PA, Spentzos D, Karlan BY, et al. Gene expression profile of BRCAness that correlates with responsiveness to chemotherapy and with outcome in patients with epithelial ovarian cancer. J Clin Oncol 2010;28(22):3555–61.
86. Rodriguez AA, Makris A, Wu MF, et al. DNA repair signature is associated with anthracycline response in triple negative breast cancer patients. Breast Cancer Res Treat 2010;123(1):189–96.
87. Mukhopadhyay A, Elattar A, Cerbinskaite A, et al. Development of a functional assay for homologous recombination status in primary cultures of epithelial ovarian tumor and correlation with sensitivity to poly(ADP-ribose) polymerase inhibitors. Clin Cancer Res 2010;16(8):2344–51.
88. Edwards SL, Brough R, Lord CJ, et al. Resistance to therapy caused by intragenic deletion in BRCA2. Nature 2008;451(7182):1111–5.
89. Sakai W, Swisher EM, Karlan BY, et al. Secondary mutations as a mechanism of cisplatin resistance in BRCA2-mutated cancers. Nature 2008;451(7182):1116–20.
90. Swisher EM, Sakai W, Karlan BY, et al. Secondary BRCA1 mutations in BRCA1-mutated ovarian carcinomas with platinum resistance. Cancer Res 2008;68(8):2581–6.
91. Norquist B, Wurz KA, Pennil CC, et al. Secondary somatic mutations restoring BRCA1/2 predict chemotherapy resistance in hereditary ovarian carcinomas. J Clin Oncol 2011;29(22):3008–15.
92. Rottenberg S, Jaspers JE, Kersbergen A, et al. High sensitivity of BRCA1-deficient mammary tumors to the PARP inhibitor AZD2281 alone and in combination with platinum drugs. Proc Natl Acad Sci U S A 2008;105(44):17079–84.
93. Bunting SF, Callen E, Wong N, et al. 53BP1 inhibits homologous recombination in Brca1-deficient cells by blocking resection of DNA breaks. Cell 2010;141(2):243–54.
94. Bouwman P, Aly A, Escandell JM, et al. 53BP1 loss rescues BRCA1 deficiency and is associated with triple-negative and BRCA-mutated breast cancers. Nat Struct Mol Biol 2010;17(6):688–95.

Role of Histone Deacetylase Inhibitors in the Treatment of Lymphomas and Multiple Myeloma

Jasmine Zain, MD

KEYWORDS

- Histone deacetylase inhibitors • Lymphoma • Multiple myeloma
- Epigenetic therapy

KEY POINTS

- Histone deacetylase inhibitors (HDACI) are epigenetic agents that affect the acetylation and deacetylation status of histones and other proteins, resulting in effects on gene expression and other important cellular functions.
- Epigenetic deregulation has been demonstrated in the pathogenesis of all types of lymphoma.
- HDACI as single agents have shown remarkable clinical activity in lymphomas, especially T cell lymphomas.
- The mechanism of the antilymphoma activity of HDACI is unknown.
- HDACI can be administered both orally and intravenously. They are well tolerated in the clinical setting, with a manageable side effect profile.
- Combining HDACI with other anticancer therapies, including cytotoxic therapies and targeted agents, is a promising new approach to the treatment of lymphomas.

Epigenetic processes are a means of affecting gene expression without altering the DNA nucleic acid sequence.[1–3] They are implicated in carcinogenesis, and epigenetic modification is an area of intense oncologic research for anticancer therapies in various human malignancies.[4] There are 3 fundamental modification processes that are of biologic significance in oncology: (1) acetylation and deacetylation of histones catalyzed by histone acetyl transferases (HATs) and histone deacetylases (HDACs); (2) genome methylation of CpG islands controlled by methylation and demethylation enzymes; and (3) small silencing RNA (siRNA)[5–7] that blocks gene expression. From a clinical perspective, biologic agents that modify the acetylation status of histones are important in the treatment of lymphoid malignancies. Presently, 2 HDACIs,

Division of Hematologic Malignancies and Medical Oncology, NYU Langone Medical Center, 7th Floor, 160 East 34th Street, New York, NY 10016, USA
E-mail address: Jasmine.zain@nyumc.org

Hematol Oncol Clin N Am 26 (2012) 671–704
doi:10.1016/j.hoc.2012.01.006
0889-8588/12/$ – see front matter
hemonc.theclinics.com

vorinostat and romidepsin, are approved for the treatment of relapsed and refractory cutaneous T cell lymphomas (CTCL),[8,9] and romidepsin is also approved for the treatment of relapsed and refractory peripheral T cell lymphomas (PTCL).[10]

Histone acetyl modifications occur in the context of nucleosomes, that are recurring packaging structures of 146 base pairs of DNA wrapped around a core of 8 histone proteins.[11] The amino end of these histone proteins extends outwards and can be modified by chemical process like acetylation, methylation, and phosphorylation modulated by the respective set of opposing enzymes that control these chemical reactions. By affecting their secondary structure, these modifications change the spatial relationship of the histone proteins, with the DNA strand making it more or less poised for the transcription machinery to reach the DNA strand and start the process of gene transcription and protein expression. Specifically, acetylation of the ε-amino moiety on the lysine tails of histones leads to an open or transcriptionally active state of chromatin allowing transcription to proceed. In contrast, deacetylation of lysine results in a closed, condensed chromatin that prevents access of the transcription machinery to the DNA strand, thus silencing transcription. These reactions are catalyzed by 2 major classes of enzymes, referred to as HATs and HDACs. There is another class of enzymes, called histone deacetylase inhibitors (HDACIs), which can block the function of HDACs by binding to and inactivating the catalytically active pocket of HDACs.[12] This prevents or reverses the deacetylated state of the histone and promotes transcription just like HATs. However, HDACIs are distinct from HATs and to date several compounds have been identified as having HDACI-like properties. They have therapeutic potential as anticancer agents as discussed below. There are other posttranslational modifications that can affect lysine and other amino acid residues on histones, as well as other cellular proteins, and secondarily affect their function. These modifications include methylation, ubiquitinylation, phosphorylation, glycosylation, and sumoylation. The proteins affected include, but are not limited to, transcription factors like p53, E2F, c-Myc, nuclear factor kB(NF-kB), hypoxia inducible factor (HIF-1a), estrogen, and androgen receptor complexes; DNA repair enzymes like Ku70; heat shock proteins (HSP) like HSP-90; signaling pathway intermediaries like signal transducer and activation of transcription 3 (STAT 3); and structural proteins like α-tubulin.[13] There are several reviews on epigenetic and posttranslational modification. This article focuses on the emerging role of HDACIs in the treatment of lymphomas and multiple myeloma (MM).

BIOLOGY OF HDACs

More than 18 different HDACs have been identified to date based on their homology to yeast proteins,[14] as shown in **Table1**. Class I, II, and IV HDACs require Zn^{2+} as a cofactor in their active site and are generally inhibited by pan-HDACI, but data are now emerging regarding the newer HDACIs that have selective activity against specific isoenzymes (eg, tubacin is an HDACI that only blocks the action of HDAC6). Class III HDACs, also known as sirutins, are homologous to the yeast Sir 2 protein[15] and require nicotinamide adenine dinucleotide (NAD+) as a coenzyme and are not affected by pan-HDACI. To date, there are no data to suggest that inhibiting one HDAC rather than another has any clinical benefit. The clinical significance of selective HDACs inhibition remains unclear.

BIOLOGY OF HDACI

HDACIs are classified into 4 structural groups that vary in their potency and their ability to block various classes of HDACs, as shown in **Table 2**. Besides the effects of HDAC

Table 1
Classification of HDACs and their properties

Class	Yeast Homologous Protein	HDAC Enzymes	Cellular Location	Unique Domains	Required Cofactor
I[147]					
1a	Rpd3	1,2	Nucleus	Ubiquitously expressed	Zn^{2+}
1b		3			
1c		8			
II[14]					
IIa	Hda1	4,5,7	Shuttles between nucleus and cytoplasm	—	Zn^{2+}
IIb[148]		6,10	Shuttles between nucleus and cytoplasm, contain 2 deacetylase domains, HDAC6 has α tubule deacetylase domain	—	Zn^{2+}
III[14]	Sir2	1,2,3,4,5,6,7	Deacetylase nonhistones and transcription factors (p53)	—	NAD+
IV[149]		11	—	—	Zn^{2+}

Abbreviations: Zn^{2+}, Zinc; NAD+, Nicotine adenine dinucleotide.

inhibition on the acetylation status of histones, these enzymes can affect other cellular proteins, which can lead to a myriad of biologic effects downstream. Hence they should more appropriately be called protein deacetylase inhibitors. Some of the salient biologic effects of HDACI that have been observed in vitro include[1,13,16–18] (1) cell cycle arrest in the G1-M, G2-M phase; (2) induction of apoptosis mediated by effects on proapoptotic and antiapoptotic mechanisms for cell death affecting both the extrinsic and intrinsic apoptotic pathways; (3) inhibition of angiogenesis; (4) increased production of reactive oxygen species (ROS) and their effects on apoptosis; (5) acetylation of tubulin and disruption of aggresome formation; (6) changes in α tubulin affecting cell motility and differentiation; (7) effects on tumor immunity via effects on T cell receptor function, cytokine milieu of immune effector cells, as well as direct upregulation of proteins on malignant cells that enhance cellular recognition by antigen presenting cells (APCs) and other immune effectors. **Table 3** highlights the mechanistic pathways and proteins that are affected by HDACIs leading to the effects listed earlier. In summary, modulation of histones and other proteins alter pathways that promote proliferation, angiogenesis, differentiation, and survival in cancer cells.

RATIONALE FOR ACTIVITY IN LYMPHOID MALIGNANCIES

HDACIs have shown efficacy against the treatment of lymphomas, and T cell lymphomas in particular. From a mechanistic perspective, it has been difficult to assign a mode of action of this class of drugs to any lymphoma, let alone CTCL or PTCL. Pharmacodynamic studies have demonstrated histone acetylation in peripheral blood mononuclear cells as well as[19] tumor tissue from patients with T cell lymphoma following treatment with HDACIs; however, there is no correlation of this with clinical

Table 2
Classification of HDACI and their properties

HDACI Class Potency in Vitro (IC_{50})	Compounds	Isoenzyme Selectivity	Pharmacologic Profile
Short-chain fatty acids (mM)	Valproic acid[150]	Class I, IIa (1, 2, 3, 8, 4, 5, 7)	Short plasma half-life, rapid metabolism, nonspecific mode of action
	Phenylbutyrate[151]	Class I, IIa (1, 2, 3, 8, 4, 5, 7)	
Hydroxamic acids (nM)	Vorinostat (SAHA)[151]	Class I, II HDAC (1, 2, 3, 8, 4, 5, 6, 7, 9, 10)	—
	Belinostat (PXD 101)[151]	Class I, II HDAC (1, 2, 3, 8, 4, 5, 6, 7, 9, 10)	
	LAQ824[151]	Class I, II HDAC (1, 2, 3, 8, 4, 5, 6, 7, 9, 10)	
	Panobinostat (LBH589)[151]	Class I, II HDAC (1, 2, 3, 8, 4, 5, 6, 7, 9, 10)	
	Tubacin[24]	Class IIb HDAC 6: no effect on histones, hyperacetylates α-tubulin	
Benzamides (μM)	MGCD0103[152]	Class I HDAC (1, 2, 3, 8)	—
	CI-994	—	
	SK-7041	—	
Cyclic peptides (nM)	Romidepsin[153] MS-275[152]	HDAC 1, 2 > 4, 6 Inhibits class >HDAC3 Does not affect HDAC 6, 8	—
Sirtuin inhibitors (mM)	Niacinamide Sirtinol	Class II specific HDACI	—

Abbreviations: IC_{50}, inhibitory concentration of 50%; mM, millimolar; nM, nano molar; μM, micromolar.

response to these agents. Given the pleiotropic effects of HDACI on cellular function, it is important to delineate the mechanism of their antilymphoma effects and to link them to known pathways in lymphomagenesis. The known information is discussed below.

In general, cancer cells show a high level of expression of HDAC isoenzymes and hypoacetylation of histones.[20] This has been shown in comparisons of biopsy samples of lymphomas with normal lymphoid tissue, as well as colon cancer compared with normal colonic epithelium.[21,22] Transformed cells are more sensitive to the effect of HDACI-induced apoptosis in comparison with normal cells. Aberrant expression of HDACs has been shown in lymphoid malignancies.[23] Both cell line data and primary tissue sample studies have supported the differential expression of HDACs across reactive nodes versus lymphoma subtypes mostly involving HDAC2s.[23] How this translates into lymphomagenesis or the sensitivity of these diseases to HDACIs is unclear. More useful data come from patient samples in various lymphoma subtypes. Class 1 HDACs (1, 2, 3, 8) were expressed in all non-Hodgkin lymphoma (NHL) and Hodgkin disease

(HD) cases, whereas class II expression was variable with class 10 being present in all, but HDAC6 being present mainly in B cell lymphomas with plasmacytoid differentiation and HD.[23] The class II HDAC6 has one of the most variable expressions among lymphoid malignancies. It has several unique properties and is known to affect the acetylation status of several proteins including α-tubulin, which is important in the regulation of microtubule stability and function.[24] In addition, it may serve as a molecular chaperone, and plays a role in regulating the aggresome pathway that eliminates misfolded protein similar to the ubiquitin-proteasome pathway. Misfolded proteins are thought to be degraded either via the ubiquitin-proteasome pathway, or possibly through the aggresome.[25] Misfolded proteins destined for the aggresome are thought to be transported along microtubules, via the activity of motor proteins like dynein and adapters proteins like HDAC6, to the microtubule organizing center (MTOC), which in turn transports these proteins to the lysosome for degradation as part of the HDAC6-aggresome pathway. Pharmacologic inhibition of HDAC6 results in hyperacetylation of tubulin and disruption of the aggresome-mediated pathway resulting in apoptosis, which may also explain the mechanistic basis for their synergy with proteasome inhibitors (PI) as discussed below. Overexpression of HDACs may result in the decreased expression of tumor suppressor genes, leading to carcinogenesis. One oncogenic mechanism that may involve aberrant HDAC expression includes the recruitment of HDACs to promoter regions of key genetic sequences.[26–28] It has been shown that specific chromosomal translocations in leukemias lead to expression of oncogenic fusion proteins that form aberrant association with HDACs at promoter site genes and leading to the onset of tumorigenesis. This process is exemplified by the translocation t (15,17) in acute promyelocytic leukemia (APL) that results in the fusion promyelocytic leukemia–retinoic acid receptor (PML-RAR) (APL), that recruits the HDAC3-containing repressor complexes leading to a decreased expression for differentiation-specific genes.[29,30] Similarly chromosomal translocations resulting in the recruitment of class I HDACs to oncogenic promoter sites may underlie the pathogenesis of T cell NHL. Overexpression of repressive transcription factors that interact with HDACs and affect the promoter regions of tumor suppressor genes may also underlie the pathogenesis of hematological malignancies.

Tumor microenvironment and tumor immunology play important parts in the pathogenesis and progression of most lymphomas and HD. HDACs and HDACIs are shown to be important regulators of the immune response and induction of tolerance. Villagra and colleagues[31,32] have demonstrated that overexpression of HDAC11 inhibits interleukin (IL) 10 expression and induces inflammatory antigen presenting cells that are able to prime naïve T cells and restore the responsiveness of tolerant CD4+ cells. Disruption of HDAC11 in APCs leads to the upregulation of expression of the gene encoding for IL-10, leading to impairment of T cell responses, which may contribute to their antilymphoma effects.

There is likely to be further delineation of the effects of various HDACIs on specific cellular functions. There is currently no evidence that inhibiting one HDAC enzyme rather than another is associated with improved activity, or that more selective HDACIs will be associated with an improved adverse effects profile.

Further discussion of HDACIs in specific lymphoma subtypes is presented below.

HDAC Modulation of T Cell Lymphomas

CTCL is the disease with the highest clinical response rates with HDACIs. A large study of the expression of various HDACs in 73 patient samples has correlated this with the clinical behavior.[33] The expression of HDAC1 and HDAC6 was similar between indolent and aggressive cases but the expression of HDAC2 and acetylated histone 4 (H4) was higher in cases of aggressive disease (HDAC2 55.5% aggressive

Table 3
Salient biologic effects of HDACI in vitro

Biologic Effect	Upregulated	Downregulated	Comments
Extrinsic pathway[154] of apoptosis (activation of caspase 8, 3, 6, 7 via external receptors on cell surface. Engages the death-induced signaling complex)	Fas, Apo/TRAIL, death receptors DR4, DR5[154–156]	cFLIP, cIAP2, and XIAP[156]	Independent of p53 status,[157] can overcome the antiapoptotic effect of Bcl-2[158]
Intrinsic pathway of apoptosis (activation of caspase 9, 3 from increased mitochondrial permeability and release of cytochrome C into the cytosol: tightly managed by Bcl-2 family of proteins and the BH3-only proteins)[159,160]	Bax, Bak	Bcl-2, Bcl-xL[159,160]	—
Cell cycle arrest: G1/M, G2/M[161]	P27, p21, p16[37,161]	Cyclin A, cyclin D[161]	Affects the balance between cell cycle regulators and their inhibitors like CDK4, CDK2 causing cell cycle arrest
Inhibits angiogenesis[162,163]	Inhibitors like thrombospondin, von Hippel-Lindau factor	VEGF, hypoxia-inducible factor, surviving in vascular endothelial cells	Decreased vascularity in tumors[37,164]
Transcription regulators	RB, CREB, p 53, BcL-6[165–169]	—	Transcriptional repression of oncogenes
Proliferation	JAK/STAT pathways, b-TGF pathways, p53 (proliferation), Rel A/p65 (NF-kB), Myc family of proteins affecting proliferation, HIF-1 α[141,168,170]	—	Decreased cell growth, inhibition of oncogenes
Signaling mediators	Estrogen receptors, androgens, glucocorticoids[168,171]	—	Decreased growth signals

DNA repair	KU70, FEN1, BRCA1, RAD51[168,172]	—	Increased cellular damage and activation of the apoptotic pathways
Chaperone proteins	Hsp-90, which affects ubiquitinylation and proteasome degradation in the acetylated state[173,174]	—	Effects on proteasomes and aggresomes
Disruption of kinetosome assembly	Effects on the phosphorylation status of premitotic proteins[175]	—	Affects mitosis
ROS[176,177]		—	—
Disruption of aggresomes	Acetylation of tubulin[66]	—	—
Tumor immunity, autophagy[72]	Effects on T cell receptor function, cytokine milieu of immune effector cells, as well as direct upregulation of proteins on malignant cells that enhance cellular recognition by APCs and other immune effectors[178,179]	—	Antitumor immune response

Abbreviations: TRAIL, tumor necrosis factor–related apoptosis-inducing ligand; VEGF, vascular endothelial growth factor.

CTCL vs 15% indolent, acetylated H4 22% aggressive vs 8%). Survival correlated with the overall expression of HDAC6 (hazard ratio 0.39) independently of the CTCL subtype. Other epigenetic markers were also deregulated in CTCL. Van Doorn and colleagues[34,35] compared genome wide DNA methylation screening in samples of CTCL with benign skin disorders. They showed widespread promoter hypermethylation in malignant T cells in CTCL, suggesting epigenetic instability. Specific CpG islands of more than 35 promoter regions were hypermethylated including the tumor suppressor gene BCL7a (B cell chronic lymphocytic leukemia [CLL]/lymphoma) in 48% of samples, PTPRG (protein tyrosine phosphatase receptor γ) gene in 27% of samples and THBS4 gene thrombospondin 4) in 52% of patient samples. These genes were also hypermethylated in the CTCL cell lines but not in the control samples. BCL7, located on chromosome 12q 24.3, is of particular importance because it has been cloned as part of the chromosomal translocations seen in Burkitt lymphoma. Its expression is diminished in mycosis fungoides and PTCL compared with lymphoblastic lymphoma. Other genes that were hypermethylated in CTCL samples compared with normal skin are grouped into the following categories: cell cycle deregulation (p15, p16, p73), defective DNA repair genes (MGMT), apoptosis deregulation (TMSI, p73), and chromosomal instability (CHFR). Hypermethylation of p73 has also been described in nodal B cell lymphomas and natural killer (NK) cell lymphomas. Promoter hypermethylation of P16 has also been noted in CD30+ T cell NHL.

For further mechanistic insight into the action of HDACIs in CTCL, Duvic and colleagues[36] attempted to look at biologic correlatives of HDACI therapy in patients with CTCL by performing serial skin biopsies on patients receiving vorinostat on trial at 2 hours, 4 hours, 8 hours, and then 12 weeks after initiation of treatment. These results established the following: at 4 weeks, 39% of the patient samples showed lymphocyte depletion consistent with the antilymphoma effect of vorinostat. At 4 weeks after therapy, there was a decrease in dermal microvessel density as measured by CD31 positivity on dermal vessels in all patients, but this was significantly lower in responding patients ($P = .001$). Prior cell line data using the CTCL cell line HH indicated that a 24-hour exposure to vorinostat resulted in an 8-fold increase of the anti-angiogenic protein TSP-1 as studied by gene expression array. Consistent with the cell line data, an increase in the dermal TSP-1 staining was noted as early as 2 hours after treatment and was present at 8 weeks in 6 of the 17 paired lesions, including 4 of the 6 responders. Another important protein that is constitutively activated in CTCL is phsophorylated STAT-3 (p-STAT3), which can be detected by immunohistochemical stains either in the nucleus or cytoplasm within both the keratinocytes and the lymphocytes in the lesions. In this study, nuclear staining for p-STAT3 was prominent in both keratinocytes and lymphocytes before the start of therapy. After 4 weeks of therapy with vorinostat, the staining pattern shifted to localization within the cytoplasm (inactive state) in 9 of the 11 patients who responded, whereas this shift was noted in only 3 of the 16 nonresponders. This shift was noted as early as 2 hours after treatment in 4 of 11 paired lesions. Using a similar model of paired skin biopsies, Ellis and colleagues[37] performed gene expression profiles (GEP) and real-time quantitative polymerase chain reaction (PCR) on skin samples from 6 patients with CTCL who were being treated with panobinostat in a phase I trial. These biopsies were obtained at 0, 4, 8, and 24 hours after administration of drug. In this study, there were 10 patients with a diagnosis of relapsed CTCL who were treated at varying dose levels as part of a large phase I study in patients with hematological malignancies. Clinical efficacy was observed in 8 patients (2 achieved a complete remission-CR at both dose levels and 4 patients achieved a pa partial remission-PR, 2 patients had stable disease-SD). The skin biopsy data showed that there was hyperacetylation of histone H3 in tumor cells as early as 4 hours after treatment. Consistent with previous data, histone acetylation within mononuclear cells was shown in both responders and nonresponders up to 48 to 72 hours after the last oral dose, indicating that this could not be used as a therapeutic marker. GEP data from all 6 patients consistently showed that panobinostat induced transcriptional regression of a greater number of genes than activation. The genes that were consistently affected included genes affecting cell cycle (CCNDI, IGFI) apoptosis (septin10, TEF, SORBBS2), angiogenesis (GUCY1A1, ANGPT1), and immune modulation (LAIR1). CDKN1A, which codes for p21, was unregulated in response to HDACI therapy, although in this study upregulation of p21 was not consistently seen in all patients. Of the 23 genes, 4 were further selected for validation by QRT-PCR. These data confirmed downregulation of guanylate cyclase 1A3 (GUCY1A3), the proangiogenic gene ANGPT1a, and the transcription factor COUP-TFII (NR2F20, which is an upstream regulator of ANGPT1 and CCND1). These effects on genes controlling angiogenesis are consistent with the effects noted by Duvic and colleagues[36] and provide confirmation that the antiangiogenic effects of HDACI therapy may be important in their mechanism of action. Bates and colleagues[38] conducted a clinical trial of romidepsin in patients with PTCL and CTCL and also studied the biologic correlates of activity of HDACI in peripheral blood and tumor samples. Predetermined markers of HDACI activity included global histone acetylation and expression of the ABCB1 gene (encodes for the p-glycoprotein called mixed drug resistance) and fetal hemoglobin. The histone acetylation data correlated with pharmakokinetics parameters of area under the curve (AUC) and maximum plasma concentration C_{max}, though there was no correlation between response, histone acetylation, and the expression of either ABCB1 or fetal hemoglobin, indicating the need for improved biomarkers to predict responses with HDACI.

HDACIs an affect signaling patterns from cell surface receptors and, increasingly, T cell malignancies are associated with deregulation of the T cell receptor (TCR) signaling and the immune function. Investigations into the effects of HDACIs, particularly vorinostat have been conducted on TCR signaling and the immune system to delineate more specific mechanisms of action for this agent, as well as to understand the basis for combining it with other agents. Wozniak and colleagues[39] performed extensive studies using GEP on a panel of CTCL cell lines (HH, HUT78, MJ, Myla, SeAx) that were exposed to vorinostat at various time points. The functional analysis of these altered genes revealed pathways including cycle regulators for G1/S transition (E2F, E2F4, cyclin-dependent kinase [CDK] 4, CDK6, cyclin A2, D2, D3, E20), G2/M regulators (CDC23, CD25B, and CHEK4), apoptosis (FAS, IRAK1, CASP6, BID, BCL2), antiproliferative genes, as well as multiple mitogen-activated signaling kinase (MAPK) signaling pathway (MAPK1, MAP3K6, MAP3K14) as described earlier. However, this study also showed changes in genes that are involved in the JAK/STAT signaling pathway, cytokine-cytokine interaction, and expression of receptors belonging to the tumor necrosis factor (TNF) family, all important pathways for survival and differentiation of lymphocytes and the immune system. Vorinostat treatment was shown to shift the expression profile of cytokines, resulting in increased expression of IL-1a, IL-6, and II-9, and a decrease in the expression of IL-4, IL-5, II-10, IL-11, and their associated receptors. Overall, the cytokine profile represented a state that inhibited lymphocyte growth and proliferation and inhibited the TH2-type immune responses. The latter aspect of the drug effect is important because CTCL is a malignancy of activated T cells and is characterized by deregulation of the immune system with reversal of the Th1/Th2 cytokine profile. Vorinostat has also been shown to affect genes that affect cell migration and chemotaxis, which may affect the skin homing properties of malignant cells in CTCL including a decrease in the expression of cytokine genes like CCL1, CCL22, CXCL10, CCR4, and CCR6 and an increase in others like CCR2 and CCR6. There was also some alteration in the expression of members of the JAK/STAT pathway like STAT6, STAT5A, and SOCS2 (decrease), and STAT1, STAT3, and JAK1 (increase).

The TCR[40] signaling pathway is crucial for the survival of T cells and is altered in T cell malignancies. HDACI have been shown to modify this pathway. In general, antigen stimulation engages TCR signaling and induces the recruitment of several kinases including lymphocyte-specific protein tyrosine kinase and a protooncogne named FYN, resulting in phosphorylation of many downstream substrates including CD3 chains, TCR ε chain, and the ζ chain associated with ZAP-70 and phospholipase C. Several downstream pathways that are activated include the PKC, MAPK/p38, Jun pathway and the serine-threonine protein kinase PI3K/AKT pathway, which is important for the survival of T lymphocytes. Treatment with vorinostat induces repression of all genes associated with TCR-related signaling including ZAP-70, CD3DIL4, IL-5, Il-10, and FOXP3, and upregulates FYN, interferon γ, and IL-12A. The effects on TCR signaling were significant and were seen across all cell lines and confirmed by QT-PCR. A decrease in the phosphorylated forms of ZAP-70 and AKT after vorinostat treatment was confirmed by Western blots, confirming the inhibitory effects of this agent on TCR signaling. FYN, which is upregulated by vorinostat, is an tyrosine kinase that belongs to the SRC family kinases that phosphorylates several negative regulators of TCR signaling and ultimately adds to the negative effect of vorinostat on TCR signaling pathways.

In summary, there are many signaling pathways that may be altered in T cell NHL, and HDACI seem to affect them in a myriad of different ways. As this knowledge of this increases, it will be logical to combine multiple targeted agents to optimize the anti-lymphoma effects of these agents.

HDAC Modulation of B Cell Lymphomas

Presently, there are no HDACIs that are approved specifically for the treatment of B cell lymphomas, although there is a strong rationale for their use in B cell malignancies. Mantle cell lymphoma (MCL) is considered to be incurable with known therapies and is a unique disease characterized by marked deregulation of cyclin D1 mediated by the t(11:14) translocation and loss of the CDK inhibitors p21 and p27.[41] Two of the most prominent effects of HDACI are the downregulation of cyclin D1 and upregulation of p21/p27.[42] The clinical data of HDACI in MCL are promising and represent an interesting avenue for combination therapy to treat this disease. Similarly, the association of deregulated BCL-6 in many cases of diffuse large B cell lymphoma (DLBCL) and the effects of HDACI on BCL-6 provide a rationale for the use of HDACI either alone or in combination with other agents in cases of lymphoma in which BCL-6 is over expressed.[43] DLBCL is one of the most common subtypes of NHL and has 2 subtypes based on gene expression analysis.[44] The more common subtype is the germinal center (GC) subtype that overexpresses BCL-6 and CD10, whereas the activated B cell (ABC) subtype expresses activation markers like MUM1 and/or CD138. The ABC subtype has low levels of BCL-6 but high levels of NF-kB and STAT3 and is more chemorefractory, leading to a worse prognosis for the patients. The overexpression of the transcription factor Bcl-6 in DLBCL (GC) from chromosomal translocations leads to recruitment of several HDACs including HDAC1, 2, 4, 5, and 7, which causes the repression of growth-regulatory target genes like p53, p21,[45] and STAT3.[46] Bcl6 can be inhibited by acetylation (through HDACI therapy as well as through inhibition of SIR-2) and leads to the activation and expression of p53, resulting in downstream effects like apoptosis.[45] In ABC subtypes, HDACI can result in decreased expression of STAT3 through its association with HDAC1, resulting in inhibition of activated STAT3 and its dephosphorylation, leading to growth inhibition of this subtype as well. STAT3 is also a transcriptional target of Bcl-6 but, in contrast with p53, it functions as an onco-gene.[23,47] These data provide a rationale for the use of HDACI in DLBCL (both GC and ABC subtypes) and has formed the basis of an ongoing trial using a combination of HDACI and Sir-2 inhibitors for the treatment of GC B cell lymphomas.

HDAC Modulation of Hodgkin's Disease

In vitro data support the potential activity of HDACIs against HD cell lines. Biologically, HD is characterized by a high level of cytokine secretion from the inflammatory infil-trate surrounding the pathognomonic Reed-Sternberg (RS) cells.[48,49] Therapeutic strategies include targeting the malignant cells as well as the inflammatory milieu and cytokines including, IL-5, IL-6, IL-7, IL-9, IL-10, IL-13, and thymus activation–regulated chemokine (TARC/CCL17), which are important in the pathogenesis of HD. Many of these are part of an autocrine loop thought to activate the JAK/STAT pathways, resulting in continual activation of the STAT family of transcription proteins, in particular STAT3 and STAT6. Cytokines including IL-2, IL-6, IL-7, IL-9, IL-10, and IL-15 induce the activation of STAT3, whereas STAT6 is primarily induced by IL4 and IL-13 and may depend on an autocrine IL-13 loop secreted by RS cells.[50] Phosphorylated STAT6 localizes to the nucleus and induces the expression of STAT6 target genes that include TARC and IL-13 as well as other cytokines that attract TH2-specific lymphocytes into the tumor microenvironment.[51] These lymphocytes are involved in humoral immunity and promote allergic responses, which suggests the importance of STAT6 in the survival of RS cells as well as promoting the unique cellular and immunologic milieu that is a hallmark of HD. STAT regulation involves phosphor-ylation as well as lysine acetylation, which implies that HDACIs could play a role in regulating critical features of HD biology.[52] This is supported by data from Buglio and colleagues,[53] where they demonstrated that exposure of HD cells (L-428 and KM-H2) to vorinostat resulted in an increase in histone acetylation and p21 expres-sion, and caspase-mediated apoptosis. Vorinostat selectively inhibited STAT6 phos-phorylation and resulted in decreased mRNA levels of STAT6 seen by PCR and a reduction of TARC as a downstream effect. Changes in cytokines were evaluated in the supernatants of exposed cells showing an increase in the level of IL-13 and inter-feron inducible protein (IP)-10, and a significant decrease in the level of IL-5, confirm-ing a shift in the Th1/Th2 cytokine balance. Another target gene regulated by STAT6 is the antiapoptotic Bcl-xL, which was significantly decreased in the HD cell lines following vorinostat exposure. This reduced level of Bcl-xL could reduce the apoptotic threshold enough to allow synergistic activity with other anti-HD agents including chemotherapy. Combinations of HDACI with hypomethylating agent can also influ-ence antitumor immune responses by affecting the expression of proteins like the cancer testis antigens (CTA), which include MAGE, SSX, and NY-ESO, in a variety of tumors including Hodgkin lymphoma (HL).[54] These immunomodulatory effects may underlie the therapeutic activity of these agents in HL.

HDAC Modulation of MM

In contrast with lymphomas, there are no studies showing abnormal expression of HDACs in plasma cell malignancies like myeloma. In spite of this, several HDACIs have shown antimyeloma activity. The mechanism of this activity remains unclear but may be related to the general effects of HDACIs on cell biology, like upregulation of p21, cell cycle arrest, or apoptosis. Preclinical data support antimyeloma activity with HDACI, as shown by the modulation of gene expression in MM cells by

HDACIs.[55,56] Both suberoylanilide hydroxamic acid (SAHA) and valproic acid (VPA) alter the expression of oncogenes, cell cycle regulators, antiapoptotic transcription factors, and members of the IGF-IR and IL-6R signaling cascades, important in the pathogenesis and progression of MM. In addition, VPA has been shown to alter genes that contribute to RNA splicing and transcription as well as DNA replication, indicating effects on cell growth that are independent of cell cycle regulation and apoptotic pathways.[57,58] These data are consistent with the effects of HDACIs shown in other cell lines.

Direct cytotoxic effects of HDACIs have been reported in various myeloma cell lines, indicating differences in potency between the different agents: sodium butyrate and valproate acid being the least potent (inhibitory concentration of 50% [IC_{50}] in mM),[57,59,60] FK228 and LBH589 are the most potent in myeloma.[61,62] The antimyeloma apoptotic effect is independent of IL-6, a key growth factor for MM cells.[60,62,63] Coculturing the MM cells with bone marrow stromal cells did not protect the cells from death, indicating that HDACIs could overcome the protective effect of the stromal microenvironment, which is one of the key clinical issues in MM.[63-66] Mechanistically, the antimyeloma effects of HDACIs seems to involve both the extrinsic and intrinsic apoptotic pathways.[67,68] MM cells contain high levels of Bcl-2 and Mcl-1 and lower levels of Bax compared with normal plasma cells, making them more resistant to apoptosis.[67,69] VPA resulted in the redistribution of death receptor (DR4) to lipid rafts, resulting in improved DR4-related signaling and restoring the sensitivity of U266 MM cell lines to APO21/TNF-related apoptosis-inducing ligand (TRAIL)–induced apoptosis.[70] LBH586 resulted in the activation of caspase 8 and the downregulation of the gene TOSA, which is a negative regulator of Fas ligand (FasL).[61] Treatment with LBH589 caused apoptosis of the cell line MMIS (malignant melanoma in situ) by affecting the translocation of mitochondrial proteins like cytochrome c and apoptosis-inducing factor; upregulation of Apaf-1; and cleaving of Bid, caspase 9, and caspase 3.[62] SAHA also decreased the expression of the antiapoptotic protein FLICE-like inhibitory protein (FLIP) and other members of the inhibitors of apoptosis (IAP) family such as X-linked IAP (XIAP).[71] This process resulted in the sensitization of the MM cells (MMIS) to a Fas-activating monoclonal antibody (CH-11) and to recombinant TRAIL. Treatment of the MM cell lines U266, as well as primary myeloma cell lines, with HDACIs resulted in decreased expression of the antiapoptotic proteins Mcl-1, Bcl2, and Bcl-xL, and an increase in Bax.[62] Both LBH589 and SAHA resulted in poly-ADP-ribose (PARP) cleavage in MM cells by 2 distinct mechanisms involving caspase 3 and calpain. Overexpression of the antiapoptotic protein Bcl-2 inhibited SAHA-induced apoptosis in MM cells.[61,71] Another HDACI named KD5170 resulted in Bax activation and cleavage of caspases 9 and 3, resulting in activation of the intrinsic apoptotic system in U266 cell lines.[65] Autophagy is another method of cell death and HDACIs have been shown to affect this pathway as well.[72,73] Schwartz and colleagues[58] showed that VPA-treated myeloma cells had cleavage of caspase 3 and autophagy granules, the first observation of this nature.

All HDACIs except tubacin induce cell cycle arrest in G1/S phase by affecting cyclins, especially cyclin D, and their CDKs. The balance is maintained by the balance between these kinases and their inhibitors like p16, p21, and p27. In MM, constitutive phosphorylation of the Rb protein may be fundamental to the growth and development of the tumor, as indicated by the increased levels of cyclins in G1compared with healthy plasma cells. In MM, HDACI-associated cell cycle arrest is associated with induction of p21 as well as a reduction of cyclin D1 and D2, thus affecting the transition of cells from G1 to S and resulting in arrest at this stage.[55]

Another important antimyeloma action of HDACI involves degradation of misfolded proteins in the cell[74] via the ubiquitination-proteasome and the aggresomal protein. The aggresomal system is particularly important in MM. Aggresomes are formed by the retrograde transport of misfolded proteins on microtubules and travel to the MTOC where they are sequestered for lysosomal degradation. Movement along the microtubules involves intact microtubules and the motor dynein. HDACs deacetylate α-tubulin and play a key role in the aggresomal pathway by affecting the motility of proteins along the microtubule.[75,76] Targeting HDAC6 with tubacin or a pan-HDACI such as vorinostat or LBH586 results in hyperacetylation of the α-tubulin, accumulation of polyubiquitinated proteins, and apoptosis.[66] Tubucin can inhibit the growth of MM cell lines, both drug-sensitive (eg, MMIS, U266, INA-6, and RPMI8226) and drug-resistant cell lines (eg, RPMI-LR5 and RPMI-Dox40) with an IC_{50} between 5 and 20 μM, but no cytotoxicity is seen in normal peripheral mononuclear cells. Thus tubacin selectively targets malignant cells independently of the drug resistance state of these cells.[77] The linkage between inhibition of an HDAC and the proteasome pathway has raised a strong mechanistic rational for the combination of these agents in the clinical setting, much of which is centered on the unfolded or misfolded protein response.

Vorinostat has been shown to suppress the expression of receptor genes involved in MM cell proliferation, survival, and migration, like IGF-1R, IL-6R and its key signal transducer gp130, TNF-R, CD138 (syndecan-1), and CXCR-4.[55] Vorinostat also suppressed the autocrine IGF-1 production and paracrine IL-6 secretion of bone marrow stem cells by triggering MM (MMIS) cell binding, suggesting that it can overcome cell adhesion–mediated resistance. NaB reduced IL-6R in cell lines. Increased p21 expression and apoptosis were observed in these cell lines along with lines that were transfected with an expression vector of IL6-R, indicating that downregulation of IL-6R is not required for HDACI-induced apoptosis, again emphasizing the many pathways affected by HDACIs in MM cells.[55]

HDACIs also affects angiogenesis in MM by a direct effect on growth and differentiation of endothelial cells and the downregulation of proangiogenic genes in tumor cells. Using OPM-2 and KM3 cell lines, VPA has been shown to decrease vascular endothelial growth factor (VEGF) secretion and VEGF receptor expression, resulting in inhibition of the vascular tubule formation in endothelial cells in cocultures with myeloma cells.[60,78,79]

De Bruyne and colleagues[80] showed that CD9, a tetraspanin, shows an inverse correlation between its expression level and tumor metastasis in solid tumors. In MM, CD9 is downregulated and treatment with LBH589 could result in its upregulation, making it more susceptible to NK cell–mediated cytolysis. Its expression is correlated with nonactive MM disease. This finding indicates that the immunologically mediated effects of HDACI are also importation in MM.

PHARMACOLOGY OF HDACI

HDACIs are a chemically diverse group of naturally occurring and synthetic molecules (**Fig. 1**) that inhibit the activity of HDACs in a wide range of concentrations from low nanomolar to high millimolar,[1,81] as listed in **Table 3**. Presently, there are at least 18 different HDACI being evaluated in preclinical and early clinical trials that target the Zn^{2+}-dependent (ie, class 1, 2, and 4) HDACs. Most HDACI have a short plasma half-life (vorinostat, 2 hours[82]; romidepsin, 3 hours[83]; MGCD0103, 9 hours[84]) and undergo hepatic metabolism either via the CYP450 system (romidepsin)[83] or the glucuronidation system (vorinostat).[82] The metabolites are excreted through the biliary and fecal routes. HDACIs have varying formulations and differing side effect profiles depending on the route of administration. The 2 agents approved by the US Food and Drug Administration (FDA) to date (namely vorinostat and romidepsin) have undergone extensive pharmacokinetic monitoring as part of the clinical trials that led to their

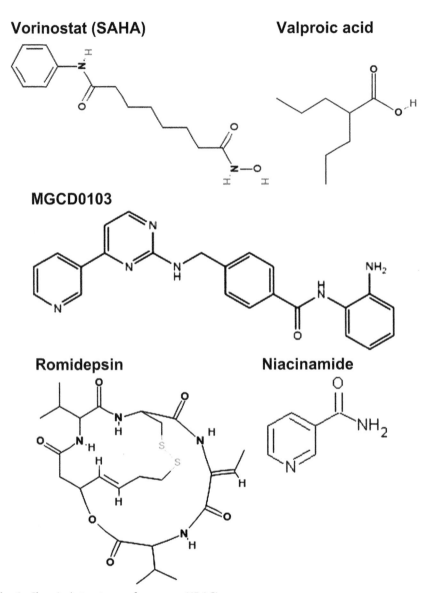

Fig. 1. Chemical structures of common HDACI.

approval. One of the earliest pharmacologic studies was performed with vorino-stat,[19,82] first with the intravenous (IV) preparation and then with the oral formulation. A direct comparison of the toxicity and pharmacokinetic profiles of IV versus oral vorinostat revealed that the C_{max} of exposure to vorinostat was higher with the IV formulation versus oral formulation (2408 ng/mL vs 658 ng/mL) but the AUC was greater with the oral route of exposure (4634 h × ng/mL vs 101,854 h × ng/mL). The toxicity profiles of these 2 regimens were also different, with more thrombocytopenia, dehydration, and diarrhea noted with the oral formulation compared with the IV. Oral vorinostat (the approved formulation) is 71% bound to proteins and is metabolized via glucuronidation and hydrolysis followed by β-oxidation into 2 inactive metabolites. Biotransformation by cytochrome P450 is negligible. It is excreted by the kidneys with less than 1% of the dose recovered as unchanged drug in the urine. The mean urinary excretion of the 2 pharmacologically inactive metabolites at steady state was 52% (±13.3%) of the vorinostat dose; 16% (±5.8%) of the dose as O-glucuronide and 36% (±8.6%) of the dose as 4-anilino-4-oxobutanoic acid. Romidepsin is highly protein bound in plasma (92%–94%) over the concentration range of 50 ng/mL to 1000 ng/mL with α1-acid-glycoprotein (AAG) being the principal binding protein. In contrast with vorinostat, it undergoes extensive metabolism in vitro, primarily by CYP3A4 with minor contributions from CYP3A5, CYP1A1, CYP2B6, and CYP2C19. At therapeutic concentrations, romidepsin did not competitively inhibit CYP1A2, CYP2C9, CYP2C19, CYP2D6, CYP2E1, or CYP3A4 in vitro.[83]

In clinical trials, the histone acetylation (H3 and H4) in mononuclear cells in the peripheral blood is considered to be a biomarker for reaching a target during administration of HDACI.[82] In the case of vorinostat, the effect can persist for up to 10 hours after the drug has cleared from the system after an oral dose. As shown by Kelly and colleagues,[82] higher doses of vorinostat did not necessarily produce more acetylated histone, but generally resulted in a longer half-life of the acetylated H3/H4. Despite the role of H3/H4 acetylation, accumulation of acetylated H3/H4 can be shown in every patient, and accumulation of the Ac-H3/H4 does not correlate with response. Identifying appropriate surrogate biomarkers of response with HDACIs continues to be a major research goal.

Side Effect Profile

The side effect profile of all HDACIs is uniform across even the diverse chemical classes of agents.[42,85–87] The most common side effects include fatigue, nausea, and diarrhea. Transient thrombocytopenia is the most common myelosuppressive effect. During the phase 1 experience with vorinostat, bone marrow examination of patients at their platelet nadir revealed a normocellular marrow with dysplastic-appearing megakaryocytes that seemed to have impaired platelet budding.[19] Subsequent studies revealed that HDAC inhibition may repress the GATA-1 gene, an important transcription factor for hematopoiesis, leading to a delay in megakaryocyte maturation and thrombocytopenia.[88]

One of the recurring themes of therapy with HDACIs is the cardiac effects of these agents. Prolongation of the corrected QT (QTc) interval has been observed as a class effect for many HDACIs and is thought to occur via the HERGK+ channels.[89,90] A systematic study of cardiac events resulting from treatment with romidepsin (282 administered cycles of romidepsin and more than 700 doses of the drug) showed that almost all patients had prolongation of the QTc interval (median 14 milliseconds) and more than half the patients had transient electrocardiogram (EKG) changes, including T wave flattening and ST depression.[91,92] These changes were clinically insignificant, with no change in cardiac enzymes or cardiac function. The agent is now approved, with the caution that the treating physician should be careful in giving the drug to patients who may have a significant cardiac history or be susceptible to prolongation of the QTc interval. It is recommended that attention be paid to maintaining the patient's potassium and magnesium levels within the normal range while receiving therapy with romidepsin. Because of the early experience with romidepsin, most trials with HDACIs now require rigorous cardiac monitoring. It is also recommended that patients with baseline prolonged QTc, significant heart disease, or patients on medications that may prolong the QTc interval be excluded from trials with HDACIs. Various HDACIs also vary in their cardiac effects. For example, vorinostat is not associated with any serious cardiac toxicity, whereas the hydroxamic acid panobinostat (LBH589) and its predecessor LAQ824 are associated with QTc interval prolongation (1 patient had torsades de pointes) There were no reported long-term changes in the EKG in any of the patients treated on trials of HDACI.

Thrombosis and pulmonary embolism are other important adverse events noted on the pivotal vorinostat trials (2 patients experienced thrombosis and pulmonary embolism). It was unclear whether this was directly related to the drug, but it is recommended that caution be used while using vorinostat in patients who may have an underlying thromboembolic disorder. An increased incidence of thromboembolic events has not been reported on the ongoing clinical trials with HDACIs.

HDACI IN LYMPHOMA (CLINICAL DATA)
B Cell Lymphoma

B cell NHL are the most common lymphomas and include subtypes that vary from some of the most aggressive tumors (Burkitt lymphoma) to some of the most indolent (follicular lymphoma [FL] and small lymphocytic lymphoma). In spite of combination cytotoxic agents, immunotherapies, and radioimmunotherapies, relapsed and refractory disease states remain a major clinical problem, particularly in indolent lymphomas. One of the earliest demonstrations of activity of an HDACI in B cell lymphoma was reported with VPA, a weak HDACI, which induced a complete remission in a patient with multiply relapsed transformed FL.[93] VPA has been more widely studied in myeloid leukemias, with little to no other experience in lymphoid malignancies. It is a potent inhibitor of STAT3 (overexpressed in the ABC type of DLBCL).[94]

In addition to VPA, there have been several early phase trials with a variety of other HDACI for the treatment of B cell NHL. Kelly and colleagues[82] reported on the first phase 1 study of intravenously administered vorinostat (previously known as SAHA) in patients with hematological malignancies. Of the 11 patients with B cell malignancies (HL n = 5, NHL n = 6), no patients with B cell NHL responded, although antitumor activity was seen in 2 patients with HD, including a 30% reduction of tumor burden in 1 patient that was maintained for 3 months, and stable disease in another patient for 8 months. A follow-up phase 1 study conducted by the same investigators[19] with an oral formulation of vorinostat revealed a favorable side effect profile and a maximum tolerated dose of 400 mg per day given for 14 consecutive days on an every-21-day cycle. This study enrolled a total of 25 patients with hematological malignancies, with the best response being a complete remission (CR) seen in a patient with transformed FL. Partial remissions (PRs) were seen in patients with transformed lymphoma and mycosis fungoides. A patient with HD had a 31% decrease in disease lasting for 10 months. These 2 studies of vorinostat in patients with solid tumors and hematological malignancies were among the first to show the potential activity of these compounds in B cell malignancies and HL. Another phase 1 trial of oral vorinostat was conducted in patients with B cell malignancies, as reported by investigators in Japan.[95] This trial enrolled 10 patients with B cell lymphomas at 2 dosing levels: 100 mg and 200 mg twice a day for 14/21 days. Four of the 10 patients responded, including 2 CRs and 1 PR seen in patients with FL and 1 PR in a patient with MCL. A dedicated phase 2 study of vorinostat in patients with relapsed DLBCL at a dose of 300 mg twice a day (14 days per 3 weeks or 3 days per week) has been reported.[96] Eighteen patients were enrolled, with 1 patient obtaining a CR lasting 468 days, and 1 patient who attained stable disease for 301 days. Based on this study and the collective experience from the phase 1 studies, it was concluded that vorinostat did not exhibit impressive single-agent activity in large B cell lymphoma. However, the maximal tolerated dose (MTD) that is now given on the label for vorinostat was not used to assess response in these studies and, based on the phase 1 experience by Duvic and colleagues,[36] this dose was poorly tolerated. A second phase II study evaluated vorinostat at a dose of 200 mg twice a day for 14/21 days in patients with relapsed and refractory indolent NHL.[97–99] This trial enrolled 33 patients (FL, 20; MCL, 8; marginal zone lymphoma [MZL], 7), of whom 6 patients achieved a CR, 4 attained a PR, and 4 had stable disease for an overall response rate (ORR) of 29% (CR+PR). Responses were limited to FL (40%) and MCL (28%), with no responses seen in MZL. Although the single-agent activity of vorinostat in DLBCL is variable, and probably low, these experiences raise 2 questions: (1) why do select patients achieve CR, whereas others do not; and (2) is the optimal pharmacokinetic profile and dosing of this agent different for these diseases?

One strategy to improve the efficacy of HDACIs in B cell lymphomas has been to evaluate more potent HDACI in the treatment of B cell lymphomas to look for stronger signals of activity. Most phase I trials are conducted to include the broad category of lymphoid diagnoses that initially encompass both B and T cells with the idea of expanding the trial to a specific subtype if a positive signal is found in a specific diagnostic group. Belinostat, a potent hydroxamic acid HDACI, is currently in development for the treatment of lymphoma, in particular peripheral T cell lymphoma (PTCL). Similarly to vorinostat, it has an oral and IV formulation, although most data collected to date are with the IV formulation.[99] The initial phase I trial of belinostat in advanced solid tumors established an MTD of 1000 mg/m^2 given intravenously for 5 days as a 30-minute infusion. This dose was confirmed as the MTD in a parallel study of the same agent in hematological malignancies, with no additional toxicity seen in this group of patients.[98] This study enrolled 11 patients (DLBCL n = 7, transformed CLL n = 2, transformed FL n = 4, CLL n = 2). No objective responses were seen in any patients, although some patients experienced stabilization of disease (DLBCL n = 2, CLL n = 3). For ease of administration, the oral formulation of belinostat is being developed and a phase 1 study of oral belinostat in patients with all subtypes of NHL is underway. The starting dose was 750 mg/m^2, with planned escalations until the MTD is reached. Interim results are to reported at ASH (American Society of Hematology) 2011.[100] The MTD has been established at 1500 mg a day for 14 days in a 21-day cycle. Results have shown 1 CR (duration 2+ cycles) in patients with NHL, 1 PR (duration 8 cycles) in patients with HD, and stable disease has been noted in 12 patients (duration 1–24 cycles, median 1.5). Aside from the 1 CR and 1 PR, tumor shrinkage between 25% and 50% was noted in 8 patients. PCI-2478 is an orally administered HDACI belonging to the class of hydroxamic acid. Evans and colleagues[101] reported the results of the initial phase I data at ASH 2010. One patient with FL achieved a CR, whereas 4 PRs and 7 stable disease responses were noted in 20 other evaluable patients. This study showed that there are no cardiac effects or prolongation of the QTc interval noted with this agent. A phase II portion of the trial is planned.

Although the experience with HDACIs as single agents in B cell lymphoma has been disappointing, these drugs have important potential activity, and the future will probably involve rational combinations. It is important to gain a better understanding of how the various classes of HDACIs work in B cell lymphoma, and to try to develop reasonable hypotheses around how these agents are likely working in these DLBCL. With this experience, potentially important HDACI are likely to emerge in the near future.

T Cell Lymphoma

Mature T cell NHL and NK cell neoplasms comprise 12% of all NHL and 15% to 20% of aggressive lymphomas worldwide. They are characterized by great morphologic diversity and genetic variation even within individual disease entities. The current 2008 World Health Organization classification recognizes more than 20 types of mature T cell and NK T cell lymphomas (PTCL).[102] CTCLs are malignancies that arise in the skin and are classified as a separate entity based on their distinct clinical behavior and prognosis.[103] Among the aggressive lymphomas, a T cell phenotype confers a worse clinical outcome compared with their B cell counterparts, with the exception of ALK-positive anaplatic large cell lymphoma. Long-term survival at 5 years remains at 10% to –30% for most histologies with present treatment strategies,[104] and relapsed/refractory disease remains a significant clinical dilemma.

For reasons that are not clear, HDACIs have shown consistent and promising activity in the treatment of many types of T cell lymphoma. Two agents of this class, vorinostat (Zolinza) and romidepsin (Istodax), have been approved for the treatment of relapsed or refractory CTCL in the United States.[8,9] In addition, romidepsin is also approved for the treatment of relapsed and refractory T cell lymphoma,[105,106] whereas belinostat and panobinostat are in clinical trials for T cell malignancies.[107]

Vorinostat was the first HDACI approved for the treatment of cancer. In the United States, this agent is approved for the treatment of CTCL in patients who have failed at least 2 prior systemic therapies.[8] Based on early signals of activity and a favorable toxicity profile in patients with lymphoma in the phase 1 experience, Duvic and colleagues[36] conducted a restricted phase I/II study of oral vorinostat in patients with CTCL. This phase 2 experience enrolled 33 patients with advanced, heavily pre-treated CTCL. Three different orally administered dosages and schedules were sequentially evaluated: 400 mg daily; 300 mg twice daily for 3 days followed by 4 days of rest; and 300 mg twice daily for 14 days with a week of rest followed by 200 mg twice daily. The ORR was 24.4%, with 8 patients having a partial remission (PR), including 4 patients with Sézary syndrome (SS). More importantly, 14 of the 33 patients (42%) reported significant pruritus relief. The median time to response was 11.9 weeks, and the median duration of response was 15.1 weeks. The major side effects included fatigue, thrombocytopenia, and gastrointestinal symptoms (predominantly diarrhea and nausea). Within the different cohorts, more thrombocytopenia was noted in the third cohort in which patients received a higher dose (300 mg twice a day for 14 days straight). However, most of the responses were seen in groups 1 and 3. Thus, based on the response rate and toxicity criteria, the dose of 400 mg per day was established as having the best safety profile. This study affirmed the findings in the original phase 1 experience, supporting the daily dosing of 400 mg of vorinostat by mouth, which was associated with the most favorable side effect profile and highest response rate of any of the explored schedules. Based on these data, a registration-directed phase II study using the dose of 400 mg by mouth was initiated by Olsen and colleagues.[8] This study included 74 patients with CTCL who had failed at least 2 prior systemic therapies. Disease assessment was by modified skin-weighted assessment tools (m-SWAT).[108] This study showed an ORR of 29.7%, with 1 patient achieving CR after 281 days of therapy. Median time to objective response was 56 days (28–171 days); some patients took up to 6 months to respond and the median duration of response was not reached in the study, although it was greater than 185 days. Nonprogressing patients continued on the study with 15 patients receiving the drug for more than a year and 6 patients receiving it for more than 2 years. In addition, another 29 patients had clinical benefit manifested by stable disease for more than 24 weeks. Pruritus relief was found in 35 patients, including responders and nonresponders, again pointing to the effect of vorinostat on cytokine profiles. These data supported the approval of vorinostat by the FDA in October 2006, making it the first HDACI to be approved for the treatment of cancer.

Romidepsin (formerly known as depsipeptide, FK228) is a cyclic peptide originally isolated from the broth culture of *Chromobacterium violaceum*.[109] It was initially studied at the National Cancer Institute (NCI) in patients with refractory or relapsed solid tumors by Piekarz and colleagues[110] reported a patient with refractory PTCL that responded to depsipeptide. Because the drug began to show a consistent signal in patients with T cell lymphoma, the study was expanded to separate patients with CTCL from those with PTCL, and then it further stratified patients based on the amount of prior therapy they received.[105] Overall, it had a stratification that consisted of 7 different treatment arms, with the intention of separating different cohorts of patients with T cell lymphomas based on histology and prior number of therapies. All patients received drug as an intravenous infusion at a dose of 14 mg/m^2 once a week in a three out of a four-week cycle. The 2 major cohorts were CTCL and PTCL and the data from these 2 groups of patients was analyzed and presented separately. Piekarz and colleagues[110] reported the results of 71 patients with relapsed CTCL that was treated with depsipeptide. The ORR was 34% (24/71) with complete remissions observed in 4 patients. The median duration of response was 13.7 months. Based on the data generated by the NCI, the drug was eventually acquired by Gloucester Pharmaceuticals, and 2 registration-directed clinical trials were launched, 1 in CTCL and 1 in PTCL. In the preparation of the new drug application to the FDA, data from the 2 studies (NCI plus Gloucester) were pooled and patients were analyzed using a composite end point to assess response using skin assessment, lymph node and visceral involvement, and abnormal circulating Sézary cells.[9,111,112] One-hundred and thirty-five patients were evaluable, with a median age of 57 years, and who had received a median of at least 2 (1–8) prior systemic therapies. One-hundred and three patients (76%) had at least a stage IIB or higher disease and 19 patients had SS. The ORR was 41%, with a complete remisson (CR) rate of 7% and duration of response of 14.9 months. On subanalysis, the response rate was 58% in patients with Sézary syndrome, which is impressive in a disease that is notoriously chemoresist-ant.[113] In addition, this study objectively evaluated pruritus using the visual scale analog (VSA), a tool that has been validated in other clinical trials,[112] and reported a relief of pruritus in more than 60% of the patients, including nonresponders. This agent was approved by the FDA for the treatment of relapsed CTCL following failure of 1 line of systemic therapy. For PTCL, the NCI trial included patients with PTCL who had failed at least 1 prior systemic therapy, further stratified into less than 2 or more than 2 prior systemic therapies.[10] There were 48 evaluable patients, and all pathology was reviewed centrally. The patients had received a median of 3 prior therapies, including 18 patients (38%) who had received a prior stem cell transplant. ORR was reported as 31% with 4 (8%) CRs. Patients who received more than 2 cycles of therapy had a response rate of 44%. Median duration of response was 9 months, with a median time to progression of 12 months. Coiffier and colleagues[106] reported the results of a second large multicenter phase II study of romidepsin in PTCL conducted by Gloucester Pharmaceuticals. The study enrolled 131 patients with histologically confirmed PTCL who had failed or were refractory to more than 1 systemic therapy and had measurable disease. The dosing schedule was the same as the NCI study (ie, weekly dosing of romidepsin at 14 mg/m^2 on days 1, 8, and 15 every 28 days). The median age of patients was 59.4 years and they had received a median of 2 prior systemic therapies. In this study, 21 patients (16%) had received a prior stem cell transplant, ORR was reported as 34%, with 19 (15%) CRs and 15 (12%) PRs. Median duration of response was not reached because 16 patients with CR had not progressed at the time of analysis. These 2 studies established impressive single-agent activity of romidepsin in PTCL, and presentation of the collective data to the FDA has led to the approval of this agent in the setting of relapsed PTCL in which patients have failed at least 1 line of systemic therapy.

Belinostat is a hydroxamic acid with pan-HDACI activity that is currently in clinical trials for solid tumors and hematological malignancies, and is available in both oral and intravenous formulations. A phase I trial of the intravenous formulation was performed in parallel with the solid tumor phase and an MTD of 1000 mg/m^2 was established.[98,114] This formulation is being studied in a large phase II trial at a dose of 1000 mg/m^2 for patients with relapsed PTCL. The oral formulation has also been developed and, as with vorinostat, it has been better tolerated than the IV formulation. In the ongoing phase I trial of oral belinostat in hematological malignancies, an MTD of 1500 mg given daily on days 1 to 14 in a 21-day cycle has been established and its activity is being explored in a variety of lymphomas.

Oral panobinostat, also known as LBH589, is a pan-HDACI belonging to the hydroxamic acid group that has shown activity in patients with CTCL in early-phase trials.[37] Six of 10 patients with CTCL showed a response in the original phase 1 trial at a dose of 20 mg and 30 mg given on Monday, Wednesday, and Friday (MWF) on a weekly basis. The trial has now been expanded to a dedicated phase II trial in patients with CTCL at a dose of 20 mg a day MWF given weekly. The interim results of this trial were reported at ASH 2010.[115] Ninety-five patients were enrolled with advanced (stage 1B–1VA) mycosis fungoides or Sézary syndrome. Of 62 patients, 11 responded by SWAT criteria, including 2 CRS. The trial is ongoing and further results are awaited.

HD

HD is one of the most curable of lymphomas, but 20% to 30% of patients relapse after attaining remission, or have primary refractory disease.[116] Approximately 50% of these patients can be cured with second-line chemotherapy and autologous stem cell transplantation (ASCT). Treatment options are limited for patients who relapse beyond second-line therapy or have primary refractory disease. The median survival for patients after relapse following ASCT is 26 months, and there are an estimated 1300 deaths annually from HD in the United States.[117,118] Novel therapies for these patients are needed.

There are several studies that consistently show that HDACIs have activity in HL. One of the earliest insights into this signal was revealed in the phase 1 experience with vorinostat. In the IV and oral phase 1 experiences with vorinostat,[19,82] 12 patients with relapsed or refractory HD were treated with escalating doses of vorinostat, with 4 patients responding as follows: on the IV study, 1 patient attained a PR that lasted for approximately 9 months; 1 patient experienced a 14% decrease in her lung disease, resulting in significant improvement of her performance status; and a third patient achieved a 42% reduction of the tumor, lasting for 2 months. On the oral study, 1 patient achieved a 31% decrease in tumor lasting nearly 10 months. A subsequent phase II trial of vorinostat[119] administered at 200 mg orally twice a day for 14 of 21 days produced only modest clinical activity, with only 1 patient achieving a PR. The phase 1 experience with oral vorinostat established an MTD of 400 mg given orally once daily for 14 days in a 21-day cycle.

Of the available HDACIs, panobinostat is being studied in a registration-directed phase 2 trial in HL. The initial phase IA/II trial of panobinostat (LBH589) used 2 different dose levels and schedules of this agent in patients with hematological malignancies. Patients with HD were entered onto the study at 2 dose levels: arm 1 was dosed at a starting dose of 30 mg a day given MWF every week, whereas arm 2 was initiated at 45 mg a day given on the same MWF every other week schedule. There were 13 patients with HD who were enrolled on the study, of whom 5 met the criteria for a partial response indicating evidence of HD activity. It appeared to be well tolerated, with fatigue, nausea, thrombocytopenia, and diarrhea being the most common side effects. The MTD was estimated by the logistic regression model and was defined as 40 mg a day given every MWF on the weekly schedule. Based on these data, a large international phase II trial of panobinostat is designed for patients with relapsed and refractory HD. The final results of the phase II portion were reported at ASH 2010.[120] Overall, 129 patients were enrolled, with a median age of 32 years. Patients were heavily pretreated with a median of 4 (2–7) prior regimens including autologous stem cell transplant (100%), allogeneic transplant (10%), and radiation (69%). Responses were observed in 35 of 129 evaluable patients (5 CRs, 30 PRs, and an ORR of 27%). At the time of presentation, 19 patients were still receiving treatment. Responses were durable, with a median duration of 6.9 months (4.1–51.3 months). The most notable adverse event was reversible thrombocytopenia. Another HDACI with activity in HL is MGCD0103, which belongs to the benzamide class. MGCD 0103 is classified as an isotype-selective HDACI that predominantly inhibits class 1 HDAC enzymes and is administered as an oral formulation. A phase II trial of MGCD0103 was conducted at a dose level of 110 mg given orally 3 times per week in patients with relapsed and refractory HD.[121] Responses were seen in 7 of the 20 patients who were treated at this dose level, including complete remissions; however, the dose was considered too toxic, requiring frequent interruptions and dose reductions. The protocol was then revised to lower the dose to 85 mg per day given on the same schedule. Another 10 patients were enrolled on the lower dose and partial responses were seen in 3 of the 10 patients. The agent was well tolerated, with the main side effects being fatigue and thrombocytopenia, although 2 patients developed pericardial effusions requiring an interruption of the protocol. Collectively, these data suggest that there is a signal of efficacy of some of the more potent HDACI in HD, but the biologic correlates of this activity are still unclear.

HDACI in MM

MM represents about 1% of all cancers and is the most commonly diagnosed hematological malignancy. The median age at diagnosis is 67 years, with an increasing incidence noted with older age groups. The clinical outcome of MM has improved greatly in the last decades. Novel agents like bortezomib, IMIDs, and stem cell transplantation have improved the median survival of patients with MM from an average of 2 to 3 years to more than 8 to 10 years. However, in spite of a plethora of treatment options, including stem cell transplantation, most patients with myeloma are destined to relapse and remain incurable because of the development of drug resistance governed by the bone marrow microenvironment. Therefore, newer targeted therapies are needed and HDACIs represent a new class of antimyeloma therapy, as discussed later.

Single-agent activity of HDACIs in MM has been disappointing. Richardson and colleagues[122] reported the first phase 1 study of SAHA in MM at various doses and schedules in 13 patients. One patient had a minor response and 1 had stable disease. In a study of PXD101 in patients with advance myeloma, only 1 patient with MM was found to have stable disease. Niesvizky and colleagues[123] reported on a phase 2 trial of the potent HDACI romidepsin for the treatment of refractory MM. Thirteen patients were enrolled and were treated at 14 mg/m^2 given as a 4-hour IV infusion on days 1, 8, and 15 of a 28-day cycle. No patients had an objective response but 4/12 patients with secretory myeloma had evidence of M-protein stabilization and several patients experienced improvement of their bone pain and hypercalcemia, indicating some biologic effects of clinical benefit. Correlative studies were designed in this study of cell cycle kinetics as well as evaluation of several proteins including BCL-2, MCL-1, CD31, and cleaved caspase 3, and the results revealed no detectable modulation in vivo in these patient samples. The focus has now shifted to rationally based combinations of HDACI in MM, which are discussed later.

Combination Therapy in MM

Both preclinical and clinical data support the use of HDACl in combination with other agents. The most striking combination is with proteasome inhibitors (PI). Bortezomib an important antimyeloma drug that targets the proteasome system and NF-kB may target HDACs as well and may function as HDACl, further strengthening the rationale to use it in combination with HDACl.[124] Kikuchi and colleagues[125] reported that bortezomib can downregulate the expression of class 1 HDACs (HDAC1, HDAC2, and HDAC3) in MM cell lines and primary MM cells at the transcriptional level accompanied by histone hyperacetylation. Short interfering RNA-mediated knockdown of HDAC1 enhanced bortezomib-induced apoptosis, and its overexpression inhibited it. HDAC1 overexpression conferred resistance to bortezomib in MM cells and administration of the HDACl romidepsin restored sensitivity to bortezomib in HDAC overexpressing cells. Thus bortezomib targets HDACs via distinct mechanisms from conventional HDACls.

Pei and colleagues[126] first showed that, in vitro, the combination of HDACl with bortezomib resulted in enhanced cellular toxicity compared with their effects as single agents. This synergy was associated with a reduction of NF-kB DNA binding activity, modulation of Jun N-terminal kinase (JNK) activation, and a ROS-dependent downregulation of cyclin D1, Mcl-1, and XIAP. Combining bortezomib with PXD101 caused oxidative stress accompanied by enhanced expression of Bim, DNA damage, MAPK p38 activation, and p53 phosphorylation.[127] Inhibition of aggresomal pathway by tubacin, together with proteasomal inhibition by bortezomib, also resulted in an accumulation of the ubiquitinated proteins followed by synergistic anti-MM activity.[77] The cytotoxicity was mediated by stress-induced JNK activation, caspase, and PARP cleavage. Bortezomib led to aggresome formation and further combining it with LBH586 or SAHA (both inhibit HDAC6) resulted in disruption of the aggresome and apoptosis.[66,128] Bortezomib and SAHA resulted in an induction of the proapoptotic proteins BH3, Noxa, and endoplasmic reticulum (ER) stress, indicated by the disruption of calcium homeostasis and caspase 4 activation. Knockdown studies have shown that caspase 4 and Noxa play an important role in Myc-driven sensitivity of MM to the combination of bortezomib and SAHA. In MM, Myc expression is correlated with the intracellular ER content and protein synthesis rate. Anti-MM activity of the combination of PI with HDACl was shown in primary MM samples and cell lines.

The combination of vorinostat and boretezomib was first reported in 2 multicenter phase 1 studies and the results were presented at ASH 2008.[129–131] In the first trial, 34 patients with relapsed and refractory myeloma were enrolled. Patients received escalating doses of vorinostat (200 mg twice a day, 300–400 mg daily for 4 days) and bortezomib (0.7, 0.9, 1.1, or 1.3 mg/m^2 on days 1, 4, 8, and 11). Cycles were repeated every 21 days. The highest doses of vorinostat (400 mg daily for 14 days and bortezomib 1.3 mg/m^2) were given together and an MTD could not be reached. Nausea, diarrhea, thrombocytopenia, and vomiting were the most common adverse events. Results revealed that the best response was a PR in 9 (26%) patients, minimal response in 7 (21%) patients, and stable disease in 18 (53%) patients. The responders included previous bortezomib failures. The second trial enrolled 23 patients who received vorinostat (100–500 mg on days 4–11) and bortezomib (1–1.3 mg/m^2 on days 1, 4, 8, and 11). Dexamethasone was added later in the cycles for varying degrees of responses (< PR, PD). The main toxicities were hematological. Of the 21 evaluable patients, 2 achieved a good PR, 7 PR, 10 stable disease, and 2 had progressive disease. Again noted were the responses amongst bortezomib-refractory patients and the acceptable[129] toxicity profile.

A study reporting the results of the combination of romidepsin, bortezomib, and dexamethasone for the treatment of MM was reported in *Blood* in August 2011. This phase 1 study was designed to determine the MTD of the triple drug combinations with a secondary objective of OR, TTP, and overall survival (OS). The final MTD-defined doses were as follows: bortezomib 1.3 mg/m^2 on days 1, 4, 8, and 11; dexamethasone, 20 mg on days 1, 2, 4, 5, 8, 9, 11, and 12; and romidepsin 10 mg/m^2 on days 1, 8, and 15 every 28 days. Main toxicities were thrombocytopenia and peripheral neuropathy. There were 2 (8%) CR and 13 (52%) PRs, including 7 very good PRs (VGPR). Median time to progression was 7.2 months and the median OS was 36 months.

Panobinostat is being studied in combination with velcade and dexamethasone. The phase 1 study of the combination with bortezomib enrolled 47 patients who received drugs at 5 different dose combinations. ORR was more than 70% and responses were seen at the lowest dose levels. The recommended dose at the end of the trial was panobinostat 20 mg orally to be given 3 times a week and velcade at 1.3 mg/m^2 to be given twice a week for 2 weeks. Hematological toxicities, nausea, diarrhea, fever, fatigue, and weakness were the most commonly reported side effects. This work has led to an international phase 3 study of panobinostat in combination with velcade.

Panobinostat in combination with revilimid and dexamethasone is also a promising combination and the preliminary results of a phase 1B study were presented at ASCO 2011. Patients received panobinostat at 5, 10, 20, or 25 mg plus 25 mg of revilimid and 40 mg of dexamethasone. Forty-six patients were enrolled. Reported dose limiting toxicities (DLTs) were thrombocytopenia and a low white cell count. The final results are awaited.

Other promising combinations include hypomethylating agents and chemotherapeutic agents. Several key tumor suppressor genes are hypermethylated and hence deactivated in human malignancies. In MM, hypomethylating agents like 5-azcitidine and decitabine in combination with HDACIs can reactivate these genes, resulting in decreased tumor cell growth.[132,133] Treatment of MM cell line U266 with NaB and decitabine resulted in an increased expression of the p16 gene and protein compared with either agent alone.[134] Similarly, the upregulation of the proapoptotic protein Bim could be enhanced significantly by LBH586 in combination with decitabine, whereas decitabine alone had no effect on this.[135] Clinical trials are underway to study this combination in MM. Many HDACIs, including LAQ824, romidepsin, and LBH586, have shown powerful synergy on growth inhibition and cytotoxicity when combined with alkylators like malphalan and dexamethasone.[62,136] Enhanced apoptosis of MM cell lines has been observed with HDACIs and activators of TRAIL and Fas pathways.[137,138]

Novel Combinations of HDACI in Lymphoma

By targeting specific molecular pathways, HDACIs lend themselves to endless combinations with other targeted therapies. Combinations of HDACIs and the PI bortezomib have shown marked synergistic clinical activity in MM and MCL. Paoluzzi and colleagues[139] showed synergistic cytotoxicity of either belinostat or romidepsin in combination with bortezomib against a panel of MCL cell lines. This combination induced mitochondrial membrane depolarization and apoptosis in treated cells. A decrease in cyclin D and Bcl-xL was also shown. Combinations of vorinostat and bortezomib were also synergistic in MCL cell lines resulting in apoptosis, ROS generation, and decreased NK-kB activity.[140] The combination of vorinostat and bortezomib has also been evaluated in vitro for synergy against CTCL cell lines. This combination has shown an upregulation of p21 and p27, and an increased expression of phosphorylated p38, which participates in a signaling cascade controlling cellular responses to cytokines and stress. Decreased expression of VEGF was also shown after treatment with vorinostat and bortezomib. Similar synergy between romidepsin and belinostat with bortezomib has also been reported in CLL cell lines and has been shown to involve mechanisms of NF-kB inactivation and perturbation of the apoptotic pathways.[141] The novel PI carfilzomib is also being evaluated in combination with HDACI and has shown promising synergistic activity with vorinostat[142] in a DLBCL cell line. This activity was associated with activation of JNK and p38 MAPK, and decrease in NK-kB, AKT inactivation, and Ku70 acetylation. Clinical trials are now underway to evaluate the combination of proteasome inhibitors and HDACI for the treatment of lymphomas.

Bcl6[43] overexpression is a hallmark of DLBCL, particularly the GC subtype. In the deacetylated state, Bcl6 functions as a transcriptional corepressor of several genes that influence cell cycling and the tumor suppressor p53 activity. Sirtuin2-α, a class III HDAC, has been shown to interact and attenuate p53-mediated function.[143] The use of HDACI to acetylate and enhance the function of BCL-6 could provide a therapeutic target for antilymphoma therapy. This function can be further enhanced by combining this with nicotinamide, which can enhance p53 function to target BCL-6–addicted tumors. Clinical trials are underway to study this combination.[144]

By lowering the apoptotic threshold, HDACI lend themselves as ideal agents to be combined with chemotherapeutic agents, a strategy that is being explored in solid tumors and other malignancies and will likely be explored in lymphoproliferative disorders. A phase I clinical trial in patients with advanced CTCL consists of vorinostat and escalating doses of bexarotene given daily for 28 days. At the time of writing, 19 patients have been enrolled and accrual is ongoing because MTD has not been reached. Responses have been reported in some patients.[145]

DNA methylation is involved in malignancy and is seen, in progression, in more than 80% of all solid tumors. Methylation is one of the main physiologic processes to induce silencing of gene expression. The clinical use of demethylating agents like 5-azacitidine and decitabine has been developed in myeloid malignancies without any significant activity noted in lymphoid diseases. However, in vitro data support the combination of HDACI with hypomethylating agents to provide antilymphoma therapy, as shown by the combination of decitabine and romidepsin.[146]

SUMMARY

HDACIs have had significant effects on deregulated genes in lymphoma and MM. The clinical results of single-agent activity are promising against specific subtypes of lymphoproliferative agents.

The use of HDACIs has allowed pharmacologic manipulation of deregulated genes in cancer cells and HDACI have shown single-agent activity against T cell lymphomas, CTCL, MCLs, and HD. The bigger promise lies in the impact that these agents can have in enhancing the activity of other targeted therapies ranging from antifolates like pralatrexate to demethylating agents, proteasome inhibitors, and even cytotoxic agents. In addition, the effects of HDACIs on the immune system and cytokines, as seen in CTCL and HD, also indicate that HDACIs can be useful in the treatment of immune dysfunction underlying tumorigenesis, autoimmune disorders, and graft-versus-host disease. There is also an effort to determine whether class specificity of HDACIs has a biologic significance, and, as more information is obtained about epigenetic dysregulation in lymphoid diseases, the clinical significance of this will become clear. It is likely that in the future an HDACI-based therapy will be the backbone of both up-front and salvage therapies for most lymphomas and will lead to better outcomes compared with current cytotoxic therapies.

REFERENCES

1. Bhalla KN. Epigenetic and chromatin modifiers as targeted therapy of hematologic malignancies. J Clin Oncol 2005;23(17):3971–93.
2. Bates SE. Epigenetic therapies reach Main Street. Clin Cancer Res 2009;15(12): 3917.
3. Batty N, Malouf GG, Issa JP. Histone deacetylase inhibitors as anti-neoplastic agents. Cancer Lett 2009;280(2):192–200.
4. Esteller M. Epigenetics in cancer. N Engl J Med 2008;358(11):1148–59.
5. Hagelkruys A, Sawicka A, Rennmayr M, et al. The biology of HDAC in cancer: the nuclear and epigenetic components. Handb Exp Pharmacol 2011;206: 13–37.
6. Jenuwein T, Allis CD. Translating the histone code. Science 2001;293(5532): 1074–80.
7. Khorasanizadeh S. The nucleosome: from genomic organization to genomic regulation. Cell 2004;116(2):259–72.
8. Olsen EA, Kim YH, Kuzel TM, et al. Phase IIb multicenter trial of vorinostat in patients with persistent, progressive, or treatment refractory cutaneous T-cell lymphoma. J Clin Oncol 2007;25(21):3109–15.
9. Demierre M. Pooled analysis of two international multicenter clinical studies of romidepsin in 167 patients with cutaneous lymphoma. 45th American Society of Clinical Oncology Annual Meeting, Atlanta, December 2009.
10. Piekarz RL, Frye R, Prince HM, et al. Phase 2 trial of romidepsin in patients with peripheral T-cell lymphoma. Blood 2011;117(22):5827–34.
11. Grunstein M. Histone acetylation in chromatin structure and transcription. Nature 1997;389(6649):349–52.
12. Davie JR. Covalent modifications of histones: expression from chromatin templates. Curr Opin Genet Dev 1998;8(2):173–8.
13. Zain J, Kaminetzky D, O'Connor OA. Emerging role of epigenetic therapies in cutaneous T-cell lymphomas. Expert Rev Hematol 2010;3(2):187–203.
14. Marks PA, Dokmanovic M. Histone deacetylase inhibitors: discovery and development as anticancer agents. Expert Opin Investig Drugs 2005;14(12): 1497–511.
15. Blander G, Guarente L. The Sir2 family of protein deacetylases. Annu Rev Biochem 2004;73:417–35.
16. Zain JM, O'Connor O. Targeted treatment and new agents in peripheral T-cell lymphoma. Int J Hematol 2010;92(1):33–44.
17. Prince HM, Bishton M, Harrison S. The potential of histone deacetylase inhibitors for the treatment of multiple myeloma. Leuk Lymphoma 2008;49(3):385–7.
18. Piekarz RL, Bates SE. Epigenetic modifiers: basic understanding and clinical development. Clin Cancer Res 2009;15(12):3918–26.
19. O'Connor OA, Heaney ML, Schwartz L, et al. Clinical experience with intravenous and oral formulations of the novel histone deacetylase inhibitor suberoylanilide hydroxamic acid in patients with advanced hematologic malignancies. J Clin Oncol 2006;24(1):166–73.
20. Cotto M, Cabanillas F, Tirado M, et al. Epigenetic therapy of lymphoma using histone deacetylase inhibitors. Clin Transl Oncol 2010;12(6):401–9.
21. Yoo CB, Jones PA. Epigenetic therapy of cancer: past, present and future. Nat Rev Drug Discov 2006;5(1):37–50.
22. Nakagawa M, Oda Y, Eguchi T, et al. Expression profile of class I histone deacetylases in human cancer tissues. Oncol Rep 2007;18(4):769–74.

23. Gloghini A, Buglio D, Khaskhely NM, et al. Expression of histone deacetylases in lymphoma: implication for the development of selective inhibitors. Br J Haematol 2009;147(4):515–25.

24. Haggarty SJ, Koeller KM, Wong JC, et al. Domain-selective small-molecule inhibitor of histone deacetylase 6 (HDAC6)-mediated tubulin deacetylation. Proc Natl Acad Sci U S A 2003;100(8):4389–94.

25. Simms-Waldrip T, Rodriguez-Gonzalez A, Lin T, et al. The aggresome pathway as a target for therapy in hematologic malignancies. Mol Genet Metab 2008; 94(3):283–6.

26. Wang J, Hoshino T, Redner RL, et al. ETO, fusion partner in t(8;21) acute myeloid leukemia, represses transcription by interaction with the human N-CoR/mSin3/HDAC1 complex. Proc Natl Acad Sci U S A 1998;95(18):10860–5.

27. Lutterbach B, Westendorf JJ, Linggi B, et al. ETO, a target of t(8;21) in acute leukemia, interacts with the N-CoR and mSin3 corepressors. Mol Cell Biol 1998;18(12):7176–84.

28. Gelmetti V, Zhang J, Fanelli M, et al. Aberrant recruitment of the nuclear receptor corepressor-histone deacetylase complex by the acute myeloid leukemia fusion partner ETO. Mol Cell Biol 1998;18(12):7185–91.

29. Lin RJ, Evans RM. Acquisition of oncogenic potential by RAR chimeras in acute promyelocytic leukemia through formation of homodimers. Mol Cell 2000;5(5):821–30.

30. Minucci S, Maccarana M, Cioce M, et al. Oligomerization of RAR and AML1 transcription factors as a novel mechanism of oncogenic activation. Mol Cell 2000; 5(5):811–20.

31. Villagra A, Cheng F, Wang HW, et al. The histone deacetylase HDAC11 regulates the expression of interleukin 10 and immune tolerance. Nat Immunol 2009;10(1):92–100.

32. Villagra A, Sotomayor EM, Seto E. Histone deacetylases and the immunological network: implications in cancer and inflammation. Oncogene 2010;29(2):157–73.

33. Marquard L, Gjerdrum LM, Christensen IJ, et al. Prognostic significance of the therapeutic targets histone deacetylase 1, 2, 6 and acetylated histone H4 in cutaneous T-cell lymphoma. Histopathology 2008;53(3):267–77.

34. van Doorn R, Gruis NA, Willemze R, et al. Aberrant DNA methylation in cutaneous malignancies. Semin Oncol 2005;32(5):479–87.

35. van Doorn R, Zoutman WH, Dijkman R, et al. Epigenetic profiling of cutaneous T-cell lymphoma: promoter hypermethylation of multiple tumor suppressor genes including BCL7a, PTPRG, and p73. J Clin Oncol 2005;23(17):3886–96.

36. Duvic M, Talpur R, Ni X, et al. Phase 2 trial of oral vorinostat (suberoylanilide hydroxamic acid, SAHA) for refractory cutaneous T-cell lymphoma (CTCL). Blood 2007;109(1):31–9.

37. Ellis L, Pan Y, Smyth GK, et al. Histone deacetylase inhibitor panobinostat induces clinical responses with associated alterations in gene expression profiles in cutaneous T-cell lymphoma. Clin Cancer Res 2008;14(14):4500–10.

38. Bates SE, Zhan Z, Steadman K, et al. Laboratory correlates for a phase II trial of romidepsin in cutaneous and peripheral T-cell lymphoma. Br J Haematol 2010; 148(2):256–67.

39. Wozniak MB, Villuendas R, Bischoff JR, et al. Vorinostat interferes with the signaling transduction pathway of T-cell receptor and synergizes with phosphoinositide-3 kinase inhibitors in cutaneous T-cell lymphoma. Haematologica 2010;95(4):613–21.

40. Weiss A, Littman DR. Signal transduction by lymphocyte antigen receptors. Cell 1994;76(2):263–74.

41. Dreyling M, Hoster E, Bea S, et al. Update on the molecular pathogenesis and clinical treatment of mantle cell lymphoma (MCL): minutes of the 9th European MCL Network Conference. Leuk Lymphoma 2010;51(9):1612–22.

42. Prince HM, Bishton MJ, Harrison SJ. Clinical studies of histone deacetylase inhibitors. Clin Cancer Res 2009;15(12):3958–69.

43. Pasqualucci L, Migliazza A, Basso K, et al. Mutations of the BCL6 proto-oncogene disrupt its negative autoregulation in diffuse large B-cell lymphoma. Blood 2003;101(8):2914–23.

44. Alizadeh AA, Eisen MB, Davis RE, et al. Distinct types of diffuse large B-cell lymphoma identified by gene expression profiling. Nature 2000;403(6769): 503–11.

45. O'Connor OA. Targeting histones and proteasomes: new strategies for the treatment of lymphoma. J Clin Oncol 2005;23(26):6429–36.

46. Lemercier C, Brocard MP, Puvion-Dutilleul F, et al. Class II histone deacetylases are directly recruited by BCL6 transcriptional repressor. J Biol Chem 2002; 277(24):22045–52.

47. Ding BB, Yu JJ, Yu RY, et al. Constitutively activated STAT3 promotes cell proliferation and survival in the activated B-cell subtype of diffuse large B-cell lymphomas. Blood 2008;111(3):1515–23.

48. Skinnider BF, Mak TW. The role of cytokines in classical Hodgkin lymphoma. Blood 2002;99(12):4283–97.

49. Re D, Thomas RK, Behringer K, et al. From Hodgkin disease to Hodgkin lymphoma: biologic insights and therapeutic potential. Blood 2005;105(12): 4553–60.

50. Skinnider BF, Kapp U, Mak TW. The role of interleukin 13 in classical Hodgkin lymphoma. Leuk Lymphoma 2002;43(6):1203–10.

51. Kapp U, Yeh WC, Patterson B, et al. Interleukin 13 is secreted by and stimulates the growth of Hodgkin and Reed-Sternberg cells. J Exp Med 1999;189(12): 1939–46.

52. Yuan ZL, Guan YJ, Chatterjee D, et al. Stat3 dimerization regulated by reversible acetylation of a single lysine residue. Science 2005;307(5707):269–73.

53. Buglio D, Georgakis GV, Hanabuchi S, et al. Vorinostat inhibits STAT6-mediated TH2 cytokine and TARC production and induces cell death in Hodgkin lymphoma cell lines. Blood 2008;112(4):1424–33.

54. Shichijo S, Yamada A, Sagawa K, et al. Induction of MAGE genes in lymphoid cells by the demethylating agent 5-aza-2'-deoxycytidine. Jpn J Cancer Res 1996;87(7):751–6.

55. Mitsiades CS, Mitsiades NS, McMullan CJ, et al. Transcriptional signature of histone deacetylase inhibition in multiple myeloma: biological and clinical implications. Proc Natl Acad Sci U S A 2004;101(2):540–5.

56. Gray SG, Qian CN, Furge K, et al. Microarray profiling of the effects of histone deacetylase inhibitors on gene expression in cancer cell lines. Int J Oncol 2004; 24(4):773–95.

57. Neri P, Tagliaferri P, Di Martino MT, et al. In vivo anti-myeloma activity and modulation of gene expression profile induced by valproic acid, a histone deacetylase inhibitor. Br J Haematol 2008;143(4):520–31.

58. Schwartz C, Palissot V, Aouali N, et al. Valproic acid induces non-apoptotic cell death mechanisms in multiple myeloma cell lines. Int J Oncol 2007;30(3):573–82.

59. Lavelle D, Westside Division, Chicago, et al. Histone deacetylase inhibitors increase p21(WAF1) and induce apoptosis of human myeloma cell lines independent of decreased IL-6 receptor expression. Am J Hematol 2001;68(3):170–8.

60. Kaiser M, Zavrski I, Sterz J, et al. The effects of the histone deacetylase inhibitor valproic acid on cell cycle, growth suppression and apoptosis in multiple myeloma. Haematologica 2006;91(2):248–51.

61. Maiso P, Carvajal-Vergara X, Ocio EM, et al. The histone deacetylase inhibitor LBH589 is a potent antimyeloma agent that overcomes drug resistance. Cancer Res 2006;66(11):5781–9.

62. Khan SB, Maududi T, Barton K, et al. Analysis of histone deacetylase inhibitor, depsipeptide (FR901228), effect on multiple myeloma. Br J Haematol 2004; 125(2):156–61.

63. Golay J, Cuppini L, Leoni F, et al. The histone deacetylase inhibitor ITF2357 has anti-leukemic activity in vitro and in vivo and inhibits IL-6 and VEGF production by stromal cells. Leukemia 2007;21(9):1892–900.

64. Catley L, Weisberg E, Tai YT, et al. NVP-LAQ824 is a potent novel histone deacetylase inhibitor with significant activity against multiple myeloma. Blood 2003;102(7):2615–22.

65. Feng R, Ma H, Hassig CA, et al. KD5170, a novel mercaptoketone-based histone deacetylase inhibitor, exerts antimyeloma effects by DNA damage and mitochondrial signaling. Mol Cancer Ther 2008;7(6):1494–505.

66. Catley L, Weisberg E, Kiziltepe T, et al. Aggresome induction by proteasome inhibitor bortezomib and alpha-tubulin hyperacetylation by tubulin deacetylase (TDAC) inhibitor LBH589 are synergistic in myeloma cells. Blood 2006;108(10): 3441–9.

67. Oancea M, Mani A, Hussein MA, et al. Apoptosis of multiple myeloma. Int J Hematol 2004;80(3):224–31.

68. Ashkenazi A. Targeting death and decoy receptors of the tumour-necrosis factor superfamily. Nat Rev Cancer 2002;2(6):420–30.

69. van de Donk NW, Lokhorst HM, Bloem AC. Growth factors and antiapoptotic signaling pathways in multiple myeloma. Leukemia 2005;19(12):2177–85.

70. Gomez-Benito M, Martinez-Lorenzo MJ, Anel A, et al. Membrane expression of DR4, DR5 and caspase-8 levels, but not Mcl-1, determine sensitivity of human myeloma cells to Apo2L/TRAIL. Exp Cell Res 2007;313(11):2378–88.

71. Mitsiades N, Mitsiades CS, Richardson PG, et al. Molecular sequelae of histone deacetylase inhibition in human malignant B cells. Blood 2003;101(10):4055–62.

72. Shao Y, Gao Z, Marks PA, et al. Apoptotic and autophagic cell death induced by histone deacetylase inhibitors. Proc Natl Acad Sci U S A 2004;101(52):18030–5.

73. Yamamoto S, Tanaka K, Sakimura R, et al. Suberoylanilide hydroxamic acid (SAHA) induces apoptosis or autophagy-associated cell death in chondrosarcoma cell lines. Anticancer Res 2008;28(3A):1585–91.

74. Wickner S, Maurizi MR, Gottesman S. Posttranslational quality control: folding, refolding, and degrading proteins. Science 1999;286(5446):1888–93.

75. Bennett EJ, Bence NF, Jayakumar R, et al. Global impairment of the ubiquitin-proteasome system by nuclear or cytoplasmic protein aggregates precedes inclusion body formation. Mol Cell 2005;17(3):351–65.

76. Kopito RR. Aggresomes, inclusion bodies and protein aggregation. Trends Cell Biol 2000;10(12):524–30.

77. Hideshima T, Bradner JE, Wong J, et al. Small-molecule inhibition of proteasome and aggresome function induces synergistic antitumor activity in multiple myeloma. Proc Natl Acad Sci U S A 2005;102(24):8567–72.

78. Dong XF, Song Q, Li LZ, et al. Histone deacetylase inhibitor valproic acid inhibits proliferation and induces apoptosis in KM3 cells via downregulating VEGF receptor. Neuro Endocrinol Lett 2007;28(6):775–80.

79. Kitazoe K, Abe M, Hiasa M, et al. Valproic acid exerts anti-tumor as well as anti-angiogenic effects on myeloma. Int J Hematol 2009;89(1):45–57.

80. De Bruyne E, Bos TJ, Asosingh K, et al. Epigenetic silencing of the tetraspanin CD9 during disease progression in multiple myeloma cells and correlation with survival. Clin Cancer Res 2008;14(10):2918–26.

81. Johnstone RW, Licht JD. Histone deacetylase inhibitors in cancer therapy: is transcription the primary target? Cancer Cell 2003;4(1):13–8.

82. Kelly WK, Richon VM, O'Connor O, et al. Phase I clinical trial of histone deacetylase inhibitor: suberoylanilide hydroxamic acid administered intravenously. Clin Cancer Res 2003;9(10 Pt 1):3578–88.

83. Sandor V, Bakke S, Robey RW, et al. Phase I trial of the histone deacetylase inhibitor, depsipeptide (FR901228, NSC 630176), in patients with refractory neoplasms. Clin Cancer Res 2002;8(3):718–28.

84. Garcia-Manero G, Assouline S, Cortes J, et al. Phase 1 study of the oral isotype specific histone deacetylase inhibitor MGCD0103 in leukemia. Blood 2008; 112(4):981–9.

85. Mann BS, Johnson JR, He K, et al. Vorinostat for treatment of cutaneous manifestations of advanced primary cutaneous T-cell lymphoma. Clin Cancer Res 2007; 13(8):2318–22.

86. Lane AA, Chabner BA. Histone deacetylase inhibitors in cancer therapy. J Clin Oncol 2009;27(32):5459–68.

87. Romidepsin (Istodax) for cutaneous T-cell lymphoma. Med Lett Drugs Ther 2010;52(1339):42–3.

88. Matsuoka H, Unami A, Fujimura T, et al. Mechanisms of HDAC inhibitor-induced thrombocytopenia. Eur J Pharmacol 2007;571(2–3):88–96.

89. Bates SE, Rosing DR, Fojo T, et al. Challenges of evaluating the cardiac effects of anticancer agents. Clin Cancer Res 2006;12(13):3871–4.

90. Strevel EL, Ing DJ, Siu LL. Molecularly targeted oncology therapeutics and prolongation of the QT interval. J Clin Oncol 2007;25(22):3362–71.

91. Piekarz RL, Frye AR, Wright JJ, et al. Cardiac studies in patients treated with depsipeptide, FK228, in a phase II trial for T-cell lymphoma. Clin Cancer Res 2006;12(12):3762–73.

92. Shah MH, Binkley P, Chan K, et al. Cardiotoxicity of histone deacetylase inhibitor depsipeptide in patients with metastatic neuroendocrine tumors. Clin Cancer Res 2006;12(13):3997–4003.

93. Zain J, Rotter A, Weiss L, et al. Valproic acid monotherapy leads to CR in a patient with refractory diffuse large B cell lymphoma. Leuk Lymphoma 2007; 48(6):1216–8.

94. Zhu YF, Ye BG, Shen JZ, et al. Inhibitory effect of VPA on multiple myeloma U266 cell proliferation and regulation of histone acetylation. Zhongguo Shi Yan Xue Ye Xue Za Zhi 2010;18(3):638–41 [in Chinese].

95. Watanabe T, Kato H, Kobayashi Y, et al. Potential efficacy of the oral histone deacetylase inhibitor vorinostat in a phase I trial in follicular and mantle cell lymphoma. Cancer Sci 2010;101(1):196–200.

96. Crump M, Coiffier B, Jacobsen ED, et al. Phase II trial of oral vorinostat (suberoylanilide hydroxamic acid) in relapsed diffuse large-B-cell lymphoma. Ann Oncol 2008;19(5):964–9.

97. Kirshbaum M, Zain J, Popplewell L, et al. Phase 2 study of suberoylanilide hydroxamic acid (SAHA) in relapsed or refractory indolent non-Hodgkin lymphoma: a California Cancer Consortium Study [abstract: 18515]. J Clin Oncol 2007;25(18S).

98. Gimsing P, Hansen M, Knudsen LM, et al. A phase I clinical trial of the histone deacetylase inhibitor belinostat in patients with advanced hematological neoplasia. Eur J Haematol 2008;81(3):170–6.

99. Steele NL, Plumb JA, Vidal L, et al. Pharmacokinetic and pharmacodynamic properties of an oral formulation of the histone deacetylase inhibitor belinostat (PXD101). Cancer Chemother Pharmacol 2011;67(6):1273–9.

100. Zain J. Preliminary results of an ongoing phase I trial of oral belinostat a novel histone deacetylase inhibitor in patients with lymphoid malignancies (ASH abstract book 3710). Blood 2011.

101. Evans A. Phase 1 analysis of the safety and pharmacodynamics of the novel broad spectrum HDACi PCI-24781 in relapsed and refractory lymphoma [abstract: 2726]. Blood 2009;114.

102. Jaffe ES, Harris NL, Stein H, et al. Classification of lymphoid neoplasms: the microscope as a tool for disease discovery. Blood 2008;112(12):4384–99.

103. Willemze R, Jaffe ES, Burg G, et al. WHO-EORTC classification for cutaneous lymphomas. Blood 2005;105(10):3768–85.

104. Vose J, Armitage J, Weisenburger D. International peripheral T-cell and natural killer/T-cell lymphoma study: pathology findings and clinical outcomes. J Clin Oncol 2008;26(25):4124–30.

105. Piekarz RL, Frye R, Turner M, et al. Phase II multi-institutional trial of the histone deacetylase inhibitor romidepsin as monotherapy for patients with cutaneous T-cell lymphoma. J Clin Oncol 2009;27(32):5410–7.

106. Coiffier B. Final results from a pivotal, multicenter, international, open-label, phase 2 study of romidepsin in progressive or relapsed peripheral T-Cell lymphoma (PTCL) following prior systemic therapy. Blood 2010;114:116 (ASH abstract book).

107. Pohlman B. Final results of a phase 2 trial of belinostat in patients with recurrent or refractory peripheral or cutaneous T cell lymphomas [abstract: 920]. Blood 2009.

108. Stevens SR, Ke MS, Parry EJ, et al. Quantifying skin disease burden in mycosis fungoides-type cutaneous T-cell lymphomas: the severity-weighted assessment tool (SWAT). Arch Dermatol 2002;138(1):42–8.

109. Konstantinopoulos PA, Vandoros GP, Papavassiliou AG. FK228 (depsipeptide): a HDAC inhibitor with pleiotropic antitumor activities. Cancer Chemother Pharmacol 2006;58(5):711–5.

110. Piekarz RL, Robey R, Sandor V, et al. Inhibitor of histone deacetylation, depsipeptide (FR901228), in the treatment of peripheral and cutaneous T-cell lymphoma: a case report. Blood 2001;98(9):2865–8.

111. Whittaker SJ, Demierre MF, Kim EJ, et al. Final results from a multicenter, international, pivotal study of romidepsin in refractory cutaneous T-cell lymphoma. J Clin Oncol 2010;28(29):4485–91.

112. Olsen E, Duvic M, Frankel A, et al. Pivotal phase III trial of two dose levels of denileukin diftitox for the treatment of cutaneous T-cell lymphoma. J Clin Oncol 2001;19(2):376–88.

113. Ali CM, Sikdar TK, Sultana N, et al. Sezary syndrome. Mymensingh Med J 2011; 20(3):497–500.

114. Steele NL, Plumb JA, Vidal L, et al. A phase 1 pharmacokinetic and pharmacodynamic study of the histone deacetylase inhibitor belinostat in patients with advanced solid tumors. Clin Cancer Res 2008;14(3):804–10.

115. Duvic M. Phase II trial of oral panobinostat (LBH589) in patients with refractory cutaneous T cell lymphoma (CTCL). J Clin Oncol 2008;26(Suppl):[abstract: 8555].

116. Thompson CA, Mauck K, Havyer R, et al. Care of the adult Hodgkin lymphoma survivor. Am J Med 2011;124(12):1106–12.
117. Jemal A, Siegel R, Ward E, et al. Cancer statistics, 2009. CA Cancer J Clin 2009; 59(4):225–49.
118. Kewalramani T, Nimer SD, Zelenetz AD, et al. Progressive disease following autologous transplantation in patients with chemosensitive relapsed or primary refractory Hodgkin's disease or aggressive non-Hodgkin's lymphoma. Bone Marrow Transplant 2003;32(7):673–9.
119. Kirshbaum M. Vorinostat in relapsed or refractory Hodgkin lymphoma: SWOG 0517 [abstract: 2574]. Blood 2007;110.
120. Sureda A. Final analysis: phase II study of oral panobinostat in relapsed/refractory Hodgkin lymphoma in patients following autologous stem cell transplant [abstract: 419]. Blood 2010;116 (ASH abstract book) 2010.
121. Younes A. Isotype-selective HDAC-inhibitor MGCD0103 decreases serum TARC concentrations and produces clinical responses in heavily pretreated patients with relapsed classical HL [abstract: 2566]. Blood 2007;110.
122. Richardson P, Mitsiades C, Colson K, et al. Phase I trial of oral vorinostat (suberoylanilide hydroxamic acid, SAHA) in patients with advanced multiple myeloma. Leuk Lymphoma 2008;49(3):502–7.
123. Niesvizky R, Ely S, Mark T, et al. Phase 2 trial of the histone deacetylase inhibitor romidepsin for the treatment of refractory multiple myeloma. Cancer 2011; 117(2):336–42.
124. Adams J. The proteasome: structure, function, and role in the cell. Cancer Treat Rev 2003;29(Suppl 1):3–9.
125. Kikuchi J, Wada T, Shimizu R, et al. Histone deacetylases are critical targets of bortezomib-induced cytotoxicity in multiple myeloma. Blood 2010;116(3):406–17.
126. Pei XY, Dai Y, Grant S. Synergistic induction of oxidative injury and apoptosis in human multiple myeloma cells by the proteasome inhibitor bortezomib and histone deacetylase inhibitors. Clin Cancer Res 2004;10(11):3839–52.
127. Feng R, Oton A, Mapara MY, et al. The histone deacetylase inhibitor, PXD101, potentiates bortezomib-induced anti-multiple myeloma effect by induction of oxidative stress and DNA damage. Br J Haematol 2007;139(3):385–97.
128. Nawrocki ST, Carew JS, Maclean KH, et al. Myc regulates aggresome formation, the induction of Noxa, and apoptosis in response to the combination of bortezomib and SAHA. Blood 2008;112(7):2917–26.
129. Siegel DS, Jagannath S, Hajek R, et al. Vorinostat combined with bortezomib in patients with relapsed or relapsed and refractory multiple myeloma: update on the Vantage Study Program. Blood 2010;116(21):(ASH meeting abstract # 1952).
130. Mazumder A, Vesole DH, Jagannath S. Vorinostat plus bortezomib for the treatment of relapsed/refractory multiple myeloma: a case series illustrating utility in clinical practice. Clin Lymphoma Myeloma Leuk 2010;10(2):149–51.
131. Jagannath S, Dimopoulos MA, Lonial S. Combined proteasome and histone deacetylase inhibition: a promising synergy for patients with relapsed/refractory multiple myeloma. Leuk Res 2010;34(9):1111–8.
132. Kiziltepe T, Hideshima T, Catley L, et al. 5-Azacytidine, a DNA methyltransferase inhibitor, induces ATR-mediated DNA double-strand break responses, apoptosis, and synergistic cytotoxicity with doxorubicin and bortezomib against multiple myeloma cells. Mol Cancer Ther 2007;6(6):1718–27.
133. Ocio EM, Mateos MV, Maiso P, et al. New drugs in multiple myeloma: mechanisms of action and phase I/II clinical findings. Lancet Oncol 2008;9(12): 1157–65.

134. Zhu WG, Otterson GA. The interaction of histone deacetylase inhibitors and DNA methyltransferase inhibitors in the treatment of human cancer cells. Curr Med Chem Anticancer Agents 2003;3(3):187–99.

135. De Bruyne E. Regulation of Bim expression by IGF-1 in the 5T33MM murine model for multiple myeloma. Blood 2007;110:3512 (ASH abstract book).

136. Catley L, Tai YT, Chauhan D, et al. Perspectives for combination therapy to overcome drug-resistant multiple myeloma. Drug Resist Updat 2005;8(4):205–18.

137. Fandy TE, Shankar S, Ross DD, et al. Interactive effects of HDAC inhibitors and TRAIL on apoptosis are associated with changes in mitochondrial functions and expressions of cell cycle regulatory genes in multiple myeloma. Neoplasia 2005; 7(7):646–57.

138. Shankar S, Singh TR, Fandy TE, et al. Interactive effects of histone deacetylase inhibitors and TRAIL on apoptosis in human leukemia cells: involvement of both death receptor and mitochondrial pathways. Int J Mol Med 2005;16(6):1125–38.

139. Paoluzzi L, Scotto L, Marchi E, et al. Romidepsin and belinostat synergize the antineoplastic effect of bortezomib in mantle cell lymphoma. Clin Cancer Res 2010;16(2):554–65.

140. Heider U, von Metzler I, Kaiser M, et al. Synergistic interaction of the histone deacetylase inhibitor SAHA with the proteasome inhibitor bortezomib in mantle cell lymphoma. Eur J Haematol 2008;80(2):133–42.

141. Dai Y, Chen S, Kramer LB, et al. Interactions between bortezomib and romidepsin and belinostat in chronic lymphocytic leukemia cells. Clin Cancer Res 2008; 14(2):549–58.

142. Dasmahapatra G, Lembersky D, Kramer L, et al. The pan-HDAC inhibitor vorinostat potentiates the activity of the proteasome inhibitor carfilzomib in human DLBCL cells in vitro and in vivo. Blood 2010;115(22):4478–87.

143. Luo J, Nikolaev AY, Imai S, et al. Negative control of p53 by Sir2alpha promotes cell survival under stress. Cell 2001;107(2):137–48.

144. Amengual J. DNA methylation is involved in malignancy and is seen, in progression, in more than 80% of all solid tumours. Methylation is one of the main physiological processes to induce silencing of gene expression. Blood 2011 (ASH meeting abstract # 3733).

145. Dummer R. Phase I trial of oral vorinostat in combination with bexarotene in advanced cutaneous T-cell lymphoma [abstract 0270]. Haematologica 2008; 93(sl):110.

146. Marchi E. Combination of epigenetic agents synergistically reverse the malignant phenotype in models of T-cell lymphoma. Blood 2011 (ASH meeting abstract # 2727).

147. Gregoretti IV, Lee YM, Goodson HV. Molecular evolution of the histone deacetylase family: functional implications of phylogenetic analysis. J Mol Biol 2004; 338(1):17–31.

148. Hubbert C, Guardiola A, Shao R, et al. HDAC6 is a microtubule-associated deacetylase. Nature 2002;417(6887):455–8.

149. Gao L, Cueto MA, Asselbergs F, et al. Cloning and functional characterization of HDAC11, a novel member of the human histone deacetylase family. J Biol Chem 2002;277(28):25748–55.

150. Kramer OH, Zhu P, Ostendorff HP, et al. The histone deacetylase inhibitor valproic acid selectively induces proteasomal degradation of HDAC2. EMBO J 2003;22(13):3411–20.

151. Bolden JE, Peart MJ, Johnstone RW. Anticancer activities of histone deacetylase inhibitors. Nat Rev Drug Discov 2006;5(9):769–84.

152. Hu E, Dul E, Sung CM, et al. Identification of novel isoform-selective inhibitors within class I histone deacetylases. J Pharmacol Exp Ther 2003;307(2): 720–8.

153. Furumai R, Matsuyama A, Kobashi N, et al. FK228 (depsipeptide) as a natural prodrug that inhibits class I histone deacetylases. Cancer Res 2002;62(17): 4916–21.

154. Guo F, Sigua C, Tao J, et al. Cotreatment with histone deacetylase inhibitor LAQ824 enhances Apo-2L/tumor necrosis factor-related apoptosis inducing ligand-induced death inducing signaling complex activity and apoptosis of human acute leukemia cells. Cancer Res 2004;64(7):2580–9.

155. Nebbioso A, Clarke N, Voltz E, et al. Tumor-selective action of HDAC inhibitors involves TRAIL induction in acute myeloid leukemia cells. Nat Med 2005;11(1): 77–84.

156. Nagata S, Golstein P. The Fas death factor. Science 1995;267(5203):1449–56.

157. Newbold A, Lindemann RK, Cluse LA, et al. Characterisation of the novel apoptotic and therapeutic activities of the histone deacetylase inhibitor romidepsin. Mol Cancer Ther 2008;7(5):1066–79.

158. Lindemann RK, Newbold A, Whitecross KF, et al. Analysis of the apoptotic and therapeutic activities of histone deacetylase inhibitors by using a mouse model of B cell lymphoma. Proc Natl Acad Sci U S A 2007;104(19):8071–6.

159. Thornberry NA, Lazebnik Y. Caspases: enemies within. Science 1998; 281(5381):1312–6.

160. Hofmann K. The modular nature of apoptotic signaling proteins. Cell Mol Life Sci 1999;55(8–9):1113–28.

161. Peart MJ, Tainton KM, Ruefli AA, et al. Novel mechanisms of apoptosis induced by histone deacetylase inhibitors. Cancer Res 2003;63(15):4460–71.

162. Kim MS, Kwon HJ, Lee YM, et al. Histone deacetylases induce angiogenesis by negative regulation of tumor suppressor genes. Nat Med 2001;7(4):437–43.

163. Jeong JW, Bae MK, Ahn MY, et al. Regulation and destabilization of HIF-1alpha by ARD1-mediated acetylation. Cell 2002;111(5):709–20.

164. Duvic M, Vu J. Vorinostat: a new oral histone deacetylase inhibitor approved for cutaneous T-cell lymphoma. Expert Opin Investig Drugs 2007;16(7):1111–20.

165. Peart MJ, Smyth GK, van Laar RK, et al. Identification and functional significance of genes regulated by structurally different histone deacetylase inhibitors. Proc Natl Acad Sci U S A 2005;102(10):3697–702.

166. Zhao Y, Lu S, Wu L, et al. Acetylation of p53 at lysine 373/382 by the histone deacetylase inhibitor depsipeptide induces expression of p21(Waf1/Cip1). Mol Cell Biol 2006;26(7):2782–90.

167. Dai Y, Rahmani M, Dent P, et al. Blockade of histone deacetylase inhibitor-induced RelA/p65 acetylation and NF-kappaB activation potentiates apoptosis in leukemia cells through a process mediated by oxidative damage, XIAP down-regulation, and c-Jun N-terminal kinase 1 activation. Mol Cell Biol 2005;25(13): 5429–44.

168. Spange S, Wagner T, Heinzel T, et al. Acetylation of non-histone proteins modulates cellular signalling at multiple levels. Int J Biochem Cell Biol 2009;41(1): 185–98.

169. Bereshchenko OR, Gu W, Dalla-Favera R. Acetylation inactivates the transcriptional repressor BCL6. Nat Genet 2002;32(4):606–13.

170. Dai Y, Chen S, Wang L, et al. Disruption of IkappaB kinase (IKK)-mediated RelA serine 536 phosphorylation sensitizes human multiple myeloma cells to histone deacetylase (HDAC) inhibitors. J Biol Chem 2011;286(39):34036–50.

171. Munshi A, Kurland JF, Nishikawa T, et al. Histone deacetylase inhibitors radio-sensitize human melanoma cells by suppressing DNA repair activity. Clin Cancer Res 2005;11(13):4912–22.

172. Cohen HY, Lavu S, Bitterman KJ, et al. Acetylation of the C terminus of Ku70 by CBP and PCAF controls Bax-mediated apoptosis. Mol Cell 2004;13(5):627–38.

173. Kovacs JJ, Murphy PJ, Gaillard S, et al. HDAC6 regulates Hsp90 acetylation and chaperone-dependent activation of glucocorticoid receptor. Mol Cell 2005;18(5):601–7.

174. Wang Y, Wang SY, Zhang XH, et al. FK228 inhibits Hsp90 chaperone function in K562 cells via hyperacetylation of Hsp70. Biochem Biophys Res Commun 2007; 356(4):998–1003.

175. Robbins AR, Jablonski SA, Yen TJ, et al. Inhibitors of histone deacetylases alter kinetochore assembly by disrupting pericentromeric heterochromatin. Cell Cycle 2005;4(5):717–26.

176. Ruefli AA, Ausserlechner MJ, Bernhard D, et al. The histone deacetylase inhibitor and chemotherapeutic agent suberoylanilide hydroxamic acid (SAHA) induces a cell-death pathway characterized by cleavage of Bid and production of reactive oxygen species. Proc Natl Acad Sci U S A 2001;98(19):10833–8.

177. Butler LM, Zhou X, Xu WS, et al. The histone deacetylase inhibitor SAHA arrests cancer cell growth, up-regulates thioredoxin-binding protein-2, and down-regulates thioredoxin. Proc Natl Acad Sci U S A 2002;99(18):11700–5.

178. Weiser TS, Ohnmacht GA, Guo ZS, et al. Induction of MAGE-3 expression in lung and esophageal cancer cells. Ann Thorac Surg 2001;71(1):295–301 [discussion: 301–2].

179. Weiser TS, Guo ZS, Ohnmacht GA, et al. Sequential 5-Aza-2 deoxycytidine-depsipeptide FR901228 treatment induces apoptosis preferentially in cancer cells and facilitates their recognition by cytolytic T lymphocytes specific for NY-ESO-1. J Immunother 2001;24(2):151–61.

Index

Note: Page numbers of article titles are in **boldface** type.

Hematol Oncol Clin N Am 26 (2012) 705–714
doi:10.1016/S0889-8588(12)00055-X
0889-8588/12/$ – see front matter © 2012 Elsevier Inc. All rights reserved.

hemonc.theclinics.com

Printed and bound by CPI Group (UK) Ltd, Croydon, CR0 4YY

03/10/2024

01040449-0006